W9-DEU-966

Oncofertility
Fertility Preservation for Cancer Survivors

Cancer Treatment and Research

Steven T. Rosen, M.D., *Series Editor*

(continued after index)

Oncofertility
Fertility Preservation
for Cancer Survivors

edited by

Teresa K. Woodruff, PhD
The Thomas J. Watkins Professor of Obstetrics and Gynecology
Director, Institute for Women's Health Research
Chief, Division of Fertility Preservation
Associate Director, Basic Science Programs,
The Robert H. Lurie Comprehensive Cancer Center
Director, Center for Reproductive Research
Feinberg School of Medicine
Northwestern University
Chicago, Illinois, USA

Karrie Ann Snyder, PhD
Research Assistant Professor
Institute for Women's Health Research
Feinberg School of Medicine
Northwestern University
Chicago, Illinois, USA

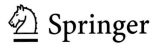 Springer

Teresa K. Woodruff, PhD
Institute for Women's Health Research
Division of Fertility Preservation
Department of Obstetrics and Gynecology
Feinberg School of Medicine
Northwestern University
Chicago, IL 60611 USA

Karrie Ann Snyder, PhD
Institute for Women's Health Research
Feinberg School of Medicine
Northwestern University
Chicago, IL 60611 USA

Series Editor:
Steven T. Rosen
Robert H. Lurie Comprehensive Cancer Center
Northwestern University
Chicago, IL
USA

Oncofertility: Fertility Preservations for Cancer Survivors

ISBN-13: 978-0-387-72292-4   e-ISBN-13: 978-0-387-72293-1

Library of Congress Control Number: 2007925436

Printed on acid-free paper.

9 8 7 6 5 4 3 2 1

springer.com

Foreword

It has been our pleasure to edit the first book on an interdisciplinary science we call oncofertility. Oncofertility bridges traditional areas of basic science and medical research, brings together oncologists and fertility specialists, and hopes to provide real options to young people who survive life-preserving but fertility-threatening treatments for cancer. The chapters in this book range from basic discovery research to reproductive medicine and from social science and the humanities to a section on stories from those who have survived cancer and have faced issues of fertility deprivation or restoration. Specifically, we have addressed three main areas: the underlying biological questions surrounding follicle growth and cryo-preservation of tissue; the application of the new technology to medical practice; and, the psychosocial implications of cancer-related infertility and oncofertility research for patients and their families. These questions are interlinking and require teams of investigators working in concert to solve a major unmet need. The book is a comprehensive initial definition of the field and we anticipate a great many more breakthroughs that will eventually provide a menu of options to those with fertility-threatening conditions.

The editors thank the Specialized Cooperative Centers Program in Reproduction and Infertility Research (U54 HD041857) and the Institute for Women's Health Research of Northwestern University for funding and support of this book.

Teresa K. Woodruff
Karrie Ann Snyder

Fundamental Question:
What regulates follicle growth and oocyte maturation?
How can eggs and follicles be preserved without damage?

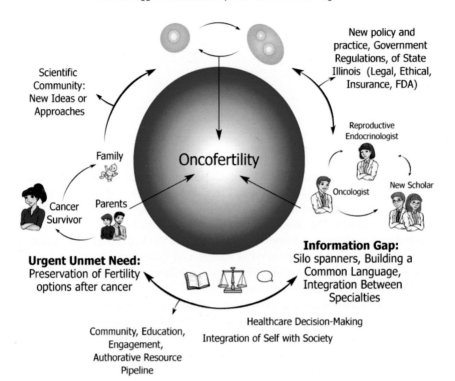

Foreword

As young women who faced both cancer and the potential loss of our ability to have children, we are extremely gratified by the efforts of the scientists, clinicians and social scientists who have come together to recognize, validate and tackle this critical issue. When we were diagnosed, there was little discussion of the physical impact of the life-preserving cancer treatments; and virtually no acknowledgement of the life-altering significance of that potential loss. It is exciting, therefore, to see the interdisciplinary, multifaceted approach that is now being put into place to meet the fertility needs of young adults diagnosed with cancer. We know that this seminal work in the field of oncofertility will set the stage for many more volumes as the field develops and the progress achieved makes more fertility-preserving options a reality for women just like us.

– Lindsay Beck
Founder and Executive Director, Fertile Hope
– Joyce Reinecke, JD
Program Director, Fertile Hope

Contents

Contributors

Sanjay K. Agarwal, University of California, San Diego

Paul Arntson, Northwestern University

Leilah E. Backhus, University of Chicago

Lindsay Beck, Fertile Hope

Robert E. Brannigan, Northwestern University

R. Jeffrey Chang, University of California, San Diego

Karen L. Clark, University of California, San Diego

Marla L. Clayman, Northwestern University

John K. Critser, University of Missouri

Christos Coutifaris, University of Pennsylvania

Aarati Didwania, Northwestern University

Kimberley J. Dilley, Northwestern University

Kathleen M. Galvin, Northwestern University

Jill P. Ginsberg, University of Pennsylvania

Yasmin Gosiengfiao, Northwestern University

Clarisa R. Gracia, University of Pennsylvania

Elizabeth A. Hahn, Northwestern University

Ralph Kazer, Northwestern University

Karen E. Kinahan, Northwestern University

Laxmi A. Kondapalli, Northwestern University

David Lee, Oregon Health & Science University

Matthew L. Loscalzo, University of California, San Diego

Steven F. Mullen, University of Missouri

Carrie L. Nieman, University of Illinois, Chicago

Joyce Reinecke, Fertile Hope

Sarah K. Rosenbloom, Northwestern University

Lonnie D. Shea, Northwestern University

Karrie Ann Snyder, Northwestern University

Timothy Volpe, Northwestern University

Teresa K. Woodruff, Northwestern University

Kathleen J. Yost, Northwestern University

Susan E. Yount, Northwestern University

Min Xu, Northwestern University

Laurie Zoloth, Northwestern University

Part I
Introduction

Chapter 1
The Emergence of a New Interdiscipline: Oncofertility

Teresa K. Woodruff, PhD

Oncofertility: The New Offensive in the War on Cancer

In 1971, the National Cancer Act was signed, providing funds to the newly established National Cancer Institute (NCI) to coordinate research and new medical advances to detect, diagnose, and treat cancer. Since then, there has been a steady increase in the number of cancer survivors, reaching 3.5% of the domestic population in 2003. The rise in the number of survivors is due to earlier detection of disease, aggressive radiation therapy, and new chemotherapeutics. Thus, while the suffering and death associated with cancer have not been eliminated, cancer has been converted, in some cases, from an acute death sentence to a disease that many people survive and live with for an extended period of time.

The war on cancer has been an aggressive one and successful treatment is associated with significant complications. These complications include a physical toll on the cardiovascular system, bone biology, movement of lymph in the appendages, and the loss of organ function. Complications can also involve psychological issues such as depression, anxiety, uncertainty, isolation, and an altered body image. The survivor can also face social and existential crises such as a fear of engaging in interpersonal relationships, problems with health and life insurance, job loss, problems with school and finances, an altered sense of purpose, and a different appreciation of life. One of the main complications of modern cancer treatment, particularly for young men, women and children is the impact of cancer treatment on future fertility.

It is the purpose of this book to review the factors impacting fertility caused by the treatment of cancer. In so doing, we will provide chapters on state-of-the-art research, clinical practice, and training that happens at the intersection of oncology, pediatrics, reproductive science and medicine, biomechanics, material science, mathematics, social science, bioethics, religion, policy research, reproductive health law, cognitive, and learning science. Taken together, this book will describe the emergence of a new discipline called "oncofertility" (Fig. 1.1).

3

T.K. Woodruff and K.A. Snyder (eds.) *Oncofertility.*
© Springer 2007

Secondary Effects of Treatment on the Health
and Quality of Life of Young Survivors of Cancer

Many people think of cancer as a disease of aging, and in many cases it is. But cancer does not impact older people alone; it also targets children and young adults, and it affects men and women of all races, socioeconomic status, political persuasions, and religious leanings. It is a disease that does not discriminate. Data collected from the NCI registry of cancer patients reports that there are 10,500,000 survivors of cancer, and 5% are between 20 and 39 years old. This means there are at least 630,000 young survivors of cancer and the number increases every year. Moreover, 25% of breast cancer patients are younger than 40 years of age. Over 12,400 children and adolescents (younger than 19 years) are diagnosed with cancer each year and the cure rate for all childhood cancers has reached 75%. In fact, the NCI reports that 1 out of every 250 adults will be a survivor of childhood cancer by 2015. This is a staggering statistic and reflects both the ability of children to survive cancer treatment and the extraordinary rise in cancer curing drugs.

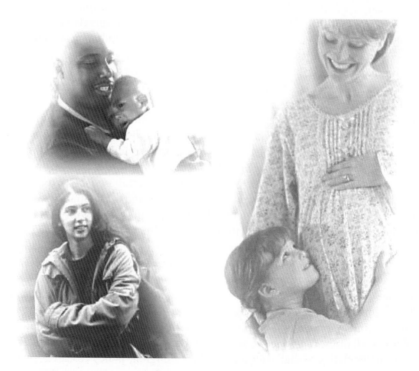

Fig. 1.1 Oncofertility is a new interdisciplinary approach to address the reproductive future of young men, women, and children facing a life-preserving but fertility-threatening cancer diagnosis

Therefore, the age of many cancer patients and the aggressive nature of the treatments they survive create a variety of new health care and quality-of-life problems for the young survivor, many of which were not anticipated at the time of diagnosis. The secondary effects of cancer treatment are exaggerated in this patient cohort because of their young age and greater life expectancy compared with the older cancer survivor. Thus, a secondary effect can become a long-term chronic issue that requires additional medical intervention. For example, patients may experience chronic pain, cognitive dysfunction, fatigue, peripheral neuropathies, cardiovascular and bone disease, or incontinence as a consequence of cancer of its treatment. The young survivor may still be in school, recently become independent, but not yet achieved the economic footing they will have later in life, or be a young parent. A cancer diagnosis can create a further tailspin because time away from education, jobs, and family for primary or ancillary treatment can derail pursuit of a degree or career advancement and can place strain on a new marriage. Moreover, access to health care coverage may be limited due to the previous cancer diagnosis. The future needs of a young cancer patient must be considered at the time of diagnosis and treatment. However, balancing survivorship and quality-of-life issues are sometimes difficult. This book details many of the questions and a roadmap toward the solution. Clearly, much more research and scholarship is needed to provide definitive answers to patients and providers. This book is the first comprehensive assessment of the field and is a call to more research and scholarship on the topic of oncofertility.

Fertility Threats Due to Cancer Treatment

While advances in radiation and chemotherapy have improved survival rates, these therapeutic options may also permanently impact the reproductive capacity of cancer survivors. For instance, systemic chemotherapy, although targeted at a specific cancer cell line, can direct toxic effects at the gonads. Consequently, the survivor may encounter immediate infertility or premature loss of reproductive function due to sublethal damage. In women, induced infertility results in a hormonal milieu similar to that seen in the natural menopause. Furthermore, pelvic radiation and alkylating agents are two known causes of induced-sterility in cancer patients. Young cancer patients are particularly susceptible to the gonadotoxic effects of these agents. However, not all treatments result in acute gonadal failure. Instead, some treatments cause subfertility, which reduces the sperm count in men and causes an accelerated loss of follicles in women. Besides their role in reproduction, the gonads produce steroid hormones that contribute signals to affect other physiologic systems, such as bone growth and maintenance, cardiovascular health, and the development of secondary sex characteristics. For young cancer survivors, the prepubertal loss of gonadal function requires hormonal intervention to recover the beneficial effects of sex steroids as well as provide a sense of normalcy. With hormone replacement therapy, young cancer survivors can achieve the same developmental milestones as their peers. In order to manage the child's transition through puberty and to ensure good bone health and cardiovascular function, boys are given the testosterone patch while girls use oral contraceptive pills to create a normal cyclic hormonal profile. However, these treatments do not restore fertility. The primary goal of treatment is to eradicate the disease, and clinicians have a full armamentarium of cancer therapies to ensure the best opportunity for survival. But even as these strategies improve survivorship, patients are now shifting their focus to understanding and managing the long-term sequelae of their cancer treatment, particularly the effect on reproductive function. Given this unmet need, new approaches to understanding the interplay between age of diagnosis and cancer treatment and its influence on fertility outcomes are essential.

Fertility threats to young women, men, children, and their families are often just as difficult to assimilate as the cancer diagnosis itself. Indeed, in a 2,000 person survey of patients at the Moores University of California – San Diego (UCSD) Cancer Center, fertility was of greatest concern, second only to mortality, and men and women were equally concerned with how cancer treatment may impact their future ability to have children (see Loscalzo and Clark, this volume). This ongoing landmark study emphasizes the importance of fertility for younger people facing cancer and its findings underscore the urgency for clinical centers to begin to provide patients with comprehensive information regarding the fertility-threat their cancer treatment poses and to ensure they provide adequate fertility-conserving options for their patients.

Moreover, post-cancer fertility is also a potential source of health disparity among cancer survivors. For example, racial and ethnic differences in access to medical care, time of cancer diagnosis, and quality of treatment have led to different outcomes across racial/ethnic lines in terms of morbidity and quality-of-life post-cancer. According to the UCSD survey, African–American patients were more concerned about fertility than other racial/ethnic groups and were also more likely to want to discuss the issue with a health care staff member, suggesting that they were less likely to discuss the issue prior to treatment. This finding is distressing because a lack of information regarding possible infertility and treatment options is the major deterrent to cancer patients not taking steps (such as sperm banking) to help safeguard their future fertility. Further research is needed on how information regarding fertility is shared with patients by health care practitioners and institutions because of the implications for later health inequities in terms of which survivors are able to meet desired parenting and family goals.

An Emerging Urgent Unment Need for Young Cancer Patients: Balancing Life-Preserving but Fertility-Threatening Cancer Treatments

Fertility preservation for men has long been an option. The most famous person who has publicized his fertility preservation and family after cancer is Lance Armstrong, the bicyclist and seven-time winner of the Tour de France. The following excerpt describes his initial realization of the impact his cancer treatment could have on future fertility:

> "I've decided Lance needs to move up his first chemotherapy treatment. He starts Monday at one o'clock. "Why?" my mother asked. ... The cancer was not just spreading, it was galloping, and Youman no longer thought I could afford to wait a week for chemo. I should begin treatment directly, because if the cancer was moving that quickly, every day might count. I hung up the phone...I would have one chance and one chance only to go to the sperm bank in San Antonio: that very afternoon. ... I was depressed and falling apart emotionally from the shock of the diagnosis. I wanted to be a father – quite badly – but I had always assumed it would happen when I was in love. I had no choice; I closed my eyes and did what I had to do." From: *'It's Not About the Bike: My Journey back to Life'*, Lance Armstrong with Sally Jenkins, 2000, Berkeley Books

At least Lance had an option. Women who face a similarly devastating diagnosis do not have the same options that men have to easily preserve fertility. This reality, which is particularly unfortunate for prepubescent girls diagnosed with cancer, means most medical oncologists do not discuss potential threats to fertility with female patients. Even more worrisome is that some physicians are less likely to discuss options with women than with men. Lance Armstrong had a very grim disease, yet he was offered the hope of a future. Clearly, good choices for fertility preservation are necessary for women, and this must be coupled with a change in physician attitudes about fertility as a part of the patient's quality of life and her expectations of a cancer-free future.

In 2002, the Lance Armstrong Foundation, the Robert H. Lurie Comprehensive Cancer Center and the Chicago chapter of Gilda's Club co-hosted an evening called *Families After Cancer* (Fig. 1.2). Nearly 600 cancer survivors attended the event. Lance and Kristin Armstrong answered questions about their experiences with a devastating cancer diagnosis and the simultaneous recommendation to bank sperm, their fertility treatments, and their hopes that women might one day have the options men have to preserve their fertility. Dr. Woodruff was part of a panel including a patient advocate (Lindsay Nohr-Beck, Founder and Executive Director of Fertile Hope) and a leading reproductive endocrinologist (Zeev Rosenwaks, MD, Cornell Medical School). The group addressed the need for more basic science at the intersection of a variety of disciplines to solve a previously intractable problem, namely, in vitro follicle growth and oocyte maturation.

There are three main gaps that create the unmet need for preserving fertility in patients with cancer: the information gap, the data gap, and the option gap. Addressing these unmet needs is the goal of many research scientists, clinical investigators, and scholars, and has become the guiding principle behind the newly created Oncofertility Research Program at the Robert H. Lurie Comprehensive Cancer Center at the Feinberg School of Medicine, Northwestern University. The problem requires a comprehensive interdisciplinary approach that will result in a new supra-disciplinary medical specialist in oncofertility and a new research discipline that addresses questions of reproductive function and conservation.

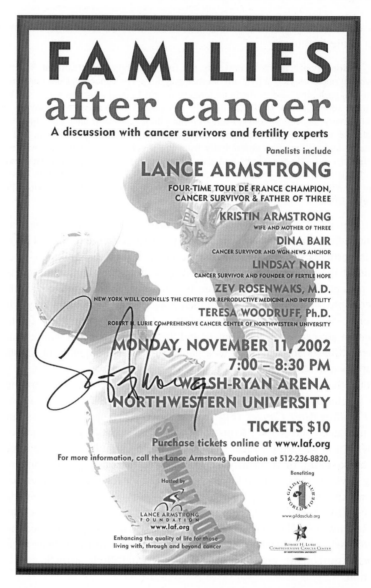

Fig. 1.2 In 2002, the Lance Armstrong Foundation, the Robert H. Lurie Comprehensive Cancer Center of Northwestern University and the Chicago chapter of Gilda's Club co-hosted an evening called *Families After Cancer*. Nearly 600 cancer survivors attended the event. Lance and Kristin Armstrong answered questions about their experiences with a devastating cancer diagnosis and the simultaneous recommendation to bank sperm, their fertility treatments and their hopes that women might one day have the options men have to preserve their fertility

Information GAP

The first gap is an information gap. Indeed, in many cases, cancer treatment will not affect the ovaries or testes and therefore doctors could relieve one of the uncertainties about the future by simply conveying this fact to the patient. In other cases, the impact on fertility is not known because valid studies have not been performed on the survivors of particular treatments. This lack of fundamental knowledge about the fertility threat of treatment is partly due to the inconsistency with which patients are treated within and between cancer centers and the need to evaluate ovarian function over an extended period of time. Clearly, the ability to advise patients about the impact of a particular treatment on fertility is important and the programs are needed to gather the data necessary to provide authoritative information to physicians and patients alike. Perhaps more problematic than the information gap is the intellectual problem medical oncologists face: a belief that there 'are no good options to offer, so why bring up the subject.'

Due to the work of Lance Armstrong and the Lance Armstrong Foundation and Lindsay Beck founder of Fertile Hope, an advocacy group dedicated to promoting fertility awareness at the time of a cancer diagnosis, patients are now, more than ever, aware that cancer treatment poses a fertility risk. Both the American Society for Reproductive Medicine (ASRM) and American Society of Clinical Oncologists (ASCO) have published guidelines that suggest that doctors talk to patients about the fertility implications of cancer treatment (guidelines published in 2005 and 2006; Brannigan, this volume and updated guidelines by Backhus et al., this volume). Nevertheless, the information delivery gap still exists because medical oncologists are not aware of the precise reproductive threats of their treatments on reproductive outcomes and clinical reproductive endocrinologists do not routinely treat cancer patients. Moreover, new drugs and multi-drug treatments pose a particular problem to clear information exchange. Therefore, it is important that we meet the need of creating new oncofertility specialists who can directly interface with practitioners and cancer patients about their fertility needs. Since it will take time for oncofertility programs to develop and train oncofertility specialists, we are simultaneously developing comprehensive, authoritative educational and outreach information that gives the traditionally trained medical oncologists badly needed information so they can confidently advise patients about the fertility threats posed by their treatment plan. If no threat is posed, cancer patients can confidently move forward with treatment. Where fertility is threatened, a new cadre of oncofertility specialists will be able to provide up-to-the-minute information on traditional and newly introduced cancer drugs on fertility. Finally, the information gap creates a tremendous amount of anxiety for a patient and his or her families and partners about choices for treatment. Understanding the needs of the patient, providing information in a way that can be understood at a time of remarkable stress, and creating corridors for support is the third way an oncofertility program will fill the information gap. Knowing that information must be packaged appropriately or the gap will remain, navigation tools for oncofertility programs must be developed, providing a means for unique scholarly inquiry about how medical information is communicated (see Kondapalli, this volume), as well as understanding the perspective of the family cluster in medical decision-making (see Clayman et al., this volume). These scholarly activities will provide the oncofertility specialist with primary information to ensure that information delivery is appropriate to the need.

Data GAP

Despite the best intentions of medical oncologists and reproductive endocrinologists, there exists a paucity of data on the precise gonadotoxicity of cancer drugs. This gap must be addressed by once again bringing the two medical disciplines together to rigorously assess the endocrinology of the cancer patient before and after treatment and during follow up. Complicating the data acquisition is that patients are treated at different ages and with different drug regimens. These variables make the studies more challenging and require knowledge of the treatment schedules, changes in drug routine, and a long-term commitment to this new field. Moreover, new drugs are introduced frequently and the fertility threat must be immediately evaluated. Traditional hormone tests over time must be conducted, and more rapid bioassays that assess risk factors used in a sophisticated way to address this problem. The new oncofertility specialist will be uniquely qualified to fill the data gap.

Option GAP

The option gap is most important to women with cancer. Recent breakthroughs in tissue cryopreservation, in vitro follicle growth, and ovarian transplants provide important new ideas that must be developed in a collective manner to ensure that these new concepts are tested in primates and are real solutions to the problem rather than simply proof-of-principle observations. In order to accomplish this goal, basic scientists, clinical investigators, and clinicians-in-practice from a variety of fields must not just collaborate, but must become fully integrated across traditional disciplinary borders representing biomedical discovery, advanced medical practice and application, and scholarship in the humanities and social science (Fig. 1.3 and see Kondapalli, Snyder, Clayman et al., Kinahan et al., this volume). This interaction is the first step in becoming interdisciplinary. Importantly, the new field of oncofertility biology must use non-human primate models and human tissue to appropriately move the ideas from the bench to the bedside. To do this, basic and clinical science must work together in ways that each group can understand the terms and concepts of the respective disciplines as well as understand patient needs and limitations. To ensure patient needs are primary, clinical coordinators and navigators trained at the intersection of disciplines will be engaged at all level of activity.

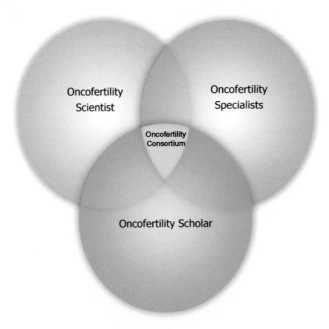

Fig. 1.3 Oncofertility represents a new interdisciplinary program that will span the known gaps and address the needs of patients with cancer by encouraging new work by newly envisioned oncofertility scientists, specialists, and scholars

Conclusion

This book and the oncofertility effort are aimed at an emerging health care crisis faced by nearly one million young people. Ironically, we coined the word "oncofertility" in February 2006 as part of a grant submission process. Clearly, the need existed for this new discipline, but to fill the need required something much larger, more comprehensive, and interdisciplinary. The term oncofertility has now entered the public sphere and we believe it has already reached a "tipping point" in public consciousness. Indeed, two years ago we were barely able to get any traction on the idea, but, now, every clinical practice we talk to is not just interested but committed to the concept. The goal of oncofertility is to meet an emerging urgent unmet need for young cancer patients: balancing life-preserving treatments with fertility-preserving options. To meet this challenge successfully, we must develop new oncofertility specialists, scientists, and scholars who will develop the tools and approaches that can best achieve this goal. Importantly, this is a problem that can be solved using a interdisciplinary approach and simply cannot be achieved in isolation.

It is hoped that future books in this series will report on significant new advances in the oncofertility field and provide new hope to those young people impacted by cancer.

Part II
Fertility Risk and Treatment Options

Chapter 2
Fertility Management for Women with Cancer

Sanjay K. Agarwal, MD and R. Jeffrey Chang, MD

Cancer is now a disease with a variety of treatment options that are leading to longer and more productive lives in survivors. More than 200,000 men and women under the age of 45 years are diagnosed with cancer annually. However, challenges remain for cancer survivors striving to return to normalcy. Infertility can be a consequence of many of the more aggressive chemo- and radiation therapies that prolong and save lives. The ability to easily preserve sperm prior to cancer treatment provides hope at the time of diagnosis to have families later in life for male survivors. A notable example is Tour de France winner Lance Armstrong, who has three children conceived by using sperm collected and frozen days before he underwent the massive chemo- and radiation therapy that saved his life. When faced with a similar devastating diagnosis, women and girls have the same hope for recovery but lack the fertility preservation options that Mr. Armstrong was given. Unlike sperm, the female germ cell, the oocyte or egg, must be retrieved surgically. Moreover, the vast majority of collected oocytes will be immature at collection and cannot be used immediately by a woman who is ready to start a family.

Many of the principles and technologies discussed in this chapter in the context of cancer patients can equally well be applied to women with benign pelvic diseases that threaten their fertility. For example, some women with severe endometriosis or pelvic infection may need to have their ovaries removed as a part of radical surgical treatment for these diseases. In others, during the process of surgically removing ovarian cysts, germ cells can be damaged, thus reducing the woman's fertility. Further, the treatment of benign diseases such as Bechet syndrome and glomerulonephropathies may require chemotherapy that could, just as with cancer patients, reduce ovarian reserve.

Ovarian Physiology

The process of germ cell (oocyte) loss from mid-pregnancy to menopause is a normal physiologic process (Fig. 2.1). At mid-pregnancy, a female fetus has about seven million germ cells that comprise the ovarian reserve. With atresia, this number is reduced to about one million per ovary at birth. The decline in germ cell

T.K. Woodruff and K.A. Snyder (eds.) *Oncofertility.*
© Springer 2007

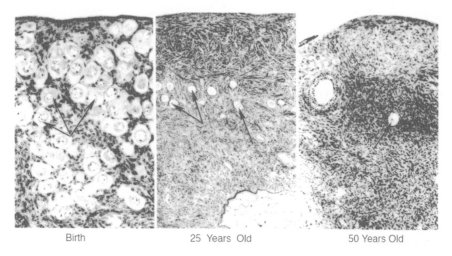

Fig. 2.1 Photomicrographs illustrating the age-related decline of primordial follicle numbers in human ovaries (From Erickson GF. An analysis of follicle development and ovum maturation. Sem Reprod Endocrinol 1986; 4:233–254 by permission of Thieme Medical Publishers, Inc.)

number continues such that by puberty there is a total of about 300,000 germ cells, and by menopause, around 1,000 remain. Thus, prior to spontaneous ovulation, there is a degenerative process of oocyte attrition, the mechanism of which is not well understood. With the onset of menstruation and normal ovulatory function, it is estimated that dozens of oocytes are consumed monthly to achieve a single ovulation. At around age 35–38, there is acceleration in oocyte atresia until the ovarian reserve is exhausted and menopause ensues (Fig. 2.2).

It is evident that, in women, the complete loss of the germ cell population is a result of both spontaneous ovulation as well as an undefined atretic mechanism. While unknown environmental and epigenetic phenomena may be harmful to germ cells, several causative factors such as cancer treatment, including chemotherapy and radiation, as well as elective social activities such as smoking, may accelerate the rate of oocyte loss, thus decreasing fertility and bringing the age of menopause forward.

The decline in germ cell number is mirrored by a decline in female fertility. With increasing age, particularly after the age of 35 years, a woman's natural fertility and chance of success with assisted reproduction declines. Since there can be quite substantial variations in fertility with age, the clinical assessment of a woman's "ovarian reserve" typically involves not just age but also changes in the release of pituitary follicle-stimulating hormone (FSH) and corresponding production of estradiol and inhibin B by granulosa cells within ovarian follicles. As the germ cell pool declines and fewer ovarian follicles are present, there is a decrease in ovarian inhibin B production. Inhibin B provides negative feedback to FSH secretion and hence an increase in FSH can be detected as a result of declining inhibin B. Since FSH values vary during the menstrual cycle, it is standard practice to obtain a measurement of serum FSH on day 3 of the menstrual cycle. An estradiol

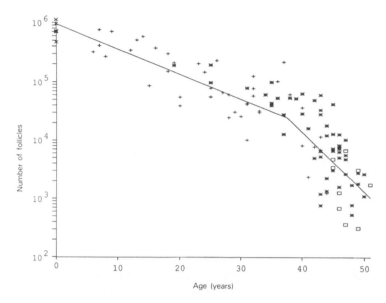

Fig. 2.2 Graph depicting the age-related decrease in primordial follicle numbers with increased rate of loss from around 35–38 years of age (From Faddy MJ, et al. Accelerated disappearance of ovarian follicles in mid-life: implications for forecasting menopause. Hum Reprod 1992; 7(10):1342–1346 by permission of Oxford University Press.)

Table 2.1 Common tools for assessing ovarian reserve in clinical practice

Female age
Day 3 serum FSH (with estradiol)
Transvaginal ultrasound determination of antral follicle count

level is determined on the same day to ensure that the FSH value is accurate and not artificially lowered by a high circulating estradiol level as may occur in the presence of premature follicular development. A more recent addition to the assessment of ovarian reserve has been the ultrasound evaluation of ovarian antral follicle count. For this, transvaginal ultrasonography is performed and the number of small antral follicles in the ovaries is documented. The number declines with age [1,2], and ideally, the observation of a total follicle count of 12 or more from both ovaries is reassuring. Table 2.1 outlines the commonly used strategies for determining ovarian reserve in current clinical practice.

For the patient with a cancer diagnosis, the implementation of treatment in a timely manner is essential in order to have optimal success with life-saving therapies. Therefore, waiting for day 3 in the menstrual cycle to determine FSH and estradiol levels for evaluation of her ovarian reserve is not always feasible. For this reason, when assessing whether or not a cancer patient is a candidate for fertility-preserving therapies, and in order to provide accurate fertility counseling, the assessment of ovarian reserve by an estimate of age and antral follicle count is of critical importance.

Ovarian reserve testing also has a role following cancer therapy in women medically suitable for pregnancy by helping to determine remaining ovarian function and hence, the appropriate degree of aggressiveness with which one should undertake fertility therapy.

Impact of Cancer Therapies on Ovarian Function

The term "ovarian failure" indicates the irreversible loss of ovarian function with failure of follicular development and ovulation. Concurrently, estrogen production by the ovaries is essentially eliminated and declines to menopausal levels. The loss of ovarian function in a woman less than 40 years of age is considered to be premature ovarian failure. Assessment of the impact of cancer therapies on ovarian function is hampered by inconsistent and varied definitions of amenorrhea and ovarian failure, and in variable time of follow up. Although most studies use a 12-month interval in evaluating post-therapy amenorrhea, it may take up to 16 months to develop in women under 40 years of age [3].

Both chemotherapy and radiation therapies used for the treatment of cancer can lead to premature ovarian failure. The likelihood of this unfortunate consequence depends on the precise therapy and increases with the age of the woman. It should be remembered that because of sporadic ovulation in women with premature ovarian failure, pregnancies have been reported. Even survivors of childhood cancer have an increased risk on premature menopause, which is dependent upon radiation dose to the ovaries, number of alkylating chemotherapy agents used and their cumulative dose, as well as a diagnosis of Hodgkin's lymphoma [4]. Radiation therapy to the pelvis can have a significant direct negative impact on ovarian function. As with chemotherapy, the extent of damage not only depends on the age of the woman but also on radiation dose and field of treatment. Doses as low as 4–6 Gy in adults and 10–20 Gy in children can lead to irreversible decrease in ovarian function with some experiencing ovarian failure [5–9]. The likelihood of ovarian damage can be reduced by surgically moving the ovaries (ovariopexy) away from the radiation field prior to radiation [10]. Total body irradiation of children is particularly likely to lead to ovarian failure, with 90% of those over 10 years of age being affected. It should be remembered that although the impact of irradiation on ovarian function is of profound importance, the uterus can also be damaged by such therapy. Uterine consequences of radiation include decrease in uterine cavity volume [11,12] and decreased blood flow, which may explain the increase in miscarriage and other pregnancy complications seen in women conceiving after pelvic irradiation.

Non-pelvic irradiation can also impact fertility. For example, cerebral irradiation may disrupt central hypothalamic-pituitary regulation of ovarian function resulting in hypogonadotropic hypogonadism [12]. Fortunately, conventional therapies such as ovulation induction with gonadotropin injections or in vitro fertilization (IVF) and embryo transfer usually suffice to restore fertility.

Breast cancer is the most prevalent cancer to affect women. Although the likelihood of developing this cancer increases with age, about 1 in 3 women are premenopausal at the time of diagnosis [13]. Fortunately, cancer related mortality for breast cancer has decreased dramatically such that with modern management, most women with this diagnosis can expect to live long, productive lives. As a result, premenopausal women with a diagnosis of breast cancer represent a sizeable population concerned about their fertility after cancer therapy [14]. Breast cancer, as well as other cancers, is commonly treated with adjuvant chemotherapeutic agents. Alkylating agents do not have a cell-specific effect and hence have a particularly high propensity for irreversibly damaging resting immature oocytes (primordial follicles). Cyclophosphamide is the chemotherapeutic agent that is most commonly implicated in decreasing ovarian function and does so in a dose-dependent manner.

Age and duration of therapy are other important factors in determining risk of ovarian failure, with older women being more vulnerable than young [15,16]. A clear example regarding the major the impact of age is provided by the study of Goldhirsch et al. [16], in which premenopausal women undergoing classic 6-month cyclophosphamide, methotrexate, and fluorouracil (CMF) adjuvant chemotherapy for breast cancer were studied and found to have a 33% risk of amenorrhea if under 40 years and an 81% risk if older. The same study also demonstrated the impact of duration of therapy, in that those treated for 1 month had less than half the rate of amenorrhea suffered by those receiving 6 months of chemotherapy. The antimetabolites 5-fluorouracil and methotrexate in the CMF regimen have not been shown to cause increased risk of amenorrhea. In combination, these two agents had a 9% amenorrhea rate compared with a 69% rate with CMF in an age-matched population [3].

Preventing chemotherapy-induced ovarian toxicity has been the largely unrealized hope of pretreatment with pharmaceutical agents such as gonadotropin releasing hormone (GnRH) agonists or oral contraceptives. The expectation was that if ovarian metabolism could be made quiescent, then any negative effect of the chemotherapy on ovarian tissue would be minimized. In practice, this theory has not been found to be as successful as once hoped. Only one randomized study has been performed that evaluated 18 women undergoing chemotherapy for Hodgkin's disease [17]. Administration of GnRH agonist prior to and for the duration of chemotherapy was not found to prevent the development of drug-induced amenorrhea during the 3 years of follow up. Incidentally, men were also included in this study, and as with the women, there was no preservation of their fertility with GnRH agonist therapy as documented by the development of oligospermia. In women, this relative lack of efficacy may be explained by the fact that since oral contraceptives and probably GnRH agonists do not preserve ovarian reserve (there is no delay in menopause in users), it is reasonable to infer that they do not prevent the physiologic atrophy of germ cells. Given that chemotherapy damages primordial follicles, it is perhaps understandable why gonadal suppression prior to and during chemotherapy does not prevent ovarian damage.

Current Techniques of Fertility Preservation

Most current methods of preserving fertility in women involve cryopreservation of ovarian tissues. The objective of cryopreservation is to maintain viability of tissue after long-term storage. It is the basis for all forms of fertility preservation for cancer sufferers. Cryopreservation requires cooling tissue from 37°C to the temperature of liquid nitrogen (−196°C), storage at this temperature, and then rewarming to 37°C at some later date. As the temperature of the tissue decreases below the freezing point, the water within the tissue forms ice crystals and expands. This expansion can damage the integrity of membranes and intracellular organelles rendering the cells non-viable. Strategies for the prevention of cell damage associated with freezing include the use of either permeating or non-permeating cryoprotectants. Permeating agents are small molecules that enter the cells and prevent ice crystal formation. Non-permeating agents remain extracellular and draw out the cellular water, hence essentially dehydrating the cells and thus preventing intracellular ice crystal formation.

The conventional method for freezing embryos is called the slow freeze method, and is a technique that can also be used for freezing oocytes and ovarian cortex strips. Cryoprotectants such as dimethyl dulfoxide (DMSO) and, more recently, sucrose are used. The temperature is lowered at a very slow rate of about 0.33°C per minute until reaching −32°C, at which point the sample is put in liquid nitrogen where it is rapidly cooled to −196°C.

Vitrification (rapid freeze) is an alternative strategy for cryopreservation and, as the name suggests, involves the rapid freezing of the sample. High doses of permeating cryoprotectants are used and once allowed to equilibrate, but before toxicity can ensue, the sample is quickly frozen in liquid nitrogen. Rapid thawing is required with this technique to prevent ice crystal formation.

The most successful and only therapeutic option that is widely available for women with cancer wanting to preserve their fertility is to undergo IVF and embryo freezing. This can take precious weeks to accomplish and requires a male partner or the use of donor sperm. The alternatives, which include freezing sections of ovarian cortex or freezing either mature or immature oocytes, still have more limited availability, though with time and increased interest in these techniques both success and availability will increase.

Embryo Freezing

The traditional, and currently the only, well established therapeutic option allowing for fertility after cancer therapy is the storage of frozen embryos. This strategy requires that the patient undergo ovarian stimulation for the in vivo maturation of oocytes and subsequent retrieval of mature oocytes prior to initiation of cancer therapy. The oocytes are fertilized on the day of egg retrieval and the resultant embryos are cryopreserved. At the time of the patient's choosing, embryos can be thawed and transferred into either the patient's own uterus, providing that her uterus is viable for pregnancy, or that of another woman (gestational surrogate).

The basic technologies necessary for embryo freezing are in clinical use throughout the world on a daily basis. Therefore, availability of services should not be an insurmountable problem. During conventional gonadotropin-stimulated ovulation induction for IVF, it is hoped that a minimum of around 4, and ideally about 10–15, dominant follicles develop. Generally, the actual number of mature follicles attainable decreases with declining ovarian reserve. During the process of ovulation induction, the development of multiple dominant follicles may give rise to substantial increases in ovarian estradiol production due to increased granulosa cell number. In these situations, circulating estradiol concentrations may exceed 3,000 pg/ml. This is substantially greater than that of a natural, unstimulated ovulatory cycle with peak estradiol levels of about 300 pg/ml. This can be a concern for women with estrogen-dependent cancers such as certain breast cancers and benign diseases such as endometriosis. A strategy to successfully induce ovulation for IVF in these women without producing high estradiol levels has been described [18]. It involves adding an aromatase inhibitor to the usual gonadotropin-based ovarian stimulation protocol. Aromatase inhibitors prevent the formation of estrogen from androgen precursors and resultant serum estradiol levels are substantially reduced compared with conventional IVF stimulation and can actually be less than that seen in a natural cycle.

Success rates with frozen embryo cycles depend primarily on the woman's age at the time the eggs were retrieved and fertilized (Table 2.2) and not the age of the woman in whose uterus they are eventually transferred. Once frozen, the embryos can be thawed and transferred years later without a time-dependent decrease in success. For the cancer patient, problems with this strategy are two-fold. First, the time required for oocyte maturation with ovulation induction is generally about 2 weeks from the onset of menses. Hence, if the decision to undergo conventional IVF and embryo freezing is made much after about day 3 of the menstrual cycle, the day of the menstrual cycle by when ovulation induction is usually initiated, the patient will have to wait until the onset of the next menstrual period prior to initiating ovulation induction. Second, because embryos rather than oocytes are frozen, there is a need for an acceptable source of sperm. This is not usually a problem if the patient is married or in some other committed relationship. However, for others not in such relationships, the difficult decision of using donor sperm has to be made.

Table 2.2 2005 National frozen cycle results – Society for Assisted Reproductive Technology

Thawed embryos from non-donor oocytes	Female age at time of embryo transfer			
	<35	35–37	38–40	41–42
Number of transfers	8,622	4,379	2,636	898
Percentage of transfers resulting in live births	31.8	27.9	23.1	15.6
Average number of embryos transferred	2.4	2.5	2.6	2.7

Ovarian Tissue Freezing

Ovarian cryopreservation has been shown to be successful in a variety of animal models and to a limited degree in humans. The technique involves the freezing of ovarian cortex segments for later thawing and transplanting either back to the ovarian site (orthotopically) or to some other location (heterotopically). The ovarian cortex is used because it is this part of the ovary that is particularly rich in primordial follicles. In order for cryoprotectants to penetrate the tissue, the cortical strips need to be no more than 2mm thick. Tissue samples from cancer patients need to be evaluated by a pathologist to detect the presence of any metastatic cancer cells. One of the problems encountered with this technique is a decrease in primordial follicles within the grafted tissue. This is due to hypoxia from a delay in revascularization. The loss of primordial follicles in cryopreserved ovarian cortex strips ranges from 50 to over 90% [19–21], which is reflected in FSH levels that usually remain elevated and inhibin B levels that remain low, even after re-transplantation. Survival of grafts after transplant depends on angiogenesis and neovascularization. As improved understanding of the mechanisms involved spur improved techniques, the outcomes will improve.

Advantages of this technique over the freezing of embryos are that sperm is not necessary at the time of freezing and no delay in cancer therapy is required for oocyte maturation and retrieval. Indeed, ovarian tissue retrieval and freezing can be performed at any time during the cycle, without delaying chemotherapy or radiation therapy. Once the frozen tissue is thawed and transplanted back in to the patient, it is possible that in addition to any fertility benefits, enough estrogen may be produced to at least temporarily treat menopausal symptoms and prevent the onset of osteoporosis. Although the technique is limited by ischemic injury to the transplant tissue, the major theoretical concern with applying this technique to cancer patients is the risk of transplanting back cancer cells with the ovarian tissue.

Pregnancy after orthotopic autotransplantation of cryopreserved human ovarian cortex may be possible naturally. Indeed, this is the ultimate goal of the technique. However, for the purposes of fertility and because of the decrease in germ cell numbers, women undergoing this technique usually require aggressive, high-dose gonadotropin stimulation of the ovarian cortex grafts and are thus usually considered to be in the category of "low responders" with a diminished ovarian reserve. If some ovarian tissue is left in situ at the time of ovarian cortex removal and pregnancy occurs some time after orthotopic ovarian tissue transplantation, it may be difficult to determine whether the source of the fertilized oocyte was the grafted ovarian tissue or the ovarian tissue that was left in situ.

There is much less experience and success with heterotopic autotransplantation. It is possible that the common subcutaneous transplant sites in the forearm or abdomen render the graft likely to fail functionally because of lower temperature and higher physical stress due to inadvertent increases in pressure than normally experienced in the pelvis [22,23]. These grafts need a degree of ovulation induction prior to the retrieval of mature oocytes, which then are used in intracytoplasmic sperm injection (ICSI) and embryo transfer.

Oocyte Freezing

Oocyte cryopreservation is developing as another technology for individuals wishing to preserve fertility but who are not willing to commit to a sperm donor. It can also be an option for those with a partner who, for time constraints, cannot defer cancer therapy for a sufficient time to undergo conventional ovulation induction for IVF and embryo freezing. Because of the complex and fragile nature of the oocyte, oocyte freezing has been technically challenging and success, although improving, has been limited. With this technology, either mature or immature oocytes are obtained and cryopreserved.

Mature oocytes can be obtained by ovulation induction and oocyte retrieval as is done for IVF. However, rather than fertilizing the oocytes prior to freezing embryos, the mature oocytes are frozen. Because of the large size of mature oocytes, they are particularly susceptible to damage during cryopreservation. Ice crystal formation, zona pellucida hardening, and meiotic spindle anomalies have been detected and are associated with reduced oocyte survival and fertilization and increased aneuploidy [24–27]. Although zona pellucida hardening can be overcome with ICSI, there are no good solutions available currently for the disruption of meiotic spindles that occurs when freezing mature oocytes. In addition, although this strategy obviously does not afford any advantage with regard to time needs as compared with conventional IVF and embryo freezing, it does allow a woman to freeze eggs without committing to the source of sperm at that time. Hence, for those not in a committed relationship and wishing to keep their sperm options open, the technology is of potential value.

In order to overcome the time requirements essential for harvesting mature oocytes, a newer strategy for oocyte freezing has evolved. This strategy involves obtaining immature oocytes from unstimulated or minimally stimulated ovaries and after in vitro maturation of the oocytes, freezing either the oocytes themselves or, if sperm is available, embryos. Because of the greater number of small follicles in the ovaries of women with polycystic ovary syndrome (PCOS), most cases described so far have been from PCOS ovaries. After retrieval, the oocytes have typically been made to undergo in vitro maturation (Fig. 2.3) prior to either freezing or fertilization. A less well explored alternative is to freeze immature oocytes soon after retrieval without significant in vitro maturation. After thawing, the oocytes would require in vitro maturation prior to fertilization and embryo transfer. The potential advantage of freezing immature oocytes is that they are smaller and metabolically less active than mature oocytes.

Oocyte freezing strategies have several potential advantages over regular IVF embryo freezing. The time for ovulation induction is not necessary, and for this reason, there is less delay in initiating chemotherapy. Additionally, patients are not exposed to pharmaceutical doses of gonadotropins and high estradiol levels during in vivo oocyte maturation, and commitment to a sperm source is not needed at the time of oocyte retrieval. The relative importance of these advantages varies from patient to patient.

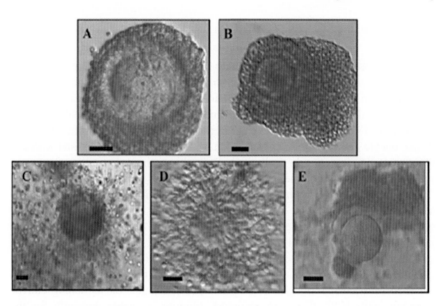

Fig. 2.3 Morphological classification of cumulus-enclosed oocytes retrieved from small antral follicles. Germinal vesicle-stage oocytes are enclosed in 3 (A) to 10 (B) layers of tightly compacted corona cells. (C) Oocytes enclosed in layers of compacted proximal granulosa cells and expanded distal granulosa cells. (D) Oocytes enclosed in expanded cumulus cells (similar to IVF-collected oocytes). (E) Atretic oocytes can be retrieved within fully enclosed cumulus-corona cell layers or partially denuded from cumulus-corona cells (as shown here), or completely naked, with or without a degenerative ooplasmic aspect. All panels, scale bar = 50 μm (From Jurema MW, Nogueira D. In vitro maturation of human oocytes for assisted reproduction. Fertil Steril 2006; 86:1277–91 by permission of Elsevier.)

One study compared chromosome configurations and meiotic spindle microtubules in oocytes that had undergone in vitro maturation to those that had been matured in vivo [28]. The investigators used confocal microscopy and fluorescent immunocytologic staining to analyze oocytes from women with PCOS following retrieval at an immature stage and in vitro maturation. These were then compared with oocytes from women with PCOS that had undergone conventional in vivo maturation with gonadotropin stimulation. The findings were that in vitro matured oocytes were more likely to have abnormal chromosome configurations and disordered meiotic spindle microtubules. Whether the same outcome will hold true for oocytes retrieved from women with a more normal endocrine profile is yet undetermined.

Although success with in vitro oocyte maturation is increasing rapidly, it is still largely limited by the available culture systems. As these and other necessary areas of expertise improve, it is expected that outcomes with this exciting new technology will also improve. Indeed, aspirating immature oocytes and performing in vitro oocyte maturation is already being touted as a useful adjunct to, and a possible replacement for, in vivo oocyte maturation in the current IVF clinic [29–31]. This is especially true for women at particularly high risk for ovarian hyperstimulation syndrome with gonadotropin-stimulated conventional IVF. With continuing refinement of oocyte freezing technology, the number of oocytes needed for a reasonable chance of pregnancy will decrease. Currently, one can expect a less than 2% chance of pregnancy per thawed oocyte [32]. Despite the current low pregnancy rate per oocyte with the use of aspirated immature oocytes that have undergone in vitro maturation, numerous pregnancies have been reported. There has only been one report of a congenital anomaly following oocyte cryopreservation: a child with an isolated ventricular septal defect [33]. It is also encouraging that, in an albeit limited evaluation, children born as a result of this technology do not appear to show developmental delay during infancy and early childhood [34].

Future Directions

Although the ability to reliably produce successful pregnancies from the harvesting of immature oocytes with subsequent in vitro maturation will likely be the easiest to achieve, there is clearly room for improved success in this and other technologies described in this chapter. Improved outcomes will only come from the deeper understanding of physiologic processes and the development of cryopreservation techniques that are less traumatic to the tissue being frozen. In addition, in the case of ovarian cortex freezing and autotransplantation, improved stimulators of angiogenesis and neovascularization will also be necessary. As these technologies mature, algorithms and guidelines will be developed to ensure that they are used appropriately. Indeed, these strategies may provide a reasonable way for women without cancer or significant fertility-threatening disease to preserve their fertility options for social reasons.

Summary

With time, great strides are being made in the care of cancer sufferers. The longevity and quality of life of these unfortunate individuals continues to improve and the word "cure" is more commonly being heard. In a similar manner, there is also much reason for optimism regarding the future fertility options for patients with cancer as well as for those with other diseases that have a high likelihood of rendering a female infertile prior to completing her family. Figure 2.4 outlines the various cryo-preservation technologies currently available. While IVF and embryo freezing remain the gold standard at the present, refinements in in vitro maturation of oocytes and cryopreservation of oocytes and ovarian cortex will lead to improved results and availability of these technologies.

Counseling patients of child-bearing age or their parents regarding future fertility when faced with a life-threatening cancer diagnosis is difficult but extremely important. With modern approaches to cancer care, survival rates have improved

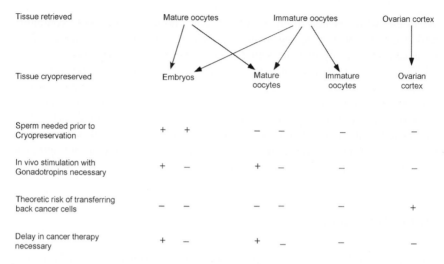

	Embryos		Mature oocytes		Immature oocytes	Ovarian cortex
Sperm needed prior to Cryopreservation	+	+	−	−	−	−
In vivo stimulation with Gonadotropins necessary	+	−	+	−	−	−
Theoretic risk of transferring back cancer cells	−	−	−	−	−	+
Delay in cancer therapy necessary	+	−	+	−	−	−

Fig. 2.4 Strategies for the preservation of fertility in women undergoing treatment for cancer or other diseases that are likely to render them infertile

significantly. Therefore, the health care team has a responsibility to provide screening to identify these patients, provide education so that an informed decision can be made as rapidly as possible, and have a team ready to preserve fertility once a decision has been made. With the improvements in fertility outcomes for these patients, appropriate education of key communities, including cancer sufferers and their health care providers, will be necessary to ensure that the issue of fertility after cancer is at least discussed and offered to those in whom it is appropriate.

References

1. Hendriks DJ, Mol BW, Bancsi LF, et al. Antral follicle count in the prediction of poor ovarian response and pregnancy after *in vitro* fertilization: a meta-analysis and comparison with basal follicle-stimulating hormone level. Fertil Steril 2005;83:291–301.
2. Erdem A, Erdem M, Biberoglu K, et al. Age-related changes in ovarian volume, antral follicle counts and basal FSH in women with normal reproductive health. J Reprod Med 2002;47:835–839.
3. Bines J, Oleske DM, Cobleigh MA. Ovarian function in premenopausal women treated with adjuvant chemotherapy for breast cancer. J Clin Oncol 1996;14:1718–1729.
4. Sklar CA, Mertens AC, Mitby P, et al. Premature menopause in survivors of childhood cancer: a report from the childhood cancer survivor study. J Natl Cancer Inst 2006;98:890–896.
5. Wallace WH, Thomson AB, Kelsey TW. The radiosensitivity of the human oocyte. Hum Reprod 2003;18:117–121.
6. Horning SJ, Hoppe RT, Kaplan HS, et al. Female reproductive potential after treatment for Hodgkin's disease. N Engl J Med 1981;304:1377–1382.
7. Lushbaugh CC, Casarett GW. The effects of gonadal irradiation in clinical radiation therapy: a review. Cancer 1976;37:1111–1125.
8. Thibaud E, Ramirez M, Brauner R, et al. Preservation of ovarian function by ovarian transposition performed before pelvic irradiation during childhood. J Pediatr 1992;121:880–884.

9. Wallace WH, Shalet SM, Hendry JH, et al. Ovarian failure following abdominal irradiation in childhood: the radiosensitivity of the human oocyte. Br J Radiol 1989;62:995–998.

10. Morice P, Juncker L, Rey A, et al. Ovarian transposition for patients with cervical carcinoma treated by radiosurgical combination. Fertil Steril 2000;74:743–748.

11. Critchley HO, Bath LE, Wallace WH. Radiation damage to the uterus – review of the effects of treatment of childhood cancer. Hum Fertil 2002;5:61–66.

12. Ogilvy-Stuart AL, Shalet SM. Effect of radiation on the human reproductive system. Environ Health Perspect 1993;101 Suppl 2:109–116.

13. Jemal A, Thomas A, Murray T, et al. Cancer statistics, 2002. CA Cancer J Clin 2002;52:23–47.

14. Partridge AH, Gelber S, Peppercorn J, et al. Web-based survey of fertility issues in young women with breast cancer. J Clin Oncol 2004;22:4174–4183.

15. Goodwin PJ, Ennis M, Pritchard KI, et al. Risk of menopause during the first year after breast cancer diagnosis. J Clin Oncol 1999;17:2365–2370.

16. Goldhirsch A, Gelber RD, Castiglione M. The magnitude of endocrine effects of adjuvant chemotherapy for premenopausal breast cancer patients. The International Breast Cancer Study Group. Ann Oncol 1990;1:183–188.

17. Waxman JH, Ahmed R, Smith D, et al. Failure to preserve fertility in patients with Hodgkin's disease. Cancer Chemother Pharmacol 1987;19:159–162.

18. Oktay K, Hourvitz A, Sahin G, et al. Letrozole reduces estrogen and gonadotropin exposure in women with breast cancer undergoing ovarian stimulation before chemotherapy. J Clin Endocrinol Metab 2006;91:3885–3890.

19. Baird DT, Webb R, Campbell BK, et al. Long-term ovarian function in sheep after ovariectomy and transplantation of autografts stored at −196 C. Endocrinol 1999;140:462–471.

20. Aubard Y, Piver P, Cogni Y, et al. Orthotopic and heterotopic autografts of frozen-thawed ovarian cortex in sheep. Hum Reprod 1999;14:2149–2154.

21. Nisolle M, Casanas-Roux F, Qu J, et al. Histologic and ultrastructural evaluation of fresh and frozen-thawed human ovarian xenografts in nude mice. Fertil Steril 2000;74:122–129.

22. Wolner-Hanssen P, Hagglund L, Ploman F, et al. Autotransplantation of cryopreserved ovarian tissue to the right forearm 4(1/2) years after autologous stem cell transplantation. Acta Obstet Gynecol Scand 2005;84:695–698.

23. Oktay K, Buyuk E, Veeck L, et al. Embryo development after heterotopic transplantation of cryopreserved ovarian tissue. Lancet 2004;363:837–840.

24. Trounson A. Spindle abnormalities in oocytes. Fertil Steril 2006;85:838; discussion 841.

25. Lanzendorf SE. Developmental potential of in vitro- and in vivo-matured human oocytes collected from stimulated and unstimulated ovaries. Fertil Steril 2006;85:836–837; discussion 841.

26. Kanaya H, Murata Y, Oku H, et al. Successful monozygotic twin delivery following in vitro maturation of oocytes retrieved from a woman with polycystic ovary syndrome: case report. Hum Reprod 2006;21:1777–1780.

27. Baka SG, Toth TL, Veeck LL, et al. Evaluation of the spindle apparatus of in-vitro matured human oocytes following cryopreservation. Hum Reprod 1995;10:1816–1820.

28. Li Y, Feng HL, Cao YJ, et al. Confocal microscopic analysis of the spindle and chromosome configurations of human oocytes matured in vitro. Fertil Steril 2006;85:827–832.

29. Dal Canto MB, Mignini RM, Brambillasca F, et al. IVM – the first choice for IVF in Italy. Reprod Biomed Online 2006;13:159–165.

30. Piquette GN. The in vitro maturation (IVM) of human oocytes for in vitro fertilization (IVF): is it time yet to switch to IVM–IVF? Fertil Steril 2006;85:833–835; discussion 841.

31. Jurema MW, Nogueira D. In vitro maturation of human oocytes for assisted reproduction. Fertil Steril 2006;86:1277–1291.

32. Sonmezer M, Oktay K. Fertility preservation in young women undergoing breast cancer therapy. Oncologist 2006;11:422–434.

33. Winslow KL, Yang D, Blohm PL, et al. Oocyte cryopreservation/a three year follow up of sixteen births. Fertil Steril 2001;76 (Suppl 1):120–121.

34. Shu-Chi M, Jiann-Loung H, Yu-Hung L, et al. Growth and development of children conceived by in-vitro maturation of human oocytes. Early Hum Dev 2006;82:677–682.

Chapter 3
Fertility Preservation in Adult Male Cancer Patients

Robert E. Brannigan, MD

Cancer is one of the most common disease states, with approximately 50% of men facing this diagnosis during the course of their lifetime. While the overriding focus for both health care professionals and patients has long been disease cure and survival, a number of factors have led to a significant change in this therapeutic perspective. With marked advances in early disease detection and therapy, patient survival for many cancers has increased dramatically over the last several decades. This, in turn, has provided many patients with the opportunity to live full lives beyond their diagnosis, allowing them to look past their cancer and consider life after treatment. Issues such as post-treatment marriage and parenthood are considered as important as the underlying disease by many patients. As such, measures to preserve sexual and reproductive health in the course of cancer treatment are increasingly important to many patients as they face a malignancy diagnosis.

In addition to improvements in cancer detection and treatment, there has been a growing demographic trend for both men and women to pursue efforts at initiating pregnancy later in life. The reasons for this are many, including initial fulfillment of educational and career goals, marriage at a later age in life, and second families started after divorce or death of a spouse. This shift has also led to a change in the traditional reproductive paradigm. Now, malignancies such as prostate, lung, and colorectal cancer are being seen in patients who may indeed wish to preserve their reproductive potential. It is specifically for these reasons that clinicians must be both vigilant and open-minded when considering the needs of patients who are facing a malignancy diagnosis. A proactive discussion with each patient regarding the possible deleterious impact of their disease state and the associated therapy must be undertaken in order to truly provide patients with comprehensive medical care. Failure to proceed in this fashion will surely lead to missed opportunities for fertility preservation in patients, some of whom may permanently lose their reproductive capability.

The Impact of Cancer on Male Reproductive Health

Cancer as a disease process can have many deleterious effects on male reproduction, even before any therapy has been initiated. These effects include disruption of the hypothalamic-pituitary-gonadal (H-P-G) axis, direct immunological or cytotoxic

T.K. Woodruff and K.A. Snyder (eds.) *Oncofertility*.

injury to the germinal epithelium within the testis, systemic processes such as fever and malnutrition, and psychological issues such as anxiety and depression. These pathological changes may individually or collectively lead to fertility impairment, which is sometimes present at the time of diagnosis [1,2].

Endocrine Effects of Tumors

Successful spermatogenesis hinges on the normal endocrine function of the hypothalamus, pituitary gland, and testis. The delicate balance maintained by these structures is often disturbed at the time of cancer diagnosis. This is particularly true in patients with testicular cancer whose tumors may produce beta-human chorionic gonadotropin (β-hCG) and alpha-fetoprotein (AFP).

In a series of 15 patients with testicular cancer, Carroll et al. reported that two-thirds had abnormalities in key reproductive hormones. These changes included a decrease in serum follicle-stimulating hormone (FSH) levels and/or elevations in luteinizing hormone (LH) and β-hCG levels [3]. In this series, FSH was decreased in 9 out of 10 patients with impaired semen parameters, and 4 of these 9 patients had elevated β-hCG levels, leading the authors to postulate a possible inhibitory effect of β-hCG on FSH in some patients. Other studies have detected markedly increased FSH levels and decreased testosterone levels in the presence of testicular tumors that produce β-hCG [4]. Larger series are needed to help further define the relationship between these hormones in patients with cancer.

Excessive levels of AFP have also been associated with disruption of spermatogenesis in testicular cancer. Hansen et al. assessed 97 men with seminomatous and non-seminomatous germ cell tumors (NSGCT), and reported an AFP elevation in 38% of these patients [4]. In the subset of men with NSGCT, increased AFP was found on multiple regression analysis to be strongly associated with impaired semen quality.

Estrogen has also been linked to impaired spermatogenesis in men with testicular cancer. Cochran et al. noted that patients with β-hCG–producing tumors exhibited increased estradiol secretion and significantly decreased FSH production, suggesting a possible endocrinopathic pathway leading to diminished sperm production [5]. Aiginger et al. suggested more broadly that increased conversion of steroid precursors to estradiol is a feature of both β-hCG positive and β-hCG negative testicular tumors, leading to inhibition of the H-P-G axis and deleterious effects on spermatogenesis [6].

Much remains to be learned about the complexities of cancer-induced disruption of the H-P-G axis. Over the last several years, the numerous cytokines that are produced by immunological cells and tumor cells alike have garnered increasing interest. In addition to direct injurious effects on germinal epithelium and Leydig cells in the testis, ample evidence suggests that cytokines may also disrupt the central nervous system (CNS) endocrine processes. Cytokine receptors are present in the CNS, and studies by several investigators suggest that some cytokines may cross the blood-brain barrier to activate central kinase systems and disturb normal endocrine pathways [7,8]. Anorexia-cachexia syndrome is an example of such a cancer-related process in which cytokines have been implicated in causing disturbances in food intake and nutrition, ultimately leading to wasting, malnourishment, and death. The cytokines implicated in this process include interleukin 1, interleukin 6, tumor necrosis factor alpha, interferon gamma, leukemia inhibitory factor, and ciliary neurotrophic factor [9].

Anorexia-cachexia syndrome, which is present in 80% of patients with advanced cancer, is relevant to reproductive health in cancer patients in two regards. First, with severe depletion of nutritional reserves, processes such as reproductive function may be detrimentally affected [8]. Second, cytokine-driven CNS endocrinopathic processes such as anorexia-cachexia syndrome should prompt consideration of the existence of similar central cytokine effects on the reproductive function of the hypothalamus and pituitary gland. Further insight into the detrimental endocrine effects of cancer is needed.

Cytotoxic Autoimmune Response

A complicated cascade of changes in the immune system occurs in the presence of cancer. While these changes may aid in battling the neoplastic process at hand, secondary detrimental changes may result in reproductive dysfunction. Lymphocytic infiltration is associated with many testicular tumors, particularly seminomas [10]. While there is a paucity of studies examining the impact of testicular inflammation on spermatogenesis in the setting of cancer, several investigators have evaluated the effects of inflammation on spermatogenesis in normal testes.

Using models of experimentally induced orchitis, several different researchers have found that inflammatory cytokines may significantly disturb spermatogenesis. Rival et al. demonstrated a link between interleukin 6 expression, germ cell sloughing, and germ cell apoptosis in a Sprague-Dawley rat model with experimentally induced orchitis [11]. Theas et al. reported increased cytochrome c, caspase 8, and caspase 9 levels with associated germ cell apoptosis also using an experimentally induced orchitis rat model [12].

Reactive oxygen species (ROS) levels may also rise in the setting of testicular lymphocytic infiltrate. Spermatozoa exposure to ROS leads to sperm membrane lipid peroxidation which, in turn, may lead to fertility impairment [13]. Martinez et al. specifically evaluated the impact of several pro-inflammatory cytokines on semen samples from normospermic donors, in particular assessing ROS effects. They found interleukin 8 and tumor necrosis factor-alpha, either alone or in the presence of leukocytes, can lead to sperm plasma membrane lipid peroxidation at levels that could significantly affect sperm function and fertility potential [14].

Cytokine excess may also have direct injurious effects on the testis by disrupting the blood-testis barrier. Guazzieri et al. noted high levels of antisperm antibodies in men with testicular cancer, suggesting violation of the normal blood-testis barrier protecting the germinal epithelium from the immune system [15]. They found a significantly higher percentage of positivity (50%) for serum antisperm antibodies in patients with advanced disease compared with patients with low-stage disease (30%), supporting the hypothesis that autoimmune pathology may play a role in impaired sperm function in testicular cancer patients.

Systemic Physiological Changes

Cancer is associated with a host of significant changes in normal physiology and homeostasis. As seen in many patients with chronic disease states, patients with cancer may suffer from a variety of comorbidities, including malnutrition [16] and opportunistic infections [17], which may independently impair reproductive health.

Endocrine changes are commonly associated with a number of cancer types [18–20]. The pathophysiology is not entirely understood, but may arise due to inhibitory effects centrally on the hypothalamus and pituitary gland (as discussed earlier) and peripherally via impairment of the testicular Leydig cells. Low testosterone in the setting of cancer may not only impact spermatogenesis, but may also decrease the desire to engage in sexual activity. Anxiety, depression, and decreased overall sense of well-being may also result.

Strasser et al. assessed men with advanced cancer who had not undergone any major intervention or treatment for 2 weeks [21]. They found that 29 out of 45 men (64%) had low free testosterone levels. LH was elevated in these men, suggesting that the low free testosterone levels were caused, at least in part, by primary testicular dysfunction. Interestingly, Strasser et al. acknowledged that central mechanisms may also play a role in their patients' overall hypogonadism.

Fever, implicated as a systemic effect of cancer leading to impaired spermatogenesis, is also a common finding in patients with Hodgkin's lymphoma. Marmor et al. evaluated a series of 57 patients with Hodgkin's disease and found semen abnormalities in 19 (33.3%) [22]. Higher fever temperatures were associated with more severe deficits in sperm production, with severely diminished sperm concentration and even azoospermia seen in some patients. Lower temperatures were associated only with deficits in motility. Of the 19 patients with fever, only 5 had normal semen analyses. In a study by Viviani et al. semen analysis was performed in 92 male patients with Hodgkin's disease prior to treatment [18]. Sixty-seven percent of these men demonstrated impaired spermatogenesis independent of disease stage.

Psychological Changes Associated with Cancer

Patients confronting a diagnosis of cancer often find themselves facing a number of difficult psychological issues. Anxiety and depression are common among male cancer patients, and both have the potential to negatively impact reproductive health.

Using questionnaires that addressed sexual health, fertility, and psychological issues, Arai et al. evaluated 85 men with testicular cancer who were disease-free one year or more after treatment [23]. Interestingly, the rates and nature of sexual dysfunction seen in the surveillance patients were similar to those seen in the other treatment groups (surgery, chemotherapy, and radiation therapy). Ejaculatory function was the only exception to this finding, with the surveillance group having better ejaculatory function than the other treatment groups. The highest rates of infertility distress were observed in chemotherapy patients. Aside from ejaculatory function, patients treated with surveillance did not have fewer sexual problems than patients in the other treatment groups [23]. The authors concluded that sexual dysfunction and infertility distress are cancer side effects possibly attributed to psychological problems, which can persist even years after malignancy diagnosis.

The Impact of Cancer Treatment on Male Reproductive Health

A number of treatment modalities are utilized in the management of cancer. Surgical therapy, cytotoxic drug therapy, radiation therapy, and stem cell transplantation are commonly used in the treatment of this broad disease state. Each treatment has its own associated risks and benefits, and these effects should be carefully considered and discussed with the patient prior to initiating therapy. Specific potential effects of treatment include disruption of the H-P-G axis, direct cytotoxic effects on the germinal epithelium within the testis, impairment of penile erectile function, damage to the sympathetic nervous system driving seminal emission and ejaculation, and injury to the genital ductal system required for normal sperm transport. As highlighted earlier in this chapter, many cancer patients have significantly impaired reproductive potential at the time of diagnosis. With this in mind, when fertility preservation is desired, therapeutic modalities that maximize clinical effectiveness while sparing reproductive potential should be selected.

Effects of Radiation Therapy

Radiation therapy has been an important and evolving form of cancer treatment for over 80 years [24]. Radiation is utilized for a variety of cancers, including cancer of the prostate, rectum, bladder, penis, and testis. Over time, the delivery of radiation treatment has improved markedly with a concurrent decrease in associated morbidity. Despite these significant advances, radiation therapy can still have detrimental and irreversible effects on the testis, particularly the germinal epithelium.

Radiation therapy causes germ cell loss in a dose-dependent fashion [25]. Damage may result from direct radiation treatment of the testis or radiation scatter from the treatment of other subdiaphragmatic organs. The testis is one of the most radiosensitive organs in the body, and the most immature cell types are the most sensitive to injury

[25]. Very small doses (as low as 0.1 Gy) can affect spermatogonia, leading to histological changes in their number and shape. Exposure to 2–3 Gy of radiation leads to significant spermatocyte damage, with a resultant drop in numbers of spermatids. Doses in the 4–6 Gy range lead to significant decreases in the numbers of spermatozoa, suggesting that doses in this range lead to spermatid injury.

The timeline for radiation injury to be reflected in semen analyses is approximately 60–70 days after exposure. As to its effect on ejaculate sperm concentration, radiation doses less than 0.8 Gy typically lead to oligospermia, doses 0.8–2 Gy often result in transient azoospermia, and exposure to doses greater than 2 Gy may lead to irreversible azoospermia [25].

Factors such as the fractionation schedule and the specific field of treatment determine the ultimate impact of radiation therapy on reproductive health. The larger the dose of radiation, the more precipitous the decline in sperm concentration and the longer the period of time required for recovery of spermatogenesis [25]. Hansen et al. evaluated pre- and post-radiation treatment semen parameters in 24 patients with seminomas and 24 patients with NSGCT. On Cox regression analysis, recovery of spermatogenesis depended on radiation dose, and use of adjuvant chemotherapy prolonged the patients' recovery period. Additionally, the return of spermatogenesis was impaired in men with low pre-treatment total motile sperm counts and those over 25 years of age [26].

Sperm concentrations usually reach nadir by 4–6 months after the conclusion of radiation therapy. Return to pretreatment levels is typically seen within 10–24 months, with patients who receive higher doses experiencing longer recovery periods. Changes in sperm concentration over time are reflected by accompanying variations in FSH level [27].

Return of spermatogenesis following radiation therapy hinges on the survival and proliferation of surviving type-A spermatogonia. Table 3.1 details the timeline for functional recovery of the human testis after single dose radiation treatment, based on a study by Rowley et al. [28]. Fractionated therapy tends to be associated with longer recovery times than single-dose therapy. Some patients who do ultimately regain spermatogenesis after radiation treatment may exhibit permanently diminished sperm concentration and motility. For these individuals, assisted reproductive techniques are often useful in facilitating achievement of pregnancy.

Table 3.1 Recovery of spermatogenesis after graded doses of ionizing radiation to the human testes

Radiation dosage	Time to complete recovery*
<1 Gy	9–18 months
2–3 Gy	30 months
≥4 Gy	≥5 years

*return to pre-irradiative sperm concentration
Source: Data from Rowley et al. [28].

Leydig cells are much less likely to sustain functional impairment from radiotherapy than are germinal epithelial cells. However, Rowley et al. demonstrated that even doses of radiation of 0.75 Gy can lead to increases in LH levels [28], suggesting some degree of Leydig cell injury. These authors detected no change in testosterone level at this dose, and LH levels gradually returned to normal within 30 months after radiation exposure [28].

Giwercman et al. evaluated men who had undergone orchiectomy and then proceeded to testicular radiation therapy for carcinoma in situ of the solitary remaining testis. These authors found that impairment in Leydig cell secretory function is generally not observed until radiation exceeds doses of 20 Gy. At this dose, not only do LH levels become elevated, but testosterone levels decline when compared with similar patients who have not undergone radiation therapy to the remaining, solitary testis [29].

External beam radiation therapy for pelvic cancers (such as colorectal, bladder, and prostate cancer) results in testicular exposure to scatter doses of 0.4–18.7% of the administered dose [30,31]. In particular, patients with rectal cancer treated with external beam radiation therapy have the highest doses of radiation reaching the testis. Herman et al. have shown that patients treated with 50 Gy for rectal cancer sustained an 85% increase in serum FSH levels and a 22% decline in serum testosterone levels [31].

Important questions regarding the impact of sperm DNA damage resulting from radiation therapy have yet to be answered. Stahl et al. have shown an increase in DNA fragmentation index in men with testicular carcinoma undergoing adjuvant radiation therapy compared with similar patients not treated with radiation. These transient changes were seen up to 2 years after treatment, but the clinical impact of the increases in sperm DNA fragmentation has yet to be fully clarified [32]. Several small studies suggest that DNA integrity of sperm returns to levels of age-matched controls over time, but additional work is needed to further clarify these findings [33,34]. A number of encouraging studies have shown no increase in congenital anomalies or other disease states in the offspring of patients treated for cancer (with radiation and/or chemotherapy) when compared with these patients' cousins and to published figures for the general population [35,36].

Radiation Therapy for Prostate Cancer

Prostate cancer, the most common cancer in men, is being increasingly diagnosed at earlier stages and younger ages due to PSA screening. As such, many men facing this diagnosis may still be interested in preserving their reproductive function. A study by Daniell et al. revealed significant differences in hormone levels between men who had received prostate external beam radiation therapy and those who had undergone radical prostatectomy [37]. Three to eight years after completion of treatment, total testosterone levels were 27.3% less, free testosterone levels were 31.6% less, LH levels were 52.7% greater, and FSH levels were 100% greater in men who had undergone external beam radiation therapy compared with men who had undergone radical prostatectomy. No semen analysis comparison is possible as one of the groups underwent radical prostatectomy, but the significant changes in hormone levels, particularly the doubling of FSH, implies a high likelihood of significant disruption of spermatogenesis in the group treated with radiation therapy.

Brachytherapy is an increasingly common modality used to treat low-grade and low-stage prostate cancer. Mydlo et al. assessed semen quality in four young men (age 39–52) treated for prostate cancer with brachytherapy [38]. Assessment of semen parameters 6 months post-treatment revealed no change, and 3 of the 4 men were able to initiate pregnancies after treatment. The fourth patient, who had not yet achieved a pregnancy, was noted to have no change in sperm concentration or motility at the 6-month postoperative time point. Scatter radiation dose with brachytherapy is typically less than 20 cGy. A subsequent study by Grocela et al. found that 3 out of 485 men who continued to be sexually active after prostate brachytherapy achieved pregnancies with their partners. Two pregnancies were carried to term and resulted in the birth of healthy children. The third pregnancy resulted in a first trimester miscarriage. All three men had low ejaculate volume and mildly decreased total sperm count [39]. Although the numbers in these studies are small, the results are encouraging from a fertility preservation standpoint and should prompt a larger study of these patients.

Radiation Therapy for Testicular Cancer

Pelvic radiation therapy is a mainstay of treatment for some patients with testicular cancer, particularly those with seminoma. Radiation in these cases is typically delivered to the para-aortic lymph nodes and the iliac lymph nodes ipsilateral to the tumor. In this setting, the testicles receive approximately 0.3–0.5 Gy due to scatter, even if testicular shielding is used [40]. Typically, spermatogenesis will be impaired for a period of 6–8 months, followed by recovery over the next 1–2 years. Despite this improvement, spermatogenesis may never return to the pretreatment baseline levels. Prognostic factors favoring more rapid or complete recovery of spermatogenesis include normal semen parameters prior to therapy and younger age at the time of treatment [41].

In comparing paternity of men with testicular cancer who underwent radiation therapy vs. those who underwent observation, Huyghe et al. found significantly lower paternity in the radiation treatment group [42]. The authors concluded that fertility in patients with testicular cancer declined by 30% after radiation treatment. They also reported that radiation therapy, when compared with chemotherapy and observation, had the most deleterious effects on reproductive potential. Huddart et al. in a study of 680 patients, did not reach similar conclusions. They found that a slightly higher percentage of patients undergoing radiation therapy were successful in conceiving when compared with patients receiving chemotherapy [43]. Given the clear link between even small doses of radiation exposure and impaired testicular function, several authors have recommended the use of protective gonadal shielding to decrease radiation scatter to the remaining testicle [26,27].

Radiation Therapy for Lymphoma

Radiation therapy is often used for the treatment of Hodgkin's lymphoma; as with other disease states, impairment of spermatogenesis occurs in a dose-dependent fashion. Kinsella et al. prospectively followed 17 men with early stage Hodgkin's disease to assess the impact of low-dose scattered irradiation in men receiving conventional fractionated therapy. In these patients, the testicular dose ranged from 6 to 70 cGy, with follow up ranging from 3 to 7 years after completion of radiation therapy. The authors concluded that if the scattered dose received was between 0.2 and 0.7 Gy, patients may experience a temporary rise in FSH and decline in sperm concentration. Return of normal FSH levels was seen in 12–24 months and resolution of transient oligospermia was observed within 18 months of therapy completion [44].

Radiation Therapy for Leukemia

Whole body radiation therapy has been used to achieve myeloablation in many patients prior to stem cell transplantation [45]. Recovery of testicular function (normal FSH, LH, testosterone, and/or sperm concentration) is seen in less than 20% of men undergoing whole body irradiation and subsequent bone marrow transplant [46]. Socie et al. in a large survey of 229 centers of the European Group for Blood and Marrow Transplantation, noted that paternity via natural means after whole body irradiation is a rare event, with only 27 such men being identified from all of the centers surveyed. In 41 pregnancies in female partners of these same male patients, no stillbirths and only 1 miscarriage were observed. The risk for either occurrence in the normal population is approximately 10%, significantly higher than observed for these patients [47].

Effects of Chemotherapy

Chemotherapy is a mainstay of treatment for many forms of cancer, and the aim is to kill rapidly proliferating cells. One of the most significant drawbacks for this form of therapy is the destruction of normal, healthy tissue. A large number of chemotherapeutic agents are available, and their effects on male reproductive health are variable. Much has been learned about the impact of various cytotoxic agents since Spitz first described testicular damage in men treated with nitrogen mustard in 1948. In that report, 27 of 30 men having undergone this type of treatment were found at the time of autopsy to be azoospermic [48]. As is the case with radiation therapy, the germinal epithelium is much more sensitive to the effects of chemotherapy than are Leydig cells. While azoospermia is seen after treatment with a variety of agents, clinical hypogonadism manifest by low serum testosterone levels is less common.

The ultimate impact of chemotherapy hinges on the specific agents used, the dosage of these medications administered, and the age of the patient. The deleterious effects of chemotherapy may act in concert with injury brought about by other forms of therapy, such as radiation therapy. Below is a brief overview of the major classes of chemotherapeutic agents and their impact on male reproductive health.

Alkylating Agents
(Includes busulfan, chlorambucil, chlormethine, cyclophosphamide, ifosfamide, and procarbazine)

Alkylating drugs are one of the most toxic classes of chemotherapeutic medications available, with a high risk of inducing post-treatment infertility. These medications disrupt DNA function via several mechanisms, including DNA base pair alkylation, formation of abnormal base cross-bridges, and mispairing of nucleotides. The end result is impaired DNA synthesis and RNA transcription leading to cellular death. These agents cause mutations in all stages of developing germinal epithelium [49].

Byrne et al. reported that severe oligospermia or azoospermia typically develop 90–120 days after alkylating agent therapy, with a significant decrease in male fertility whether or not concurrent radiation therapy was administered [50]. A number of investigators have shown that the deficits in sperm production associated with alkylating agents are often severe and irreversible. Buchanan and colleagues reported that even 4 years after treatment with cyclophosphamide, most patients had not yet regained spermatogenesis. Those patients that did resume sperm production did so at 31 months after treatment [51]. Multi-agent regimens that include procarbazine usually render patients irreversibly infertile, leading investigators such as Bokemeyer and colleagues to recommend alternative agents in its place [52].

Antimetabolites
(Includes 5-fluorouracil [5-FU], 6-mercaptopurine, gemcitabine, and methotrexate)

The antimetabolites interfere with DNA synthesis and transcription, typically resulting in reversible, transient declines in sperm concentration. Choudhury and colleagues reported that in a rat model, 5-FU induced chromosomal aberrations in spermatogonial cells. A gradual decrease in the transmission of these cytotoxic changes from spermatogonia to sperm was noted over time, with the authors postulating that the damaged spermatogonia are gradually eliminated during the cycle of spermatogenesis [53]. D'Souza et al. reported seminiferous tubule atrophy and marked changes in sperm morphology using a rat model treated with 5-FU [54,55].

Platinum Analogs
(Includes cisplatin and carboplatin)

The platinum analogs cause DNA crosslink formation, and animal studies have shown that spermatogonia and spermatocytes are the most markedly affected cell types [56]. Lampe and colleagues reported on 170 patients with testicular germ cell cancer. Approximately 25% of the men were azoospermic and approximately 25% were oligospermic prior to initiation of therapy [57]. After treatment with platinum-based chemotherapy, recovery of spermatogenesis continued over time, with approximately 50% of men with spermatogenesis at 2 years and 80% of men with spermatogenesis 5 years after completion of therapy. For the subgroup of men with normal sperm concentrations prior to therapy, 64% had normal sperm concentrations at a median of 30 months after completion of platinum-based chemotherapy. These authors found a higher likelihood of recovery of spermatogenesis with carboplatin than with cisplatin therapy.

Vinca Alkaloids
(Includes vinblastine, vincristine, vindesine, and vinorelbine)

The vinca alkaloids, which are derived from the periwinkle plant, exert their antineoplastic effects via inhibition of microtubule formation, which in turn inhibits mitosis. These agents have been implicated in arresting spermatogenesis and in decreasing spermatozoa motility [58]. Other investigators, such as Sjoblom et al. and Aubier et al. have demonstrated that spermatogenesis is relatively resistant to the effects of vinblastine, in contrast to Arnon's findings [59,60].

Topoisomerase Inhibitor Agents
(Includes doxorubicin, etoposide, and bleomycin)

Topoisomerase-inhibiting agents induce damage in a variety of ways, such as DNA binding, RNA-breaks, and RNA synthesis inhibition. Bleomycin, one such agent, has been shown to cause chromosomal abnormalities in spermatogonia and spermatocytes in an animal study by van Buul et al. [61]. Hou et al. evaluated the effects of doxorubicin in rats of various ages and found that the initiation phase of spermatogenesis is highly susceptible to doxorubicin-induced apoptosis. They discovered that gonocytes and early spermatogonia are most vulnerable to this apoptosis, leading to a decline in the number of germline stem cells [62].

Effects of Surgery

Surgical therapy of cancer can have a wide array of deleterious effects on male reproductive health. Consideration of these effects is imperative during preoperative discussions with patients.

Men suffering from testicular cancer typically sustain a significant loss of overall testicular mass when undergoing orchiectomy, which can impair reproductive health due to lower overall germ cell mass and Leydig cell mass. This may lead to reduced sperm concentration and serum testosterone levels. Some men with testicular cancer may also undergo subsequent retroperitoneal lymphadenectomy, potentially resulting in anejaculation or retrograde ejaculation as a result of disruption of the lumbar sympathetic plexus and hypogastric plexus. Modified, nerve-sparing templates for dissection have resulted in preserved ejaculatory function in the majority of these men [63].

Men with bladder or prostate cancer who require extirpative surgery will suffer disruption of the genital ductal system as the prostate gland and seminal vesicles are routinely removed. Patients undergoing these procedures typically still produce sperm normally – it is the transport and delivery of sperm to the prostatic urethra that are disrupted. As a result, normal ejaculatory function, and thus fertility, is destroyed.

While erectile function may be preserved in over 80% of men undergoing radical prostatectomy and radical cystectomy with nerve-sparing techniques [64], recovery of erections may take a year or more and may be incomplete. With the advent of PDE-5 inhibitors and other therapies for erectile dysfunction, this problem is often readily treatable.

Traditional assumptions about a patient's reproductive aspirations, based on age or other demographic traits, should be carefully considered. Changes in reproductive health are a fairly common outcome of oncological surgery and it is incumbent upon physicians to routinely discuss the potential impact of each procedure on reproductive health prior to initiating surgical therapy.

Effects of Opiods

Pain management is a critical component of cancer therapy. The use of opiods is often chronic and may involve high doses. Opiod-induced suppression of the H-P-G axis is well documented, and the resultant decrease in gonadotropins may lead to declines in libido, erectile function, and spermatogenesis. All of these factors, individually or collectively, may impair fertility. Fortunately, these negative effects are typically reversible with cessation of opiod use [65].

Fertility Preservation in Male Cancer Patients

Over 20,000 patients of childhood and reproductive age are treated with radiation therapy and/or chemotherapy each year [58]. With improving diagnostic and therapeutic modalities, overall survival for most cancers has increased significantly over the last 75 years. For patients under 15 years of age, the 5-year survival rate for cancer is approximately 75% [66], and the survival rate for men aged 15–44 facing a cancer diagnosis is 61% [67]. The prevalence of cancer survivors seeking fertility continues to grow; Bleyer reported that by 2010, one in every 250 adults will be a survivor of childhood cancer [68], and many of these individuals, if not most, will desire parenthood. Furthermore, many men are waiting until later in life to start their first families, and others start second families at an older age due to divorce or death of a spouse. As such, an increasing number of adult male cancer survivors will be pursuing fatherhood post-treatment. The end result of this phenomenon will be an increasing pool of patients striving to achieve parenthood in the wake of fertility impairing cancer treatments.

For patients, a cancer diagnosis is often devastating and overwhelming. The immediate focus is typically on therapy and cure of the underlying disease process. Thus, it is imperative that the treating physicians actively address the issue of fertility preservation as comprehensive care is administered to the patient. This concept was recently recommended by the President's Cancer Panel; specifically, the panel suggested that all reproductive-age patients and parents of children with cancer be notified in detail of the risks of infertility associated with cancer and cancer treatment [69]. While approaches such as use of donor sperm and adoption are available to facilitate paternity in cancer survivors, many patients express a strong desire to father biological children [70].

A recent study by Zapzalka et al. of American Society of Clinical Oncology (ASCO) members in Minnesota revealed that 100% of oncologists reported discussing fertility issues with their patients [71]. However, Shover et al. surveyed approximately 900 male cancer patients, and only 60% replied that they were informed about fertility issues. Furthermore, only 50% stated they had been notified about sperm banking [70]. Similar observations are anecdotally noted by physicians and patients at many centers, highlighting the significant communication barriers existing between health care providers and patients. The President's Cancer Panel acknowledged these deficits in effective communication between health care providers and patients. They recommended the use of complete culture- and literacy-sensitive information, both verbally and in writing, regarding fertility preservation options and possible effects of treatments.

There is little room for communication breakdown when treating cancer patients. Diagnostic testing and therapeutic procedures in the acute care setting occupy large amounts of time, leaving very little time to address fertility preservation. However, cryopreservation of sperm in advance of cancer treatment is essential, as even one cancer treatment can reduce semen quality and induce sperm DNA damage [72].

American Society of Clinical Oncology Guidelines

In 2006, ASCO published recommendations on fertility preservation in cancer patients [73]. The authors of this manuscript acknowledged that application of fertility preservation measures is limited by several factors, including knowledge deficits regarding fertility risks associated with cancer treatments, failure to

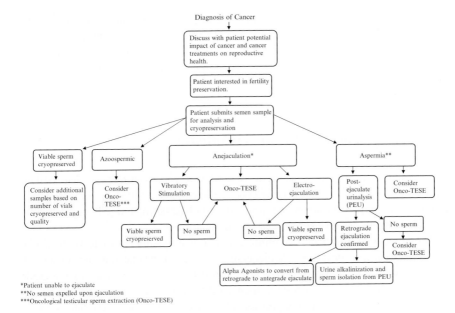

Diagnosis of Cancer

Discuss with patient potential impact of cancer and cancer treatments on reproductive health.

Patient interested in fertility preservation.

Patient submits semen sample for analysis and cryopreservation

Viable sperm cryopreserved

Azoospermic

Anejaculation*

Aspermia**

Consider additional samples based on number of vials cryopreserved and quality

Consider Onco-TESE***

Vibratory Stimulation

Onco-TESE

Electro-ejaculation

Post-ejaculate urinalysis (PEU)

Consider Onco-TESE

Viable sperm cryopreserved

No sperm

No sperm

Viable sperm cryopreserved

Retrograde ejaculation confirmed

No sperm

Consider Onco-TESE

Alpha Agonists to convert from retrograde to antegrade ejaculate

Urine alkalinization and sperm isolation from PEU

*Patient unable to ejaculate
**No semen expelled upon ejaculation
***Oncological testicular sperm extraction (Onco-TESE)

Fig. 3.1 Fertility preservation algorithm for male cancer patients

discuss fertility preserving options prior to treatment, lack of insurance coverage for these procedures, and the investigational status of some of the fertility preservation techniques. The expert panel recommended that oncologists discuss at the earliest opportunity the possible risk of fertility impairment associated with various cancer treatments. For those patients interested in pursuing fertility preservation, the prompt referral of the patient to a qualified specialist in this area was recommended. Finally, the authors advocated the participation of patients in clinical trials to advance the state of knowledge within the field of fertility preservation. Below, several methods available for fertility preservation in men are detailed. A helpful summary algorithm is also provided (Fig. 3.1).

Sperm Cryopreservation

A number of articles from the "pre-in vitro fertilization" (pre-IVF) era highlighted poor outcomes of sperm cryopreservation, with a minority of semen samples provided by cancer patients being adequate to pursue intrauterine insemination [74,75]. As such, this early literature did not advocate pretreatment sperm cryopreservation due to the low resultant pregnancy rates. Unfortunately, these historical outcomes still guide clinical decision making by some health care providers with regard to fertility preservation. With the advent of IVF and intracytoplasmic sperm injection (ICSI), literally just one sperm per oocyte is necessary to achieve possible fertilization and pregnancy. Thus, even men with extremely diminished overall semen quality should be offered sperm cryopreservation, as the above assisted reproductive techniques can often overcome severe deficits in sperm production and function.

Overview of Sperm Collection Techniques

The semen collection process itself is achieved via masturbation. The patient should be provided a sterile specimen collection cup and ample time and privacy to produce the sample. Avoidance of lubricants (such as petroleum jelly and saliva) is critical, as many of these substances are spermatotoxic.

If no ejaculate is expelled on climax, then a post-ejaculate urinalysis should be inspected to assess for retrograde ejaculation. If retrograde ejaculation is observed, alpha agonists may be administered in an effort to convert retrograde to antegrade ejaculation. If this is not successful, then alkalilization of the urine and subsequent collection and processing of the post-ejaculate urine sample may facilitate isolation of viable sperm.

If the patient is unable to climax, care should be taken to ensure that he has had ample privacy and time. If this difficulty persists, then consideration should be given to vibratory stimulation, electro-ejaculation, or surgical testicular sperm extraction techniques, all of which have a potential role in such patients.

Testicular Tissue Cryopreservation (ONCO-TESE)

Azoospermia at the time of attempted sperm cryopreservation was noted in 13.8% of cancer patients by Lass et al. in a 1998 review of their center's data [72]. When the provided sample reveals azoospermia, surgical testicular sperm extraction prior to cancer treatment is an option [76–79]. Dubbed "Onco-TESE" (Oncological Testicular Sperm Extraction) by Schrader et al. this procedure was successful in yielding sperm retrieval in 6 of 14 men with testicular germ cell tumors and in 8 of 17 patients with malignant lymphoma [79]. Given the possible irreversible damage to germinal epithelium with cancer therapy and the good overall success rates with "Onco-TESE", Schrader et al. recommend that this procedure be considered as a means of fertility preservation in azoospermic cancer patients.

Figure 3.2 illustrates the Onco-TESE procedure performed on a man with a solitary testis and azoospermia undergoing radical orchiectomy for seminoma. Critical components of this procedure include coordination of laboratory personnel with the operating room staff, availability of an operating microscope, a sterile workbench away from the operating field, and a phase contrast microscope to inspect wet prep slides.

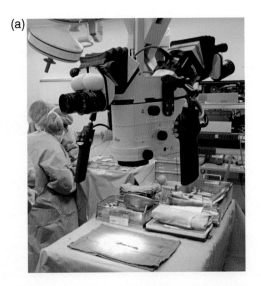

(a)

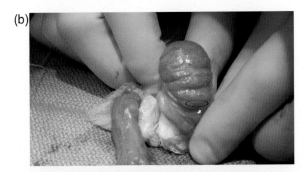

(b)

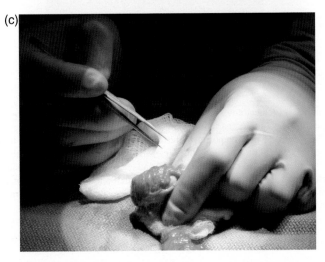

(c)

Fig. 3.2 (**a**) The operating microscope and sterile field where the Onco-TESE will be performed in the foreground. The radical orchiectomy is being performed in the background. (**b**) The radical

(continued)

(d)
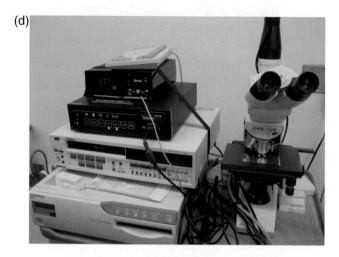

(e)
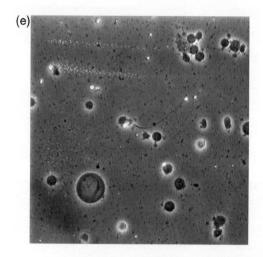

Fig. 3.2 (continued) orchiectomy specimen has been bivalved to allow microsurgical inspection and dissection of the seminiferous tubules. Seminoma with marked inflammatory change infiltrated over 90% of this testis. The postero-inferior aspect was found to be free of tumor with low levels of spermatogenesis on wet prep slide. (**c**) Microsurgical inspection and dissection of the seminiferous tubules. Selected tubules are excised and teased to make a wet prep slide. (**d**) Phase-contrast microscope with attached video recorder and microphotograph printer for wet prep slide inspection in the operating room. (**e**) Wet prep slide of testicular tissue revealing presence of viable sperm with motility. This tissue was cryopreserved

Future Directions in Fertility Preservation in Male Cancer Patients

Many investigational male fertility preserving techniques are undergoing evaluation. Some have been studied more thoroughly than others, and a number offer hope as our understanding of male reproductive physiology grows. Several of these investigational techniques are briefly described below.

Luteinizing hormone releasing hormone (LHRH) agonists have been used to achieve H-P-G axis suppression during chemotherapy. While early animal studies showed some evidence of gonadal protection during chemotherapy, several human studies have been less promising. This approach did not lead to fertility preservation or hasten the return of spermatogenesis in several studies in men [80–83].

Testicular tissue harvesting for autotransplantation has also been considered by several investigators. Effects to date have focused on successful germ cell isolation and cryopreservation [84]. The hope is that after cancer treatment, the harvested germinal epithelium may be transplanted back to the patient with resumption of spermatogenesis. This technique remains investigational, and to date has not been effectively implemented in humans.

Testicular tissue harvesting for transplantation into immunodeficient mice is another investigational technique garnering much attention. Nagano and colleagues have demonstrated that this procedure is technically feasible in these mice with successful ensuing spermatogenesis, pregnancies, and live births. To date, this approach has only been successfully performed in animal models [85,86], but it may hold promise for human application, particularly in prepubescent boys.

Conclusion

Fertility preservation in male cancer patients is an important aspect of comprehensive health care. As cancer diagnostic techniques and treatments improve, a growing number of cancer survivors will continue to look past their malignancy toward issues such as parenthood. In this chapter, we have detailed the numerous ways in which cancer itself and its associated treatments can negatively impact many aspects of normal male reproductive health. This underscores the importance of tailoring a careful discussion with each patient over the potential deleterious impact of their specific disease state and therapy prior to initiating treatment.

At the time of cancer diagnosis, patients and clinicians alike are often overwhelmed by the high volume of urgent tests and procedures that must be accomplished in a timely fashion. This situation sets the stage for a profound breakdown in communication between health care providers and patients with regard to fertility preservation. In retrospect, not only do many patients fail to recall discussions of fertility preservation, they often harbor great disappointment and regret at the perceived oversight in this aspect of their care. Fortunately, with a proactive approach, fertility preservation in men is quite feasible and will help avoid the irreversible and permanent loss of reproductive capacity that accompanies many cancer treatments today.

References

1. Meirow D, Schenker JG. Cancer and male infertility. Hum Reprod 1995;10:2017–2022.
2. Hallak J, Kolettis PN, Sekhon VS, et al. Sperm cryopreservation in patients with testicular cancer. Urology 1999;54:894–899.
3. Carroll PR, Whitmore WF, Jr., Herr HW, et al. Endocrine and exocrine profiles of men with testicular tumors before orchiectomy. J Urol 1987;137:420–423.
4. Hansen PV, Trykker H, Andersen J, et al. Germ cell function and hormonal status in patients with testicular cancer. Cancer 1989;64:956–961.
5. Cochran JS, Walsh PC, Porter JC, et al. The endocrinology of human chorionic gonadotropin-secreting testicular tumors: new methods in diagnosis. J Urol 1975;114:549–555.
6. Aiginger P, Kolbe H, Kuhbock J, et al. The endocrinology of testicular germinal cell tumors. Acta Endocrinol (Copenh) 1981;97:419–426.
7. Turrin NP, Ilyin SE, Gayle DA, et al. Interleukin-1beta system in anorectic catabolic tumor-bearing rats. Curr Opin Clin Nutr Metab Care 2004;7:419–426.
8. Ramos EJ, Suzuki S, Marks D, et al. Cancer anorexia-cachexia syndrome: cytokines and neuropeptides. Curr Opin Clin Nutr Metab Care 2004;7:427–434.
9. Inui A. Cancer anorexia-cachexia syndrome: are neuropeptides the key? Cancer Res 1999;59:4493–4501.
10. Parker C, Milosevic M, Panzarella T, et al. The prognostic significance of the tumour infiltrating lymphocyte count in stage I testicular seminoma managed by surveillance. Eur J Cancer 2002;38:2014–2019.
11. Rival C, Theas MS, Guazzone VA, et al. Interleukin-6 and IL-6 receptor cell expression in testis of rats with autoimmune orchitis. J Reprod Immunol 2006;70:43–58.
12. Theas MS, Rival C, Dietrich SJ, et al. Death receptor and mitochondrial pathways are involved in germ cell apoptosis in an experimental model of autoimmune orchitis. Hum Reprod 2006;21:1734–1742.
13. Aitken RJ, Sawyer D. The human spermatozoon – not waving but drowning. Adv Exp Med Biol 2003;518:85–98.
14. Martinez P, Proverbio F, Camejo MI. Sperm lipid peroxidation and pro-inflammatory cytokines. Asian J Androl 2007;9:102–107.
15. Guazzieri S, Lembo A, Ferro G, et al. Sperm antibodies and infertility in patients with testicular cancer. Urology 1985;26:139–142.
16. Sher KS, Jayanthi V, Probert CS, et al. Infertility, obstetric and gynaecological problems in coeliac sprue. Dig Dis 1994;12:186–190.
17. Heyns CF, Fisher M. The urological management of the patient with acquired immunodeficiency syndrome. BJU Int 2005;95:709–716.
18. Viviani S, Ragni G, Santoro A, et al. Testicular dysfunction in Hodgkin's disease before and after treatment. Eur J Cancer 1991;27:1389–1392.
19. Berthelsen JG, Skakkebaek NE. Gonadal function in men with testis cancer. Fertil Steril 1983;39:68–75.
20. Morrish DW, Venner PM, Siy O, et al. Mechanisms of endocrine dysfunction in patients with testicular cancer. J Natl Cancer Inst 1990;82:412–418.
21. Strasser F, Palmer JL, Schover LR, et al. The impact of hypogonadism and autonomic dysfunction on fatigue, emotional function, and sexual desire in male patients with advanced cancer: a pilot study. Cancer 2006;107:2949–2957.

22. Marmor D, Elefant E, Dauchez C, et al. Semen analysis in Hodgkin's disease before the onset of treatment. Cancer 1986;57:1986–1987.
23. Arai Y, Kawakita M, Okada Y, et al. Sexuality and fertility in long-term survivors of testicular cancer. J Clin Oncol 1997;15:1444–1448.
24. Mazeron JJ, Gerbaulet A. [The centenary of the discovery of radium]. Cancer Radiother 1999;3:19–29.
25. Shalet SM. Effect of irradiation treatment on gonadal function in men treated for germ cell cancer. Eur Urol 1993;23:148–151; discussion 152.
26. Hansen PV, Trykker H, Svennekjaer IL, et al. Long-term recovery of spermatogenesis after radiotherapy in patients with testicular cancer. Radiother Oncol 1990;18:117–125.
27. Gordon W, Jr., Siegmund K, Stanisic TH, et al. A study of reproductive function in patients with seminoma treated with radiotherapy and orchiectomy: (SWOG-8711). Southwest Oncology Group. Int J Radiat Oncol Biol Phys 1997;38:83–94.
28. Rowley MJ, Leach DR, Warner GA, et al. Effect of graded doses of ionizing radiation on the human testis. Radiat Res 1974;59:665–678.
29. Giwercman A, von der Maase H, Berthelsen JG, et al. Localized irradiation of testes with carcinoma in situ: effects on Leydig cell function and eradication of malignant germ cells in 20 patients. J Clin Endocrinol Metab 1991;73:596–603.
30. Budgell GJ, Cowan RA, Hounsell AR. Prediction of scattered dose to the testes in abdominopelvic radiotherapy. Clin Oncol 2001;13:120–125.
31. Hermann RM, Henkel K, Christiansen H, et al. Testicular dose and hormonal changes after radiotherapy of rectal cancer. Radiother Oncol 2005;75:83–88.
32. Stahl O, Eberhard J, Jepson K, et al. The impact of testicular carcinoma and its treatment on sperm DNA integrity. Cancer 2004;100:1137–1144.
33. Thomson AB, Campbell AJ, Irvine DC, et al. Semen quality and spermatozoal DNA integrity in survivors of childhood cancer: a case-control study. Lancet 2002;360:361–367.
34. Chatterjee R, Haines GA, Perera DM, et al. Testicular and sperm DNA damage after treatment with fludarabine for chronic lymphocytic leukaemia. Hum Reprod 2000;15:762–766.
35. Li FP, Fine W, Jaffe N, et al. Offspring of patients treated for cancer in childhood. J Natl Cancer Inst 1979;62:1193–1197.
36. Hawkins MM, Smith RA, Curtice LJ. Childhood cancer survivors and their offspring studied through a postal survey of general practitioners: preliminary results. J R Coll Gen Pract 1988;38:102–105.
37. Daniell HW, Clark JC, Pereira SE, et al. Hypogonadism following prostate-bed radiation therapy for prostate carcinoma. Cancer 2001;91:1889–1895.
38. Mydlo JH, Lebed B. Does brachytherapy of the prostate affect sperm quality and/or fertility in younger men? Scand J Urol Nephrol 2004;38:221–224.
39. Grocela J, Mauceri T, Zietman A. New life after prostate brachytherapy? Considering the fertile female partner of the brachytherapy patient. BJU Int 2005;96:781–782.
40. Jacobsen KD, Olsen DR, Fossa K, et al. External beam abdominal radiotherapy in patients with seminoma stage I: field type, testicular dose, and spermatogenesis. Int J Radiat Oncol Biol Phys 1997;38:95–102.
41. Aass N, Fossa SD, Theodorsen L, et al. Prediction of long-term gonadal toxicity after standard treatment for testicular cancer. Eur J Cancer 1991;27:1087–1091.
42. Huyghe E, Matsuda T, Daudin M, et al. Fertility after testicular cancer treatments: results of a large multicenter study. Cancer 2004;100:732–737.
43. Huddart RA, Norman A, Moynihan C, et al. Fertility, gonadal and sexual function in survivors of testicular cancer. Br J Cancer 2005;93:200–207.
44. Kinsella TJ, Trivette G, Rowland J, et al. Long-term follow-up of testicular function following radiation therapy for early-stage Hodgkin's disease. J Clin Oncol 1989;7:718–724.
45. Socie G, Salooja N, Cohen A, et al. Nonmalignant late effects after allogeneic stem cell transplantation. Blood 2003;101:3373–3385.
46. Sanders JE, Hawley J, Levy W, et al. Pregnancies following high-dose cyclophosphamide with or without high-dose busulfan or total-body irradiation and bone marrow transplantation. Blood 1996;87:3045–3052.

47. Salooja N, Szydlo RM, Socie G, et al. Pregnancy outcomes after peripheral blood or bone marrow transplantation: a retrospective survey. Lancet 2001;358:271–276.
48. Spitz S. The histological effects of nitrogen mustard on human tumours and tissues. Cancer 1948;383–398.
49. Witt KL, Bishop JB. Mutagenicity of anticancer drugs in mammalian germ cells. Mutat Res 1996;355:209–234.
50. Byrne J, Mulvihill JJ, Myers MH, et al. Effects of treatment on fertility in long-term survivors of childhood or adolescent cancer. N Engl J Med 1987;317:1315–1321.
51. Buchanan JD, Fairley KF, Barrie JU. Return of spermatogenesis after stopping cyclophosphamide therapy. Lancet 1975;2:156–157.
52. Bokemeyer C, Schmoll HJ, van Rhee J, et al. Long-term gonadal toxicity after therapy for Hodgkin's and non-Hodgkin's lymphoma. Ann Hematol 1994;68:105–110.
53. Choudhury RC, Misra S, Jagdale MB, et al. Induction and transmission of cytogenetic toxic effects of 5-fluorouracil in male germline cells of Swiss mice. J Exp Clin Cancer Res 2002;21:277–282.
54. D'Souza UJ, Narayana K. Induction of seminiferous tubular atrophy by single dose of 5-fluorouracil (5-FU) in Wistar rats. Indian J Physiol Pharmacol 2001;45:87–94.
55. D'Souza UJ. Re: 5-Fluorouracil-induced sperm shape abnormalities in rats. Asian J Androl 2003;5:353.
56. Choudhury RC, Jagdale MB, Misra S. Potential transmission of the cytogenetic effects of cisplatin in the male germline cells of Swiss mice. J Chemother 2000;12:352–359.
57. Lampe H, Horwich A, Norman A, et al. Fertility after chemotherapy for testicular germ cell cancers. J Clin Oncol 1997;15:239–245.
58. Arnon J, Meirow D, Lewis-Roness H, et al. Genetic and teratogenic effects of cancer treatments on gametes and embryos. Hum Reprod Update 2001;7:394–403.
59. Sjoblom T, Parvinen M, Lahdetie J. Stage-specific DNA synthesis of rat spermatogenesis as an indicator of genotoxic effects of vinblastine, mitomycin C and ionizing radiation on rat spermatogonia and spermatocytes. Mutat Res 1995;331:181–190.
60. Aubier F, Flamant F, Brauner R, et al. Male gonadal function after chemotherapy for solid tumors in childhood. J Clin Oncol 1989;7:304–309.
61. van Buul PP, Goudzwaard JH. Bleomycin-induced structural chromosomal aberrations in spermatogonia and bone-marrow cells of mice. Mutat Res 1980;69:319–324.
62. Hou M, Chrysis D, Nurmio M, et al. Doxorubicin induces apoptosis in germ line stem cells in the immature rat testis and amifostine cannot protect against this cytotoxicity. Cancer Res 2005;65:9999–10005.
63. Foster RS, Bennett R, Bihrle R, et al. A preliminary report: postoperative fertility assessment in nerve-sparing RPLND patients. Eur Urol 1993;23:165–167; discussion 168.
64. Schlegel PN, Walsh PC. Neuroanatomical approach to radical cystoprostatectomy with preservation of sexual function. J Urol 1987;138:1402–1406.
65. Rajagopal A, Vassilopoulou-Sellin R, Palmer JL, et al. Symptomatic hypogonadism in male survivors of cancer with chronic exposure to opioids. Cancer 2004;100:851–858.
66. Landis SH, Murray T, Bolden S, et al. Cancer statistics, 1999. CA Cancer J Clin 1999;49:8–31, 1.
67. Sant M, Aareleid T, Berrino F, et al. EUROCARE-3: survival of cancer patients diagnosed 1990–94 – results and commentary. Ann Oncol 2003;14 Suppl 5:v61–v118.
68. Bleyer WA. The impact of childhood cancer on the United States and the world. CA Cancer J Clin 1990;40:355–367.
69. Schover LR, Brey K, Lichtin A, et al. Knowledge and experience regarding cancer, infertility, and sperm banking in younger male survivors. J Clin Oncol 2002;20:1880–1889.
70. Living Beyond Cancer: Finding a New Balance, President's Cancer Panel 2003–2004 Annual Report, U.S. Department of Health and Human Services, 2004, 1–87.
71. Zapzalka DM, Redmon JB, Pryor JL. A survey of oncologists regarding sperm cryopreservation and assisted reproductive techniques for male cancer patients. Cancer 1999;86:1812–1817.

72. Lass A, Akagbosu F, Abusheikha N, et al. A programme of semen cryopreservation for patients with malignant disease in a tertiary infertility centre: lessons from 8 years' experience. Hum Reprod 1998;13:3256–3261.
73. Lee SJ, Schover LR, Partridge AH, et al. American Society of Clinical Oncology recommendations on fertility preservation in cancer patients. J Clin Oncol 2006;24:2917–2931.
74. Bracken RB, Smith KD. Is semen cryopreservation helpful in testicular cancer? Urology 1980;15:581–583.
75. Sanger WG, Armitage JO, Schmidt MA. Feasibility of semen cryopreservation in patients with malignant disease. JAMA 1980;244:789–790.
76. Rosenlund B, Westlander G, Wood M, et al. Sperm retrieval and fertilization in repeated percutaneous epididymal sperm aspiration. Hum Reprod 1998;13:2805–2807.
77. Res U, Res P, Kastelic D, et al. Birth after treatment of a male with seminoma and azoospermia with cryopreserved-thawed testicular tissue. Hum Reprod 2000;15:861–864.
78. Kohn FM, Schroeder-Printzen I, Weidner W, et al. Testicular sperm extraction in a patient with metachronous bilateral testicular cancer. Hum Reprod 2001;16:2343–2346.
79. Schrader M, Muller M, Sofikitis N, et al. "Onco-tese": testicular sperm extraction in azoospermic cancer patients before chemotherapy-new guidelines? Urology 2003;61:421–425.
80. Johnson DH, Linde R, Hainsworth JD, et al. Effect of a luteinizing hormone releasing hormone agonist given during combination chemotherapy on posttherapy fertility in male patients with lymphoma: preliminary observations. Blood 1985;65:832–836.
81. Waxman JH, Ahmed R, Smith D, et al. Failure to preserve fertility in patients with Hodgkin's disease. Cancer Chemother Pharmacol 1987;19:159–162.
82. Brennemann W, Brensing KA, Leipner N, et al. Attempted protection of spermatogenesis from irradiation in patients with seminoma by D-Tryptophan-6 luteinizing hormone releasing hormone. Clin Invest 1994;72:838–842.
83. Kreuser ED, Hetzel WD, Hautmann R, et al. Reproductive toxicity with and without LHRHA administration during adjuvant chemotherapy in patients with germ cell tumors. Horm Metab Res 1990;22:494–498.
84. Brook PF, Radford JA, Shalet SM, et al. Isolation of germ cells from human testicular tissue for low temperature storage and autotransplantation. Fertil Steril 2001;75:269–274.
85. Nagano M, Patrizio P, Brinster RL. Long-term survival of human spermatogonial stem cells in mouse testes. Fertil Steril 2002;78:1225–1233.
86. Schlatt S, Honaramooz A, Ehmcke J, et al. Limited survival of adult human testicular tissue as ectopic xenograft. Hum Reprod 2006;21:384–389.

Chapter 4
Managing Fertility in Childhood Cancer Patients

Kimberley J. Dilley, MD, MPH

The scope of potential fertility issues for pediatric cancer patients is broad and difficult to predict. Both genders are susceptible to central dysregulation of the hypothalamic axis. For boys, chemotherapy and radiation can affect production of both sex hormones and sperm. These effects can be reversible or permanent. For girls, the ovary can be similarly affected, with inadequate or absent hormone production and depletion of ovarian follicle reserve. Additionally, even in a young woman with normal puberty and early fertility, premature menopause is a possibility after certain exposures. Finally, the uterus can be affected by radiation and create problems in carrying a normal pregnancy to term, even if hormonal fertility is achieved.

Radiation is a clearly established risk to the hormone- and gamete-producing tissues. What is more difficult to predict are the fertility outcomes after chemotherapeutic exposures. The main exposures implicated for pediatric patients are cyclophosphamide and other alkylating agents; large cumulative doses have been shown to irreversibly impair fertility in both male and female patients. However, the variability in gonadal function between different individuals after therapy with an alkylating agent is quite large, making prediction of fertility outcomes after many protocols extremely difficult. Furthermore, evidence suggests that males are more susceptible than females, and spermatogenesis is impaired at lower doses than is testosterone production.

Many pediatric patients who are survivors of cancer are never offered fertility-sparing interventions, so it is important for health care personnel to monitor the fertility status of survivors of childhood cancers. Management should focus on assessment of gonadal function via patient history, physical examination, and laboratory screening. Below, I discuss guidelines from the Children's Oncology Group (COG) that identify high-risk patients who should receive more careful monitoring and counseling regarding long-term issues such as premature menopause and bone density concerns. Future challenges include better definition of patients at risk of infertility pretreatment in order to target fertility preservation schemes accordingly. (For further discussion of fertility risk among pediatric cancer patients, see Garcia and Ginsburg, this volume.)

T.K. Woodruff and K.A. Snyder (eds.) *Oncofertility*.
© Springer 2007

Follow-up Guidelines Related to Male Fertility

Risk Factors

Radiation, even without concomitant chemotherapy, can impact the gonadal axis in a number of ways. Radiation doses of 40 Gy or more to a field that includes the hypothalamus can lead to gonadotropin deficiency [1]. Radiation directly to the testes, including pelvic irradiation and total body irradiation (TBI), can cause germ cell failure. After doses of 1–3 Gy, azospermia may be reversible, but reversibility is unlikely at higher doses, especially >6 Gy [2]. Pelvic or testicular radiation at doses of 20 Gy or higher, especially if combined with alkylating agents or head/brain irradiation, is a risk factor for Leydig cell dysfunction leading to delayed or arrested puberty and hypogonadism [3].

Use of alkylating agents can place the male gonads at risk of delayed or arrested puberty, hypogonadism, oligospermia or azospermia, and infertility [4]. The risk factors include higher cumulative doses, particularly of cyclophosphamide or busulfan, and combinations with other alkylators or with radiation in a field that affects the testes directly or that affects the neuroendocrine axis. Leydig cell dysfunction can occur after alkylating agent exposure at any age [5].

Finally, surgical procedures related either to tumor removal or to complications during treatment can also affect fertility. Bilateral or unilateral orchiectomy can cause hypogonadism or infertility if combined with radiation or alkylating agents [6]. Pelvic surgery could also place a male patient at risk for mechanical sexual dysfunction including retrograde ejaculation, anejaculation, or erectile dysfunction.

Surveillance and Screening

After any of the exposures discussed above, a yearly patient history should monitor the onset and timing of puberty, sexual function as age appropriate, including erections and nocturnal emissions, and medications that may impact sexual function. Frothy white urine at first void after intercourse suggests retrograde ejaculation [7].

The annual physical examination should include overall assessment of growth and development. A genitourinary exam specifically involves Tanner stage (sexual maturity rating or SMR), including testicular volume, until sexual maturity (SMR 5) has been reached.

In patients at risk for hypogonadism, laboratory screening should include measurement of follicle-stimulating hormone (FSH) and luteinizing hormone (LH), as well as testosterone at age 14 as a baseline. These studies should be repeated as clinically indicated due to signs of delayed puberty or testosterone deficiency [1,3,4]. Semen analysis should be performed for evaluation of infertility or at the request of the patient in family planning [2–4,6].

Additional Management Issues

Those males at risk of azospermia and their sexual partners should be counseled to use appropriate birth control methods as sperm production can resume spontaneously up to 10 years after treatment. For this same reason, periodic reassessment by semen analysis may be indicated for those desiring to start a family. Patients who have testosterone deficiency will also be at risk for low bone mineral density (BMD) in addition to abnormal development of secondary sexual characteristics, so testosterone replacement is warranted.

In the current treatment era, optimal care for pediatric patients with cancer would include fertility-preservation options at diagnosis prior to therapeutic exposures that can cause azospermia. Sperm banking can be offered to even early pubertal patients, while development of methods to preserve spermatogonia from prepubertal patients represents an area of active research.

Follow-up Guidelines Related to Female Fertility

Risk Factors

The number of ways in which female fertility can be affected by exposure to cancer therapies is quite large and complex. Not only are there potential effects parallel to those seen in males on the hypothalamic-gonadal axis, on the gonads themselves, and on sexual function, even in a "fertile" female with functioning gonads there are potential problems carrying a pregnancy to term due to direct effects on the uterus.

Radiation doses to the head of ≥40 Gy confer a risk for gonadotropin deficiency in females [1]. Radiation fields that expose the ovaries, including TBI, can also cause ovarian dysfunction, resulting in delayed or arrested puberty (both secondary sexual characteristic development and menstruation) as well as infertility [8]. Of additional concern for females is that even if puberty development and early fertility were normal, premature menopause can occur. While surgical premature menopause is the most common etiology in cancer survivors, as well as in patients never treated for cancer, the risk of nonsurgical premature menopause for a cancer survivor is 13 times higher than in sibling controls [9]. Cumulative incidence is highest in those women who, when treated for cancer as children, received both radiation to the ovaries and alkylating agent chemotherapy.

Radiation can also affect the vascular supply to and growth of the uterus [10]. The highest risk is conferred by prepubertal age at treatment and by radiation dose ≥30 Gy or TBI. In addition, girls with Wilm's tumor are at high risk of congenital uterine anomalies that would further impact uterine sufficiency. The implications for uterine vascular insufficiency can include adverse pregnancy outcomes, such as spontaneous abortion, premature labor, and low birth weight. An additional treatment effect, particularly from radiation to the vagina or from chronic graft vs. host disease in stem cell transplant recipients, can include vaginal fibrosis or stenosis, which in turn lead to problems such as dyspareunia and post-coital pain, as well as possible psychosocial consequences of sexual functioning difficulties [11].

Chemotherapy effects on ovarian function can be highly variable. Alkylating agents, particularly cyclophosphamide, busulfan, and procarbazine, have been implicated in different patient populations and different studies [12]. Older age at treatment appears to be a risk for girls as well, especially when combined with high cumulative doses of cyclophosphamide [13]. Ovarian failure can be temporary or permanent, and chemotherapy is also implicated, as discussed above, in premature menopause even for those women who experienced some post-treatment period of normal gonadal function.

The surgical procedures that can impact fertility for girls include hysterectomy and oophorectomy. Hysterectomy not only prevents a woman from carrying her own pregnancy, it can also cause problems with pain or urinary leakage that may impact a survivor's psychological well-being [14]. Bilateral oophorectomy is a cause of hypogonadism and infertility, but these women may still be able to carry a pregnancy with hormone replacement therapy (HRT) if the uterus is intact [15]. Unilateral oophorectomy, particularly in patients who smoke or had other treatments that affect gonadal function, can increase the risk for premature meno-pause [16]. Oophoropexy is sometimes used to shield the ovaries from radiation to nearby structures, but it can result in late effects such as the inability to conceive even with normal ovarian function [17]. Spinal or pelvic surgery can also impact sexual functioning in females with an indirect impact on fertility [18].

Surveillance and Screening

For females, a yearly patient history should monitor the onset and timing of puberty, including menstrual and pregnancy history, sexual function as age appropriate, including vaginal dryness, and medications that may impact sexual function. Family history of pubertal development timing may also be helpful in judging whether puberty is delayed. Physical examination should include overall assessment of growth and development. SMR should be documented yearly until sexual maturity has been reached.

In female patients at risk for hypogonadism, laboratory screening should include FSH and LH, as well as estradiol at age 13 as a baseline. These studies should be repeated as clinically indicated due to signs of delayed puberty, irregular menses, primary or secondary amenorrhea, or clinical signs of estrogen deficiency [1,8,12,16].

The various potential genitourinary tract abnormalities that may be due to radiation are generally found by history and physical examination. When contemplating pregnancy, high-level ultrasound can be considered for female patients who received radiation in a field impacting the uterus [10]. High-risk obstetrical care is warranted for a patient who conceives after abdominopelvic or lumbosacral spine radiation or TBI.

Additional Management Issues

Recovery of fertility and normal gonadal function is highly variable in females as well as males. Patients should be counseled to use birth control to avoid unintended pregnancy because recovery of fertility can occur even years after therapy ends. For patients with ovarian failure who have been on HRT, clinicians should consider a 2-month trial off of hormones to assess whether ovarian function has resumed. Conversely, patients who experience normal gonadal function and fertility after treatment with potentially gonadotoxic therapy should be counseled to be cautious about deliberately delaying childbearing as premature menopause can also occur [1,8,12,16].

Patients with abnormal hormone levels or delayed puberty should be referred to endocrinology. Estrogen deficiency is also a risk factor for osteoporosis, so assessment of bone density is important and hormone replacement should be at least partially protective. Reproductive endocrinology referral is warranted for patients who experience infertility [1,8,12,16].

For female patients with sexual dysfunction due to treatment, including dyspareunia or vaginal dryness, gynecologic consultation for symptom management can be helpful, but psychological distress due to these difficulties may also need attention. Referral to a psychologist may also be warranted for patients experiencing infertility.

Fertility preservation options that can be offered to female patients prior to gonadotoxic therapy are more invasive and time-consuming than the options for males. Adult women with a male partner or who choose to use donor sperm and who can safely delay cancer therapy can undergo stimulation and in vitro fertilization with a high efficiency of pregnancy using cryopreserved embryos. However, the ability to cryopreserve oocytes with successful fertilization and implantation later has been technically difficult. Many programs are currently focusing on cryopreservation of intact ovarian tissue, which requires surgical removal of all or part of an ovary. However, newer methods such as reimplantation and in vitro follicle maturation that would allow clinical use of oocytes after freezing are still in the experimental stage. (For further discussion of cryopreservation, see Mullen and Critser, this volume and see Appendix A for currently available oncofertility options.)

Optimal Care for Pediatric Cancer Patients

Dealing with fertility preservation upon diagnosis of cancer is challenging even for a young adult patient. This issue is even more complex for pediatric patients where decision making generally falls to the parents but where high cancer survival rates increase the possibility of survivors needing to confront infertility later in life (See Clayman, Galvin, and Arntson, this volume). Parents and adolescent patients report that achieving a healthy state is most important, and that while they are interested in fertility preservation options, they may not be willing to delay treatment for pursuit of those options [19] (for further discussion, see Kinahan, Didwania, and Nieman, this volume).

Fertility preservation options will only be offered to patients if the knowledge of oncology providers leads them to appropriately identify patients at risk and if they have appropriate resources to support their patients in fertility preservation decision making. Most pediatric clinicians in one pediatric hematology/oncology clinic were aware that radiation and chemotherapy can affect fertility, but only half were aware of gender differences in toxicity, and only about one third currently consult with specialists regarding fertility preservation [20].

Optimal care of pediatric cancer patients undergoing gonadotoxic therapy should include enrollment in available trials that will continue to refine knowledge of the effects of therapy on fertility for both male and female patients. Patients and families need information at diagnosis regarding the potential impact of therapy on fertility as well as referral to appropriate specialists for fertility preservation when desired. Studies and resources that allow potentially fertility-sparing interventions such as ovarian cryopreservation will not only need to be expanded, but adequate education and support for oncology providers who screen for patients at risk will be key. For patients that did not undergo fertility-sparing procedures prior to treatment, careful monitoring of reproductive function is warranted and current technologies will still allow many of those patients to parent their own biological children.

References

1. Children's Oncology Group. Children's Oncology Group Long-Term Follow-Up Guidelines for Survivors of Childhood, Adolescent, and Young Adult Cancers. Version 2.0 – March 2006. Available at: http://www.survivorshipguidelines.com. Accessed March 16, 2007. Page 61.
2. Children's Oncology Group. Children's Oncology Group Long-Term Follow-Up Guidelines for Survivors of Childhood, Adolescent, and Young Adult Cancers. Version 2.0 – March 2006. Available at: http://www.survivorshipguidelines.com. Accessed March 16, 2007. Pages 96, 118.
3. Children's Oncology Group. Children's Oncology Group Long-Term Follow-Up Guidelines for Survivors of Childhood, Adolescent, and Young Adult Cancers. Version 2.0 – March 2006. Available at: http://www.survivorshipguidelines.com. Accessed March 16, 2007. Page 97.
4. Children's Oncology Group. Children's Oncology Group Long-Term Follow-Up Guidelines for Survivors of Childhood, Adolescent, and Young Adult Cancers. Version 2.0 – March 2006. Available at: http://www.survivorshipguidelines.com. Accessed March 16, 2007. Page 9.
5. Kenney LB, Laufer MR, Grant FD, et al. High risk of infertility and long term gonadal damage in males treated with high dose cyclophosphamide for sarcoma during childhood. Cancer 2001;91:613–621.
6. Children's Oncology Group. Children's Oncology Group Long-Term Follow-Up Guidelines for Survivors of Childhood, Adolescent, and Young Adult Cancers. Version 2.0 – March 2006. Available at: http://www.survivorshipguidelines.com. Accessed March 16, 2007. Page 154.
7. Children's Oncology Group. Children's Oncology Group Long-Term Follow-Up Guidelines for Survivors of Childhood, Adolescent, and Young Adult Cancers. Version 2.0 – March 2006. Available at: http://www.survivorshipguidelines.com. Accessed March 16, 2007. Page 157.
8. Children's Oncology Group. Children's Oncology Group Long-Term Follow-Up Guidelines for Survivors of Childhood, Adolescent, and Young Adult Cancers. Version 2.0 – March 2006. Available at: http://www.survivorshipguidelines.com. Accessed March 16, 2007. Pages 94, 117.
9. Sklar CA, Mertens AC, Mitby P, et al. Premature menopause in survivors of childhood cancer: A Report from the Childhood Cancer Survivor Study. J Natl Cancer Inst 2006;98:890–896.

10. Children's Oncology Group. Children's Oncology Group Long-Term Follow-Up Guidelines for Survivors of Childhood, Adolescent, and Young Adult Cancers. Version 2.0 – March 2006. Available at: http://www.survivorshipguidelines.com. Accessed March 16, 2007. Pages 93, 116.

11. Children's Oncology Group. Children's Oncology Group Long-Term Follow-Up Guidelines for Survivors of Childhood, Adolescent, and Young Adult Cancers. Version 2.0 – March 2006. Available at: http://www.survivorshipguidelines.com. Accessed March 16, 2007. Pages 95, 105.

12. Children's Oncology Group. Children's Oncology Group Long-Term Follow-Up Guidelines for Survivors of Childhood, Adolescent, and Young Adult Cancers. Version 2.0 – March 2006. Available at: http://www.survivorshipguidelines.com. Accessed March 16, 2007. Page 10.

13. Chemaitilly W, Mertens AC, Mitby P, et al. Acute ovarian failure in the Childhood Cancer Survivor Study. J Clin Endocrinol Metab 2006;91:1723–1728.

14. Children's Oncology Group. Children's Oncology Group Long-Term Follow-Up Guidelines for Survivors of Childhood, Adolescent, and Young Adult Cancers. Version 2.0 – March 2006. Available at: http://www.survivorshipguidelines.com. Accessed March 16, 2007. Page 140.

15. Children's Oncology Group. Children's Oncology Group Long-Term Follow-Up Guidelines for Survivors of Childhood, Adolescent, and Young Adult Cancers. Version 2.0 – March 2006. Available at: http://www.survivorshipguidelines.com. Accessed March 16, 2007. Page 153.

16. Children's Oncology Group. Children's Oncology Group Long-Term Follow-Up Guidelines for Survivors of Childhood, Adolescent, and Young Adult Cancers. Version 2.0 – March 2006. Available at: http://www.survivorshipguidelines.com. Accessed March 16, 2007. Page 152.

17. Children's Oncology Group. Children's Oncology Group Long-Term Follow-Up Guidelines for Survivors of Childhood, Adolescent, and Young Adult Cancers. Version 2.0 – March 2006. Available at: http://www.survivorshipguidelines.com. Accessed March 16, 2007. Page 151.

18. Children's Oncology Group. Children's Oncology Group Long-Term Follow-Up Guidelines for Survivors of Childhood, Adolescent, and Young Adult Cancers. Version 2.0 – March 2006. Available at: http://www.survivorshipguidelines.com. Accessed March 16, 2007. Pages 150,157.

19. Burns KC, Boudreau C, Panepinto JA. Attitudes regarding fertility preservation in female adolescent cancer patients. J Pediatr Hematol Oncol 2006;28:350–354.

20. Goodwin T, Oosterhuis BE, Kiernan M et al. Attitudes and practices of pediatric oncology providers regarding fertility issues. Pediatr Blood Cancer 2007;48:80–85.

Chapter 5
Fertility Risk in Pediatric and Adolescent Cancers

Clarisa R. Gracia, MD, MSCE and Jill P. Ginsberg, MD

Recent diagnostic and therapeutic advances in pediatric oncology have led to greater survival rates in children with malignancies. However, while childhood and adolescent cancer therapies improve long-term survival, such treatments may lead to abnormal pubertal development, infertility, and gonadal failure. As more children and young adults survive childhood cancer and lead productive lives, these concerns are becoming increasingly important. Clinicians and researchers must be aware of current research in the area of fertility preservation in order to best guide patients through cancer treatment towards a healthy, fulfilled life. This chapter will review the effects of cancer treatments on reproductive potential, describe current methods of monitoring reproductive potential, and describe the fertility-sparing options available to young cancer patients of reproductive age. Specific attention will be paid to gaps in research pertinent to this topic.

Scope of the Problem

The number of childhood cancer survivors has increased dramatically over the last 25 years as substantial therapeutic advances have been made. Today, 75% of children with cancer can be expected to survive. Since the prevalence of cancer in children and adolescents up to 20 years of age is approximately 1 in 300, survivors can be expected to comprise 1 of 450 individuals in the young adult population [1]. Improvements in cancer treatments have prolonged survival and hence the focus has shifted from treating the cancer to improving the long-term health and quality of life among childhood cancer survivors [2].

The Importance of Fertility to Cancer Patients

The ability to lead full reproductive lives is very important to young cancer survivors [3–5] (for further discussion, see Kinahan, Didwania and Nieman, this volume). Web sites devoted to young cancer survivors contain patient testimonials related to fertility concerns and other quality-of-life issues after cancer. In fact, three fourths of cancer

T.K. Woodruff and K.A. Snyder (eds.) *Oncofertility*.

patients surveyed discussed fertility issues with their physician. One third of young women with breast cancer admitted that infertility concerns influenced their treatment decisions. Sadly, however, only 51% of cancer survivors surveyed felt that their concerns were addressed adequately, highlighting the need to focus counseling efforts on fertility preservation and treatment [3]. While childbearing is often considered a "woman's issue", there is evidence to suggest that this issue is important to males as well. Indeed, a retrospective survey of testicular cancer survivors and a small qualitative study of young male cancer survivors have demonstrated that infertility among cancer survivors can cause substantial distress [6,7].

Common Cancers in Children and their Treatment

The most common cancers of childhood in the order of decreasing incidence include: leukemia, central nervous system (CNS) malignancies, lymphomas, soft tissue sarcoma, renal cancer, and bone tumors. Leukemia is by far the most common cancer in children, accounting for 31% of all cancer cases in children under 15 years of age. Acute lymphocytic leukemia (ALL) commonly occurs in children ages 2–6. Treatment involves multi-agent chemotherapy, including a small dose of alkylating agent given over a 2–3–year period. The incidence of acute myelogenous leukemia (AML) peaks at 2 years and again at 16 years. Most effective therapy for AML involves chemotherapy with anthracyclines. Allogenic bone marrow transplantation is the best treatment option for AML patients in first remission.

Central nervous system malignancies are the second most frequent malignancy in children, accounting for 17% of childhood cancers. Treatment is multimodal and often involves surgery and chemotherapy.

Lymphomas account for 15% of childhood cancer cases. Therapy for Hodgkin's lymphoma includes combination chemotherapy with alkylating agents such as cyclophosphamide. The need for radiation is based on response to chemotherapy, tumor burden, and potential complications. Similarly, therapy for non-Hodgkin's lymphoma includes multiple chemotherapeutic agents including alkylator therapy with cyclophosphamide. Radiation is generally reserved for emergent therapy only.

With respect to other childhood malignancies, 7% of children with cancer are diagnosed with soft tissue sarcomas, 6.3% have renal cancer (most commonly Wilm's tumor), and 6% have bone tumors such as osteosarcoma and Ewing's sarcoma [8].

Fertility Risks for Young Females

Gonadotoxicity of Cancer Treatments

In the female, the ovary is particularly sensitive to the adverse effects of chemotherapy and radiation due to its finite number of unrenewable germ cells [9,10]. A woman's reproductive lifespan is determined by the size of the follicular pool. Cancer treatments that cause follicular atresia and destruction of the follicular pool can lead to premature menopause and infertility [11]. Such decreased reproductive potential can be unpredictable and can lead to long-term health problems, including osteoporosis, cardiovascular disease, and sexual problems.

Limited data exist that provide reliable estimates of female infertility and premature ovarian failure for counseling pediatric cancer survivors. The Childhood Cancer Survivor Study (CCSS) recently reported findings from a study of over 3,000 childhood and adolescent cancer survivors and their siblings. They found that 6.3% of childhood survivors experienced acute ovarian failure, that is, ovarian failure that occurred during or immediately after cancer treatment [12]. A comparison of the incidence of non-acute premature ovarian failure in childhood cancer survivors compared with their siblings revealed a significantly higher incidence of premature menopause in survivors (8% vs. 0.8%). Specifically, the risk of premature menopause was 13-fold higher in survivors compared with siblings. Risk factors identified in this study for premature menopause included increased age, exposure to pelvic radiation, increased number of cycles and cumulative dose of alkylating agent therapy, and a diagnosis of Hodgkin's disease. Women who had undergone treatment with alkylating agents and pelvic irradiation had a 30% incidence of premature menopause [13].

Chemotherapy

Ovarian function is affected by chemotherapy. Alkylating agents such as cyclophosphamide and ifosfamide are particularly toxic to the oocyte [14–17]. Alkylating agents are commonly used in treating childhood sarcomas, leukemia, and lymphomas. By cross-linking DNA and introducing single-stranded DNA breaks, alkylating agents destroy cells in a dose-dependent fashion [18]. In patients with chemotherapy-related ovarian failure, histological sections of the ovary show a spectrum of changes ranging from decreased numbers of follicles to complete absence of follicles and stromal fibrosis [19–21]. Age is strongly associated with gonadotoxicity of chemotherapy. In particular, the effects are more pronounced in post-pubertal females than in prepubertal females. This can be explained by the presence of fewer primordial oocytes in the ovaries at baseline and hence, less ovarian reserve to offset the cytotoxicity of cancer treatment. For instance, the risk of ovarian failure in women treated for Hodgkin's disease is 13% in girls treated before the age of 15, 60% in women less than 30 years of age, and close to 100% of women over 30 years of age [22].

Radiation

Females who receive abdominal, pelvic, or spinal radiation are at risk of developing ovarian failure, especially if the ovaries are within the treatment field. Data suggests that the ovary of an older individual is more susceptible to damage from radiation than is the ovary of a young individual. In women over 40 years of age, radiation doses of 600 cGy may be sufficient to produce ovarian failure, whereas in the majority of females treated during childhood, doses in excess of 2,000 cGy are needed to induce permanent ovarian failure [23–25]. The effect of radiation on ovarian function is compounded if radiation is given in conjunction with alkylator-based chemotherapy. In this case, ovarian dysfunction may occur despite the use of lower doses of radiation [26].

Using mathematical models that assume the age of natural menopause to be 51 years, 2,000 cGy represents a critical dose at which 50% of primordial oocytes are destroyed, and ovarian failure risk is increased [27]. Similar to the trends seen with alkylating chemoagents, older ovaries are more vulnerable to radiation damage than younger ovaries in that much smaller doses of radiation will render sterility in the setting of a diminishing primordial oocyte pool [28]. Taking into account different ages at treatment and various doses ranging from 3 to 9 Gy, Wallace et al. devised a table for predicting the age of ovarian failure and the maximum doses at any age that would render a patient sterile. These tools can be valuable in counseling patients about their reproductive potential.

Girls treated with whole abdominal and/or pelvic irradiation (total dose 2,200–3,000 cGy) for Hodgkin's disease or another solid tumor were evaluated by Wallace et al. Twenty-seven of 38 girls failed to undergo or complete pubertal development. An addiitonal 10 girls experienced early menopause at a median of 23.5 years of age [24]. Patients who receive a bone marrow transplant (BMT) with total body irradiation (TBI) are at the greatest risk of developing permanent ovarian failure. Almost all female patients who undergo a marrow transplant after age 10 will develop premature ovarian failure, whereas 50% of girls transplanted before age 10 will suffer acute loss of ovarian function [29].

Other effects of pelvic irradiation on pelvic organs can also contribute to infertility, namely, a damaged, scarred uterus with severely diminished blood flow potentially compromised in its capacity to accommodate implantation and a growing gestation. The degree of uterine damage depends on the total irradiation dose and the site of irradiation [30]. Prepubertal girls in whom the uterus has not yet developed in response to rising levels of sex steroids seem the most vulnerable to pelvic irradiation and the most resistant to physiologic sex steroid replacement. Overall, average uterine volume following TBI is 40% smaller than normal adult size [31]. Bath et al. [32] showed that in a group of survivors who received TBI as children or adolescents, some uterine volume was gained with sex steroid replacement (from 6.8 to 17.3 ml^3), but still remained significantly smaller than healthy controls and survivors who did not receive pelvic irradiation (41.5 ml^3). While the endometrial lining can be cycled using exogenous sex steroids, suggesting adequate exposure and response to exogenous estrogen, it still remains thinner than normal uteri assessed at matched cycle time (5.9 vs. 8.7 mm). With the larger doses used in abdominopelvic irradiation, these sequelae are even more profound, and there is a subset of patients in whom the uterine musculature and vasculature have been so damaged that no restoration will be achieved with hormonal replacement [33]. In women treated with abdominopelvic radiation after puberty, limited data suggest that fertility is decreased 23% [34]. In addition, there is an increased risk of spontaneous abortion, preterm labor, and delivery of low birthweight infants among women who have received pelvic irradiation [35,36].

Effects on the Hypothalamic-Pituitary-Ovarian Axis

Cranial irradiation can affect the hypothalamic-pituitary-ovarian axis. With respect to reproductive function, changes in gonadotropin secretion may lead to precocious or delayed puberty. Specifically, Bath et al. demonstrated ovulatory dysfunction in subjects who had cranial irradiation and chemotherapy for childhood ALL [37]. At times, it can be difficult to determine whether reproductive dysfunction is a result of impaired hypothalamic-pituitary function vs. evolving gonadal failure [38–40].

Time Course of Ovarian Dysfunction

Limited data exist that document the effects of chemotherapeutic agents on endocrine function prior to, during, and immediately following cancer treatment. In particular, there are no longitudinal studies assessing ovarian function in adolescents and young adults. Nonetheless, a recent study conducted in 50 adult breast cancer patients is informative. This longitudinal study collected endocrine and ultrasound measures of pituitary and ovarian function in women (median age 41) before treatment and every 3 months during chemotherapy for a total of 12 months. During this time, a significant fall in anti-Mullerian hormone (AMH) levels and inhibin B occurred, while an increase in follicle-stimulating hormone (FSH) and luteinizing hormone (LH) levels were observed by 3 months. Estradiol (E2) levels remained relatively unchanged during therapy. Ovarian volume and antral follicle counts declined over 12 months. Most women experienced irregular menstrual cycles [41]. This study and others support the theory that small preantral follicles are destroyed primarily by chemotherapy while larger follicles that produce E2 are less affected [41–43]. No longitudinal studies have been conducted assessing similar measures of ovarian function in adolescent and young cancer survivors. Presumably, the ovaries in such patients are more resistant to the effects of chemotherapy and smaller differences in measures would be detected. Being able to identify and predict when ovarian failure is expected to occur in particular patients would be helpful in determining fertility potential for family planning and the onset of menopause for bone and cardiovascular health.

Clinical Signs Occur after Fertility is Severely Compromised

Currently, it is difficult to predict whether, and to what extent, cancer survivors will experience infertility. Once clinical symptoms of ovarian dysfunction occur, such as irregular menses and vasomotor symptoms, pregnancy is usually not possible even with aggressive fertility treatments. Even women who maintain cyclic menses after therapy are at risk of infertility, early menopause, and long-term health problems related to early ovarian failure [14,17,44–48]. Therefore, early detection of compromised ovarian function is necessary in order to offer cancer survivors viable fertility options and improve quality of life. Most exciting is the possibility of identifying women at highest risk for infertility and cryopreserving ovarian tissue for future use.

Ovarian Function Markers

Over the past decade, several clinical tests have been developed to evaluate a woman's fertility potential in the infertility clinic setting [49]. Serum levels of several reproductive hormones and ultrasound-based ovarian measurements are utilized routinely as counseling tools to select treatment protocols for infertility. Such ovarian reserve testing includes isolated serum measures of basal FSH, E2, inhibin B, and AMH; dynamic serum measures, such as the Clomiphene Citrate Challenge Test; and ultrasound measures of the ovary, including antral follicle count (AFC) and ovarian volume [49–57]. If premature ovarian failure secondary to gonadotoxic treatment is preceded by ovarian and hormonal changes analogous to those seen with age-related changes, such surrogate measures should reflect fertility potential in cancer survivors as well.

While somewhat inconsistent, the findings of several small studies conducted in European centers suggest that surrogate measures of fertility potential in cancer survivors are promising. Bath et al. compared measures of fertility potential in 10 cancer survivors and found that FSH levels were higher, AMH levels were lower, and ovarian volume was smaller in cancer survivors compared with controls. No differences in basal or stimulated inhibin B or AFC were observed [58]. However, when Larsen et al. compared hormone profiles and ultrasound measures in 70 cancer survivors with spontaneous menses and 21 controls, he was able to demonstrate lower inhibin B levels, smaller ovarian volumes, and decreased AFC in the cancer survivors [59]. In a follow-up study, he found that cancer survivors with normal FSH levels and regular menses reported shorter menstrual cycles and had smaller ovarian volumes and a lower AFC compared with controls, but that the two groups had similar hormone profiles [60].

It is important to emphasize that these studies are limited by several factors that may have substantially biased the results: small sample sizes, age disparities between cases and controls, diverse gonadotoxic treatments, and inclusion of subjects taking exogenous hormones. In addition, no study has simultaneously tested several measures, assessed novel markers of ovarian aging, or assessed changes in measures during and after cancer therapy. Such data would help to elucidate which test(s) may best predict the otherwise "invisible transition" toward decreased ovarian reserve and/or premature ovarian failure.

Pregnancy Outcomes in Cancer Survivors

A large-scale epidemiologic study, the CCSS, included over 20,000 childhood cancer survivors and offers some optimism in pregnancy outcomes. Comparing outcomes of over 4,000 pregnancies in survivors with 1,900 of their siblings, the authors found a small but significant decrease in live births in cancer survivors regardless of cancer diagnosis or treatment regimen received (relative risk, RR 0.52–0.87). The authors explained the decrease in live births with the finding that survivors were more likely to choose termination of pregnancy, perhaps due to concerns regarding pregnancy outcome or maternal medical effects. Importantly, risk for stillbirth was not increased across all cancer diagnoses and treatments. No specific chemotherapy agent was identified that contributed more to adverse pregnancy outcomes, including alkylating agents. Radiation to the ovaries, either directly or indirectly through scatter and inadequate shielding, resulted in higher risk of miscarriage, but no effect on live births. The CCSS found that low birth weight infants (<02,500 g) were twice as likely to be born to survivors compared with their siblings, and particularly to those who received pelvic irradiation. The increased risk of low birth weight infants primarily related to a history of pelvic irradiation has been confirmed by several other studies [34,61].

Fortunately, studies demonstrate that cancer survivors who conceive at least 5 years following cancer treatment are not at increased risk of having a child with major congenital abnormalities when compared with the general population [61–64]. In addition, children of cancer survivors do not appear to be at higher risk of developing cancer themselves [65]. While this data is reassuring, the majority of studies assessing pregnancy outcomes cannot be generalized to current populations, since some studies date as far back as the 1940s, when treatment protocols were drastically different than those of today. Future investigations of large, current databases of cancer survivors are needed to provide more information for patient counseling. At present, however, evidence suggests that if ovarian function is preserved and pregnancy is achieved, outcomes are encouraging enough to actively pursue fertility [65]. The prenatal and obstetrical care of the cancer survivor should be multi-disciplinary, since the spectrum of medical complications resulting from cancer treatment would certainly benefit from diverse expertise.

Options for Preserving Fertility in Girls and Young Women

Unfortunately, limited options are currently available for girls and young women suffering from cancer to ensure future reproductive capacity (see Table 5.1). The most successful option for fertility preservation in post-pubescent girls facing cancer is emergency in vitro fertilization (IVF) and embryo cryopreservation prior to chemotherapy. The pregnancy rate with this technique averages 30–40% [66,67]. While

Table 5.1 Options for fertility preservation in cancer patients

Before cancer treatment
- Medical
  GnRH agonist concurrent with chemotherapy
- Surgical
  Oophoropexy prior to pelvic irradiation
- Cryopreservation
  Sperm cryopreservation*
  Embryo cryopreservation*
  Oocyte cryopreservation
  Ovarian tissue cryopreservation
  Testicular tissue cryopreservation

After cancer treatment
- IVF*donor oocyte*

*denotes established procedures

often successful, this option requires time for ovarian stimulation, oocyte retrieval, and in vitro embryo development, which delays cancer treatment 2–5 weeks [68]. Complications from IVF include ovarian hyperstimulation syndrome, which occurs in 5% of cycles. Embryo cryopreservation is ideally used when there is a male partner involved, but it can be performed in single, young cancer patients who are willing to use donor sperm. In addition, this procedure is not successful in prepubescent girls [34]. While emergency IVF is the preferred way to preserve fertility for young adults, the emotional and physical demands of the process, the duration of stimulation, and the financial burden often make it a suboptimal choice for fertility preservation.

Other options for minimizing the damaging effects of cancer treatments include oophoropexy or fertility-sparing cancer surgery [69–71]. In addition, co-administration of GnRH agonists may provide some protection against ovarian damage during chemotherapy, although prospective controlled trials are needed to establish any real benefit [72–76]. Anti-apoptotic agents like S1P have substantial promise and are currently under investigation [77–79]. While still considered experimental, other potential options for fertility preservation include cryopreservation of oocytes or ovarian tissue [80–84]. These options are particularly desirable for young single women and will be discussed in detail in Agarwal and Chang, this volume. After reproductive potential has been significantly compromised by cancer treatments, aggressive treatment with IVF may improve pregnancy rates. Oocyte donation and embryo donation offer excellent chances of pregnancy after ovarian failure has occurred, but may not be acceptable to many couples.

Fertility Risks for Young Men

Cancer therapy can interfere with reproductive ability and libido in men. The differential sensitivity of spermatozoa-producing Sertoli cells compared with the testosterone-producing Leydig cells allows for greater effects in on the reproductive capacity of men than effects on their sexual function. Moreover, since the testes are more sensitive than the ovary to cytotoxic therapies, the ensuing injury is more damaging to male fertility than to female fertility. Comparison of fertility in treated men and women revealed a 0.76 adjusted relative fertility [85]. The testes are extremely sensitive to chemotherapy, radiation, and surgical interventions.

Chemotherapy

Testicular dysfunction is among the most common long-term side effects of chemotherapy in men. Testicular damage is agent-specific and dose-related. The germinal epithelium is particularly susceptible to injury by cytotoxic drugs secondary to a high mitotic rate. In contrast, Leydig cells appear relatively resistant to the effects of chemotherapy [86]. In 1948, azoospermia after exposure to an alkylating agent (nitrogen mustard) was described in 27 of 30 men treated for lymphoma [87]. Subsequently, it has become apparent that all alkylating agents such as cyclophosphamide, ifosfamide, and procarbazine are gonadotoxic [88–90]. Conversely, antimetabolite therapy, such as methotrexate and mercaptopurine, does not have an adverse impact on male fertility. Cisplatin-based regimens including velban, bleomycin, and etoposide result in temporary impairment of spermatogenesis in all patients but with recovery in a significant percentage [91].

Initial reports suggested that the younger the boy the more resistant he was to the gonadotoxicity of the chemotherapy [92]. More recently, however, it has become apparent that both the prepubertal and pubertal testes are vulnerable to cytotoxic drugs [93–95]. Impairment of spermatogenesis may be irreversible in the months to years following chemotherapy. However, late recovery of spermatogenesis up to 14 years following chemotherapy has been reported [96,97]. The chance of recovery of spermatogenesis following cytotoxic chemotherapy and the extent and speed of recovery are related to the agent used and the dose received [97–100]. In contrast to the germinal epithelium, Leydig cells appear relatively resistant to the effects of chemotherapy [101]. However, a few studies have demonstrated a reduction in testosterone concentrations following treatment with gonadotoxic agents, and there is evidence to suggest that Leydig cell impairment following chemotherapy may be relevant clinically.

While chemotherapy lowers sperm counts and may disrupt DNA integrity, it appears that sperm integrity is re-established over time [102,103]. In addition, as reviewed previously, there does not appear to be any increased risk of congenital anomalies among children born of cancer survivors [104].

Radiotherapy

Spermatogenesis is exquisitely sensitive to radiation [105]. The testes are directly irradiated in rare situations, such as testicular relapse of ALL. Although the testes are usually not directly in the radiation field, they can still receive irradiation via body scatter. The amount of scattered radiation is a function of the proximity of the radiation field to the target, the field size and shape, the X-ray energy, and the depth of the target. Of these, distance from the field edge is the most important factor. Scatter dose to the testes becomes a real issue when treating a field that extends into the pelvis, as in some cases of Hodgkin's disease, seminoma, or soft tissue sarcoma of the thigh. Small children, because of their short trunk length, can be at greater risk from scattered radiation than larger individuals.

The germinal epithelium is most sensitive to radiation effects and some effect on spermatogenesis will be seen at doses of 10 cGy. Permanent sterilization may be seen with doses as low as 100 cGy [105]. Ash summarized data from several older studies that examined testicular function following radiation in patients who were treated for a range of cancers, including Hodgkin's disease, prostate cancer, and testicular cancer [105]. The author found that oligospermia occurred at doses as low as 10 cGy and azoospermia at 35 cGy, which was generally reversible. However, 200–300 cGy could result in azoospermia that did not reverse even years after irradiation. Leydig cells in the testes are more resistant to radiation than germ cells. The available data indicate that chemical changes in Leydig cell function are observable following direct testicular irradiation, with the effect more pronounced with 2,400 cGy than with 1,200 cGy [106]. The severity of the effect is more marked the younger the patient is at the time of radiotherapy [107]. In general, progression through puberty and testosterone production proceeds normally in males subjected to radiation therapy.

Options for Preserving Fertility in Boys and Young Men

Sperm cryopreservation after masturbation remains the best option for fertility preservation in the post-pubertal male diagnosed with cancer. All adolescents and young adults facing cancer therapy should be offered sperm cryopreservation as a way to preserve future fertility. Multiple samples should be cryopreserved before cancer treatment begins. Since sperm production begins around the age of 12–13, adolescent boys who are unable to produce a specimen via ejaculation can undergo electroejaculation or testicular sperm extraction under anesthesia [108]. Although sperm banking is a relatively simple process, there is evidence that oncologists do not routinely discuss this option with their patients [109]. In addition, even when sperm is banked, many men do not use the specimens. A study of 422 testicular cancer survivors with cryopreserved semen reported that while only 29 (7%) used the cryopreserved samples for artificial reproductive techniques, 48% (14/29) were successful [110].

Unfortunately, at this time there are no feasible options for preserving fertility of prepubertal male patients. There has been no demonstrated protective effect of using GnRH analogues with and without testosterone to suppress testicular function during chemotherapy [111,112]. In cooperation with pediatric oncologists, we must continue to attempt to reduce the gonadotoxicity of treatment regimens while maintaining superior cure rates.

   Fertility preservation in prepubertal boys remains problematic and is an active area of investigation. Extracting and cryopreserving spermatogonial stem cells from boys in order to use later in autografts, xenografts, or maturation in vitro are exciting and promising avenues of investigation. While transplantation of cryopreserved testicular tissue has been successful in mice and rats, data in humans is lacking [113,114].

Ethical Issues in Pediatric Patients

The use of novel methods of assisted reproductive technologies (ART), such as oocyte and ovarian tissue cryopreservation, raise ethical challenges for the informed consent process in the pediatric and adolescent patient. As discussed, while these methods are experimental and may offer no guarantee of future fertility, they involve invasive procedures that have a small but significant potential for medical complications. The decision-making process is complex since it involves the need to weigh complex options (ovarian tissue, oocyte, and embryo cryopreservation; future donor oocyte; future adoption), in order to achieve a potential future goal (childbearing). Whether the authority to make such a decision rests with the parent or the cancer patient is not clear and depends on the age and maturity of the patient and state law. It is possible that parental judgment may not reflect the future best interests of the patient, but the patient may not have the capacity to truly consent or refuse the fertility-preserving procedures. Informed choice is also challenging in this area since there is limited evidence on the safety and efficacy of novel fertility-preserving technologies (for further discussion, see Zoloth and Backhus, this volume).
   Another issue that must be considered is ownership of cryopreserved tissue in the case of a pediatric patient's death. Who should decide on ownership? Should parents or guardians be permitted to use this tissue to undergo ART in the case of the child's death? Such ethical issues must be carefully considered when counseling patients and families about fertility preserving options [115].

Conclusion

The scope of the "problem" of fertility preservation in cancer survivors will only continue to grow as cancer treatments improve disease-free survival. Therefore, quality-of-life issues, including reproduction and avoiding premature menopause, will certainly become even more prominent concerns, and much of pre-cancer treatment counseling will need to broaden to cover these issues. We must work together in the medical and research community to find ways to minimize the gonadotoxicity of cancer treatments, develop novel and effective fertility preserving techniques, improve the detection of impaired fertility potential in cancer survivors, improve patient counseling about available fertility options, and assist those interested in pursuing fertility preserving therapies prior to treatment. Ultimately, a multi-faceted team approach that includes the expertise of a reproductive endocrinologist and oncologist will culminate in the best treatment plan possible, encompassing not just cancer treatment but also fertility preservation. We are optimistic that more choices will soon be available to help cancer survivors lead full reproductive lives.

References

1. Hewitt M, Breen N, Devesa S. Cancer prevalence and survivorship issues: analysis of 1992 National Health Interview Survey. J Natl Cancer Inst 1999;91:1480–1486.
2. Jemel A, Clegg LH, Ward E, et al. Annual report to the nation on the status of cancer, 1975–2001, with a special feature regarding survival. Cancer 2004;101:3–27.
3. Partridge AH, Gelber S, Peppercorn J, et al. Web-based survey of fertility issues in young women with breast cancer. J Clin Oncol 2004; 22:4174–4183.
4. Wenzel L, Dogan-Atles A, Habbal R, et al. Defining and measuring reproductive concerns of female cancer survivors. J Natl Cancer Inst Monogr 2005;34:94–98.
5. Burns KC, Boudreau C, Panepinto JA. Attitudes regarding fertility preservation in female adolescent cancer patients. J Pediatr Hematol Oncol 2006;28:350–354.
6. Rieker PP, Fitzgerald EM, Kalish LA. Adaptive behavioral responses to potential infertility among survivors of testis cancer. J Clin Oncol 1990;8:347–355.
7. Green D, Galvin H, Norme B. The psycho-social impact of infertility on young male cancer survivors: a qualitative investigation. Psycho-oncology 2003;12:141–152.
8. Ries LAG, Smith MA, Gurney JG, et al. Cancer Incidence and survival among children and adolescents: United States SEER Program 1975–95. National Cancer Institute, SEER Program. NIH pub. No. 99-4649. Bethesda, MD, 1999.
9. Johnson J, Canning J, Kaneko T, et al. Germline stem cells and follicular renewal in the postnatal mammalian ovary. Nature 2004;428:145–150.
10. Forbasco AS, de Pol A, Vizzotto L, et al. Morphometric study of the human neonatal ovary. Anat Rec 1991;231:201–208.
11. Faddy MJ, Gosden RG, Gougeon A, et al. Accelerated disappearance of ovarian follicles in mid-life: implications for forecasting menopause. Hum Reprod 1992;7:1342–1346.
12. Chemaitilly W, Mertens AC, Mitby P. Acute ovarian failure in the childhood cancer survivor study. J Clin Endocrinol Metab 2006;91:1723–1728.
13. Sklar CA, Mertens AC, Mitby P, et al. Premature menopause in survivors of childhood cancer: a report from the childhood cancer survivor study. J Natl Cancer Inst 2006;98:890–896.
14. Hensley ML, Reichman BS. Fertility and pregnancy after adjuvant chemotherapy for breast cancer. Crit Rev Oncol Hematol 1998;28:121–128.
15. Wallace WH, Blacklay A, Eiser C, et al. Developing strategies for long term follow up of survivors of childhood cancer. BMJ 2001;323:271–274.
16. Thomson AB, Critchley HO, Wallace WH. Fertility and progeny. Eur J Cancer 2002;38:1634–1644.
17. Damewood MD, Grochow LB. Prospects for fertility after chemotherapy or radiation of neoplastic disease. Fertil Steril 1986;45:443–459.
18. Meirow D, Epstein M, Lewis H, et al. Administration of cyclophosphamide at different stages of follicular maturation in mice: effects on reproductive performance and fetal malformations. Hum Reprod 2001;16:632–637.
19. Warne GL, Fairley KF, Hobbs JB, et al. Cyclophosphamide-induced ovarian failure. N Engl J Med 1973;289:1159–1162.
20. Koyama H, Wada T, Nishizawa Y, et al. Cyclophosphamide-induced ovarian failure and its therapeutic significance in patients with breast cancer. Cancer 1977;39:1403–1409.

21. Familiari G, Caggiati A, Nottola SA, et al. Ultrastructure of human ovarian primordial follicles after combination chemotherapy for Hodgkin's disease. Hum Reprod 1993;8:2080–2087.
22. Chapman RM, Sutcliffe SB, Malpas JS. Cytotoxic-induced ovarian failure in women with Hodgkin's disease. I. Hormone function. JAMA 1979;242:1877–1881.
23. Wallace WH, Shalet SM, Hendry JH, et al. Ovarian failure following abdominal irradiation in childhood: the radiosensitivity of the human oocyte. Br J Radiol 1989;62:995–998.
24. Wallace WH, Shalet SM, Crowne EC, et al. Ovarian failure following abdominal irradiation in childhood: natural history and prognosis. Clin Oncol 1989;1:75–79.
25. Thibaud E, Ramirez M, Brauner R, et al. Preservation of ovarian function by ovarian transposition performed before pelvic irradiation during childhood. J Pediatr 1992;121:880–884.
26. Sklar C. Reproductive physiology and treatment-related loss of sex hormone production. Med Pediatr Oncol 1999;33:2–8.
27. Wallace WH, Thomson AB, Kelsey TW. The radiosensitivity of the human oocyte. Hum Reprod 2003;18:117–121.
28. Wallace WH, Thomson AB, Saran F, et al. Predicting age of ovarian failure after radiation to a field that includes the ovaries. Int J Radiat Oncol Biol Phys 2005;62:738–744.
29. Sklar C. Growth and endocrine disturbances after bone marrow transplantation in childhood. Acta Paediatr Suppl. 1995;411:57–61; discussion 62.
30. Critchley HO, Wallace WH. Impact of cancer treatment on uterine function. J Natl Cancer Inst Monogr 2005;34:64–68.
31. Holm K, Nysom K, Brocks V, et al. Ultrasound B-mode changes in the uterus and ovaries and Doppler changes in the uterus after total body irradiation and allogeneic bone marrow transplantation in childhood. Bone Marrow Transplant 1999;23:259–263.
32. Bath LE, Critchley HO, Chambers SE, et al. Ovarian and uterine characteristics after total body irradiation in childhood and adolescence: response to sex steroid replacement. Br J Obstet Gynaecol 1999;106:1265–1272.
33. Larsen EC, Schmiegelow K, Rechnitzer C, et al. Radiotherapy at a young age reduces uterine volume of childhood cancer survivors. Acta Obstet Gynecol Scand 2004;83:96–102.
34. Chiarelli AM, Marrett LD, Darlington G. Early menopause and infertility in females after treatment for childhood cancer diagnosed in 1964–1988 in Ontario, Canada. Am J Epidemiol 1999;150:245–254.
35. Chritchley HO, Bath LE, Wallace HB. Radiation damage to the uterus – review of the effects of treatment of childhood cancer. Hum Fertil 2002;5:61–66.
36. Bath LE, Anderson RA, Critchley HO, et al. Hypothalamic-pituitary-ovarian dysfunction after prepubertal chemotherapy and cranial irradiation for acute leukaemia. Hum Reprod 2001;16:1838–1844.
37. Cicognani A, Pasini A, Pession A, et al. Gonadal function and pubertal development after treatment of childhood malignancy. J Pediatr Endocrinol Metab 2003;16:321–326.
38. Spoudeas HA, Charmandari E, Brook CG. Hypothalamo-pituitary-adrenal axis integrity after cranial irradiation for childhood posterior fossa tumors. Med Pediatr Oncol 2003;40:224–229.
39. Kanumakala S, Warne GL, Zacharin MR. Evolving hypopituitarism following cranial irradiation. J Paediatr Child Health 2003;39:232–235.
40. Kim S.S. Fertility preservation in female cancer patients: current developments and future directions. Fertil Steril 2006;85:1–11.
41. Anderson RA, Themmen APN, Al-Qahtani A, et al. The effects of chemotherapy and long-term gonadotrophin suppression on the ovarian reserve in premenopausal women with breast cancer. Hum Rep Advance Access. July 2006.
42. Chatterjee R, Mills W, Katz M, et al. Prospective study of pituitary-gonadal function to evaluate short-term effects of ablative chemotherapy or total body irradiation with autologous or allogenic marrow transplantation in post-menarcheal female patients. Bone Marrrow Transplant 1994;13:511–517.
43. Wallace EM, Groome NP, Riley SC, et al. Effects of chemotherapy-induced testicular damage on inhibin, gonadotrophin and testosterone secretion: a prospective longitudinal study. J Clin Endocrinol Metab 1997;82:3111–3115.

44. Kreuser E, Felsenberg D, Behles C, et al. Long-term gonadal dysfunction and its impact on bone mineralization in patients following COPP/ABVD chemotherapy for Hodgkin's disease. Ann Oncol 1992;3:105–110.
45. Mills JL, Fears TR, Robison LL, et al. Menarche in a cohort of 188 long-term survivors of acute lymphoblastic leukemia. J Pediatr 1997;131:598–602.
46. Byrne J, Fears TR, Gail MH, et al. Early menopause in long-term survivors of cancer during adolescence. Am J Obstet Gynecol 1996;166:788–793.
47. Sklar C. Reproductive physiology and treatment-related loss of sex hormone production. Med Pediatr Oncol 1999;33:2–8.
48. Meirow D. Reproduction post-chemotherapy in young cancer patients. Mol Cell Endocrinol 2000;169:123–131.
49. Scott RT Jr, Hofmann GE. Prognostic assessment of ovarian reserve. Fertil Steril 1995;63:1–11.
50. Muasher SJ, Oehninger S, Simonetti S, et al. The value of basal and/or stimulated serum gonadotripin levels in prediction of stimulation response and in vitro fertilization outcome. Fertil Steril 1988;50:298–307.
51. Toner JP, Philput CB, Jones GS, et al. Basal follicle-stimulating hormone level is a better predictor of in vitro fertilization performance than age. Fertil Steril 1991;55:784–791.
52. Bancsi LF, Broekmans FJ, Mol BW, et al. Performance of basal follicle-stimulating hormone in the prediction of poor ovarian response and failure to become pregnant after in vitro fertilization: a meta-analysis. Fertil Steril 2003;79:1091–1100.
53. Hendriks DJ, Mol BW, Bancsi LF, et al. Antral follicle count in the prediction of poor ovarian response and pregnancy after in vitro fertilization; a meta-analysis and comparison with basal follicle-stimulating hormone level. Fertil Steril 2005;83:291–301.
54. Seifer DB, Scott RT Jr, Bergh PA, et al. Women with declining ovarian reserve may demonstrate a decrease in day 3 serum inhibin B before a rise in day 3 follicle-stimulating hormone. Fertil Steril 1999;72:63–65.
55. Seifer DB, Lambert-Messerlian G, Hogan JW, et al. Day 3 serum inhibin-B is predictive of assisted reproductive technologies outcome. Fertil Steril 1997;67:110–114.
56. Seifer CB, MacLaughlin DT, Christian BP, et al. Early follicular serum mullerian-inhibiting levels are associated with ovarian response during assisted reproductive technology cycles. Fertil Steril 2002;77:468–471.
57. Sharara FI, McClamrock HD. The effect of aging on ovarian volume measurements in infertile women. Obstet Gynecol 1999;94:57–60.
58. Bath LE, Wallace WH, Shaw MP, et al. Depletion of ovarian reserve in young women after treatment for cancer in childhood: detection by anti-Mullerian hormone, inhibin B and ovarian ultrasound. Hum Reprod 2003;18:2368–2374.
59. Larsen EC, Muller J, Schmiegelow K, et al. Reduced ovarian function in long-term survivors of radiation and chemotherapy-treated childhood cancer. J Clin Endocrinol Metab 2003;33:5302–5314.
60. Larsen EC, Muller J, Rochnitzer C, et al. Diminished ovarian reserve in female childhood cancer survivors with regular menstrual cycles and basal FSH < 10 IU/l. Hum Reprod 2003;18:417–422.
61. Hawkins MM, Smith RA. Pregnancy outcomes in childhood cancer survivors: probable effects of abdominal irradiation. Int J Cancer 1989;43:399–402.
62. Li FP, Fine W, Jaffe N, Holmes GE, Holmes FF. Offspring of patients treated for cancer in childhood. J Natl Cancer Inst 1979;62:1193–1197.
63. Byrne J, Rasmussen SA, Steinhorn SC, et al. Genetic disease in offspring of long-term survivors of childhood and adolescent cancer. Am J Hum Genet 1998;62:45–52.
64. Green DM, Zevon MA, Lowrie G, et al. Congenital anomalies in children of patients who received chemotherapy for cancer in childhood and adolescence. N Engl J Med 1991;325:141–146.
65. Nagarajan R, Robison LL. Pregnancy outcomes in survivors of childhood cancer. J Natl Cancer Inst Monogr 2005;34:72–76.
66. Lobo RA. Potential options for preservation of fertility in women. N Engl J Med 2005;353:64–73.

67. Ginsburg ES, Yanushpolsky EH, Jackson KV. In vitro fertilization for cancer patients and survivors. Fertil Steril 2001;75:705–710.
68. Kim SS. Fertility preservation in female cancer patients: current developments and future directions. Fertil Steril 2006;85:1–11.
69. Ray GR, Trueblood HW, Enright LP, et al. Oophorepexy: a means of preserving ovarian function following pelvic megvoltage radiotherapy for Hodgkin's disease. Radiology 1970;96:175–180.
70. Scott SM, Schlaff W. Laparoscopic medial oophoropexy prior to radiation therapy in an adolescent with Hodgkin's disease. J Pediatr Adolesc Gynecol 2005;18:355–257.
71. Hadar H, Loven D, Herskovitz P, et al. An evaluation of lateral and medial transposition of the ovaries out of radiation fields. Cancer 1994;74:774–779.
72. Gunthert AR, Grundker C, Bottcher B, et al. Luteinizing hormone-releasing hormone (LHRH) inhibits apoptosis induced by cytotoxic agent and UV-light but not apoptosis mediated through CD95 in human ovarian and endometrial cancer cells. Anticancer Res 2004;24:1727–1732.
73. Ataya K, Rao LV, Lawrence E, et al. Luteinizing hormone-releasing hormone agonist inhibits cyclophosphamide-induced ovarian follicular depletion in rhesus monkeys. Biol Reprod 1995;52:365–372.
74. Blumenfeld Z, Eckman A. Preservation of fertility and ovarian function and minimization of chemotherapy-induced gonadotoxicity in young women by GnRH-a. J Natl Cancer Inst Monogr 2005;34:40–43.
75. Blumenfeld Z, Avivi I, Linn S, et al. Prevention of irreversible chemotherapy-induced ovarian damage in young women with lymphoma by a gonadotrophin-releasing hormone agonist in parallel to chemotherapy. Hum Reprod 1996;11:1620–1626.
76. Pereyra Pacheco B, Mendez Ribas JM, Milone G, et al. Use of GnRH analogs for functional protection of the ovary and preservation of fertility during cancer treatment in adolescents: a preliminary report. Gynecol Oncol 2001;81:391–397.
77. Tilly JL, Kolesnick RN. Sphingolipids, apoptosis, cancer treatments and the ovary. Investigating a crime against female fertility. Biochem Biophys Acta 2002;1585:135–138.
78. Morita Y, Perez GI, Paris F, et al. Oocyte apoptosis is suppressed by disruption of the acid sphingomyelinase gene or by sphingosine-1 phosphate therapy. Nat Med 2000;6:1109–1114.
79. Perez GI, Jurisicova A, Matikainen T, et al. A central role for ceramide in the age-related acceleration of apoptosis in the female germline. FASEB J 2005;19:860–862.
80. Donnez J, Dolmans MM, Demylle D, et al. Livebirth after orthotopic transplantation of cryopreserved ovarian tissue. Lancet 2004;364:1405–1410.
81. Oktay T, Tilly J. Livebirth after cryopreserved ovarian tissue autotransplantation. Lancet 2004;364:2091–2092; author reply 2092–2093.
82. Meirow D, Levron J, Eldar-Geva T, et al. Pregnancy after transplantation of cryopreserved ovarian tissue in a patient with ovarian failure after chemotherapy. N Engl J Med 2005;353:318–321.
83. Van der Elst J. Oocyte freezing: here to stay. Hum Reprod Update 2003;9:463–470.
84. Borini A, Bonu MA, Coticchio G, et al. Pregnancies and births after oocyte preservation. Fertil Steril 2004;82:601–605.
85. Byrne J, Mulvihill JJ, Myers MH, et al. Effects of treatment on fertility in long-term survivors of childhood or adolescent cancer. N Engl J Med 1987;19:1315–1321.
86. Tsatsoulis A, Shalet SM, Morris ID, et al. Immunoactive inhibin as a marker of Sertoli cell function following cytotoxic damage to the human testis. Horm Res 1990;34254–34259.
87. Spitz S. The histological effects of nitrogen mustards on human tumors and tissues. Cancer 1948;1:383–398.
88. Heikens J, Behrendt H, Adriaanse R, et al. Irreversible gonadal damage in male survivors of pediatric Hodgkin's disease. Cancer 1996;78:2020–2024.
89. Mackie EJ, Radford M, Shalet SM. Gonadal function following chemotherapy for childhood Hodgkin's disease. Med Pediatr Oncol 1996;27:74–78.
90. Papadakis V, Vlachopapadopoulou E, Van Syckle K, et al. Gonadal function in young patients successfully treated for Hodgkin disease. Med Pediatr Oncol 1999;32:366–372.

91. Hansen PV, Hansen SW. Gonadal function in men with testicular germ cell cancer: the influence of cisplatin-based chemotherapy. Eur Urol 1993;23:153–156.
92. Sherins RJ, Olweny CL, Ziegler JL. Gynaecomastia and gonadal dysfunction in adolescent boys treated with combination chemotherapy for Hodgkins disease. N Engl J Med 1978;299:12–16.
93. Aubier F, Flamamant F, Brauner R, et al. Male gonadal function after chemotherapy for solid tumors in childhood. J Clin Oncol 1989;7:304–309.
94. Ben Arush MW, Solt I, Lightman A, et al. Male gonadal function in survivors of childhood Hodgkin and non-Hodgkin lymphoma. Pediatr Hematol Oncol 2000;17:239–245.
95. Howell S, Shalet S. Gonadal damage from chemotherapy and radiotherapy. Endocrinol Metab Clin North Am 1998;27:927–943.
96. Buchanan JD, Fairley KF, Barrier JU. Return of spermatogenesis after stopping cyclophosphamide therapy. Lancet 1975;2:156–157.
97. Watson AR, Rance CP, Bain J. Long-term effects of cyclophosphamide on testicular function. Br Med J 1985;291:1457–1460.
98. da Cunha MF, Meistrich ML, Fuller LM. Recovery of spermatogenesis after treatment for Hodgkin's disease: limiting dose of MOPP chemotherapy. J Clin Oncol 1984;2:571–577.
99. Howell SJ, Shalet SM. Testicular function following chemotherapy. Hum Reprod Update 2001;7:363–369.
100. Pryzant RM, Meistrich ML, Wilson G. Long-term reduction in sperm count after chemotherapy with and without radiation therapy for non-Hodgkin's lymphomas. J Clin Oncol 1993;11:239–247.
101. Shalet SM, Tsatsoulis A, Whitehead E, et al. Vulnerability of the human Leydig cell to radiation damage is dependent upon age. J Endocrinol 1989;120:161–165.
102 Chatterjee R, Jaines GA, Perera DM, et al. Testicular and sperm DNA damage after treatment with fludarabine for chronic lymptocytic leukaemia. Hum Reprod 2000;15:762–766.
103. Thomson AB, Campbell AJ, Irvine DC, et al. Semen quality and spermatozoal DNA integrity in survivors of childhood cancer: a case–control study. Lancet 2002;360:361–367.
104. Meistrich ML, Byrne J. Genetic disease if offspring of long-term survivors of childhood and adolescent cancer treated with potentially mutagenic therapies. Am J Hum Genet 2002;70:1069–1071.
105. Ash P. The influence of radiation on fertility in man. Br J Radiol 1980;53:271–278.
106. Sklar CA, Robison LL, Nesbit ME, et al. Effects of radiation on testicular function in long-term survivors of childhood acute lymphoblastic leukemia: a report from the Children Cancer Study Group. J Clin Oncol 1990;8:1981–1987.
107. Castillo LA, Craft AW, Kernahan J, Evans R.G. and Aynsley-Green A. Gonadal function after 12-Gy testicular irradiation in childhood acute lymphoblastic leukaemia. Med Pediatr Oncol 1990;18:185–189.
108. Schmiegelow ML, Sommer P, Carlsen E, et al. Penile vibratory stimulation and electroejaculation before anticancer therapy in two pubertal boys. J Pediatr Hematol Oncol 1998;20:429–430.
109. Shover LR, Brey K, Lichtin A, et al. Oncologists' attitudes and practices regarding banking sperm before cancer treatment. J Clin Oncol 2002;20:1890–1897.
110. Magelssen H, et al. Twenty years experience with semen cryopreservation in testicular cancer patients: who needs it? Eur Urol 2005;48:779–785.
111. Johnson DH, Linde R, Hainsworth JD, et al. Effect of luteinizing hormone releasing hormone agonist given during combination chemotherapy on posttherapy fertility in male patients with lymphoma: preliminary observations. Blood 1985;65:832–836.
112. Waxman JH, Ahmed R, Smith D, et al. Failure to preserve fertility in patients with Hodgkin's disease. Cancer Chemother Pharmacol 1987;19:159–162.
113. Brinster LR, Avarbock MR. Germline transmission of donor haplotype following spermatogonial transplantation. Proc Natl Acad Sci 1994;91:11303–11307.
114. Zhang Z, Renfree MB, Short RV. Successful intra- and inter-specific male germ cell transplantation in the rat. Biol Reprod 2003;68:961–963.
115. Nisker J, Baylis F, McLeod C. Choice in fertility preservation in girls and adolescent women with cancer. Cancer 2006;107:1686–1689.

Part III
Oncofertility Techniques and Research

Chapter 6
Bioengineering and the Ovarian Follicle

Min Xu, PhD, Teresa K. Woodruff, PhD, and Lonnie D. Shea, PhD

Three-dimensional scaffolds are widely used in the field of tissue engineering, which combines the principles and methods of the life sciences with those of engineering to provide a fundamental understanding of structure–function relationships in normal and diseased tissues, to develop materials and methods to repair damaged or diseased tissues, and to create entire tissue replacements [1]. A synthetic scaffold can serve as a stroma that creates a cellular environment designed to provide the factors that stimulate maturation of ovarian follicles, but lacks the factors found in the native stroma that inhibit follicle maturation.

In the area of follicle maturation, synthetic scaffolds have been employed to maintain the appropriate size, shape, and architecture of the tissue while providing the necessary signals to direct cellular responses [2–7]. These scaffolds maintain the intimate physiological connections between the oocytes and somatic cells within the follicle, which are essential for normal development. Additionally, a three-dimensional scaffold is more durable and poses fewer concerns regarding jolting the cultures, which can be problematic in two-dimensional systems [5]. Finally, the scaffold-encased follicle can be individually manipulated, providing an extraordinary level of control. The development of scaffold materials, in combination with basic studies of follicle biology, will ultimately lead to the development of a synthetic ovarian stroma and the optimal media conditions to support follicle development and maturation in vitro, which will enable women to preserve their fertility in the face of various insults, including chemotherapy- or radiation therapy-induced infertility.

In this chapter, we discuss the application of bioengineering principles to the emerging field of oncofertility. We will summarize current knowledge of and achievements in the development of in vitro systems for culture of preantral follicles. Then, we will discuss the concept of application of biomaterials on in vitro follicle development and principles of hydrogel selection and modification. Finally, we will address the transplantation of ovarian tissue as an alternative to in vitro maturation. Though the approach is early in its development, it has successfully yielded live offspring. Biomaterial scaffolds, combined with drug delivery technology, may facilitate engraftment and function of the transplanted tissue [8,9].

75

T.K. Woodruff and K.A. Snyder (eds.) *Oncofertility*.
© Springer 2007

Follicle Growth In Vivo

Follicle formation begins between week 16 and 18 of fetal life in humans, and neonatally in rodents. Soon after the initial formation of primordial follicles in the ovary, and in response to an unknown signal, follicles are gradually and continuously recruited to enter the growth process. From this time onward, growth appears to be continuous until menopause. Follicle growth is a complex, multi-stage process that involves multiple cell types, cell–cell and cell–substrate interactions, and a variety of soluble stimuli (e.g., hormones, growth factors) (Fig. 6.1) [10–14]. During the growth of primary and secondary follicles, the oocyte increases in volume, a zona pellucida composed of 3 glycoproteins (ZP1, ZP2, ZP3) is synthesized, and the granulosa cells multiply to form several layers. To complete the follicle unit, thecal cells from the surrounding stroma differentiate to form a cell layer outside the granulosa cells. Oocyte growth is dependent upon gap junction-mediated communication between the oocyte and the supporting granulosa cells [15], and the rate of growth is related to the number of granulosa cells coupled to the oocyte [16]. Later in development, follicles are stimulated by growth and differentiation factors and pituitary hormones, such as follicle-stimulating hormone (FSH) and luteinizing hormone (LH). FSH acts on a subset of follicles, causing them to begin explosive growth leading to a fully mature follicle. At the end of growth, the gonadotrophin surges stimulate many events, including oocyte maturation, cumulus expansion, degradation of the surface epithelial cells, and ovulation. Oocyte maturation involves progression from prophase of the first meiotic division to metaphase of the second meiotic division. Throughout the life cycle of the follicle, growth factors, hormones, and environmental cues (O_2, matrix, and cell–cell contacts) change to orchestrate the developmental process. If the oocyte is not fertilized, new follicles are recruited, and the cycle of follicular maturation and hormone activation continues. Within the ovary, the process of follicle maturation is highly regulated, with inhibitory factors that restrict follicle recruitment and maturation. Isolating follicles from the ovary removes these inhibitory stimuli, and can allow follicle development given the appropriate culture environment.

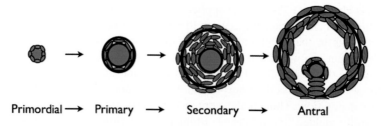

Fig. 6.1 Ovarian follicle maturation demonstrating the progression of primordial follicles to antral follicles

Culture Systems for Follicle Growth

Several follicle culture systems that support oocyte development in vitro have been developed and the appropriate use of these approaches, alone or in combination, could permit the growth of any stage follicle. Thus far, live births have been achieved using follicles grown in vitro from either fresh [17–20] or cryopreserved [21,22] ovarian tissues only in mice. Nevertheless, recent reports that successful transplantation of cryopreserved ovarian tissue in women led to pregnancy and birth of healthy offspring [23–25] raises the possibility that in vitro follicle culture techniques may become another option for preserving fertility.

Two types of in vitro culture systems, termed non-spherical (two-dimensional) and spherical (three-dimensional), have been developed to support oocyte maturation in cultured preantral follicles. Non-spherical culture systems include that of Eppig and O'Brien, which cultured enzymatically isolated follicles on a collagen membrane [11,18,20,26], and Smitz and Cortvrindt, which grew attached primary and secondary follicles that were mechanically isolated from mice [27–29]. Although these two-dimensional culture systems supported growth of meiotically competent eggs that could be fertilized and produce live birth in mice, such systems have been unable to support normal follicle development in larger mammalian species, including cows [30], sheep [31], and humans [32,33]. Loss of follicle architecture and the critical cellular interactions between adjacent somatic cells and between somatic and germ cells may lead to uncoordinated growth and differentiation of granulosa and thecal cells and the oocyte, as illustrated in Fig. 6.2b. A spherical culture system was originally developed by Nayudu and Osborn [34] and was later modified by other groups [17,35–38] in an effort to optimize preservation of follicle integrity. Most researchers used later stage preantral follicles (~170–240 μm) that were only able to remain viable in culture for short periods of time (4–6 days). Other studies have reported follicle culture using the inverted drop [35] or rotating-wall vessel [39] suspension system to maintain spherical structure. However, it is

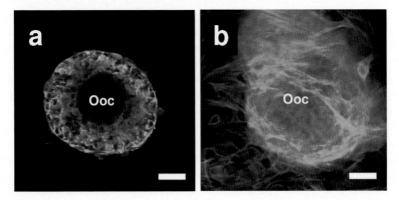

Fig. 6.2 Follicles cultured (**a**) in three-dimensional hydrogels or (**b**) on polystyrene. Scale bar: 30 μm

unclear whether oocyte development and maturation was supported in these systems, as only somatic cell growth was measured.

Recently, we developed a three-dimensional in vitro follicle culture system that utilizes an alginate hydrogel matrix as a scaffold for follicle growth. The application of biomaterials to the culture of immature ovarian follicles has enabled in vitro phenocopying of the in vivo microenvironment for follicle development (Fig. 6.2a). Three-dimensional culture within hydrogels applies the principles of tissue engineering to maintain the tissue architecture and cellular organization of the follicle and promote the coordinated growth of the germ and somatic cells [2–4,7]. This application of tissue engineering to reproductive biology provides an enabling technology to maintain follicular architecture while presenting a combination of diffusible, insoluble, and mechanical signals, which combine to influence the development of the follicle. Immature mouse follicles can be cultured to produce mature oocytes that fertilize at rates similar to in vivo matured eggs, and transferred embryos are viable, with healthy male and female in vitro-derived offspring that retain fertility [2,3,7]. These results demonstrate the efficacy of three-dimensional culture that may provide a core technology to support the creation of human egg banks.

Hydrogels for Three-Dimensional Culture In Vitro

Hydrogel encapsulation of a follicle maintains the communication between the cellular compartments by preserving the cell–cell interactions and paracrine signaling through secreted diffusible factors. Hydrogels are composed of hydrophilic polymers, either natural (e.g., collagen) or synthetic (e.g., alginate, polyethylene glycol [PEG]), that can self-assemble or be crosslinked into three-dimensional structures. Follicles are suspended within the hydrophilic solution (e.g., 0.2–5%) and are entrapped upon gelation. Alginate, in particular, has been employed for follicle culture as it undergoes gelation under mild conditions (50 mM Ca^{2+}) that do not adversely affect cell viability or function [40]. Alginate, a polysaccharide isolated from algae, supports limited protein adsorption and thus provides minimal cellular interactions, evidenced by the minimal adhesion of mammalian cells on alginate hydrogels. For follicle culture, alginate primarily provides a physical support to maintain the three-dimensional architecture of the follicle (Fig. 6.3). However, the carboxylic acid functional groups on the polysaccharide can be modified to attach functional chemical moieties, such as cell adhesion peptides or proteins. These cell adhesion proteins or peptides can be attached at controlled densities to interact with the follicle and stimulate growth or differentiated cell function, while retaining follicle architecture [3].

An important aspect of the hydrogel culture system for follicle maturation is the mechanical properties and stability of the hydrogel itself [6,41]. The hydrogel must provide a support to retain the follicle's three-dimensional architecture, yet it must not restrict follicle growth (Fig. 6.3). The mechanical properties of the hydrogel can be regulated through properties such as the percentage of polymer,

Fig. 6.3 The three-dimensional follicular architecture is maintained by the supporting hydrogel (*blue*), yet must allow expansion (*red*)

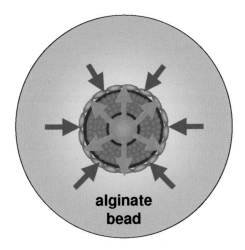

extent of crosslinking, and polymer molecular weight [42]. We have published reports indicating that these factors influence follicle growth and maturation and oocyte quality. In addition, hydrogel mechanical properties may influence follicle access to macromolecules contained in the culture media necessary for follicle growth as well as access to factors produced and secreted by the follicle [43]. As follicles from larger species are cultured, hydrogels will need to be developed that can accommodate the increases in diameter and longer culture times. For example, alginate is not degraded by mammalian cells and thus the follicle can expand against the alginate. Long culture periods or extensive changes in follicle size could require that the alginate be removed and replaced, which would require additional handling of the follicle. An alternative approach involves the incorporation of components within the hydrogel that degrade in response to cell-secreted enzymes, which would create space as the follicle develops. The quantity of degradable and non-degradable components must be balanced to support follicle growth with retention of the three-dimensional architecture of the follicle [41,42].

Ovarian Transplantation Using Biomaterials

The hydrogels developed for in vitro follicle growth may be adapted to support the strategy of ovarian transplantation by providing factors that enhance engraftment of the transplanted tissue. The transplanted tissue requires a vascular supply to provide the necessary nutrients and waste removal, along with the necessary endocrine stimulation. Though this research has not yet been performed, several design issues are evident based on research with other tissues. First, the hydrogels must support cellular infiltration, which will allow blood vessels to provide the necessary nutrients. Many hydrogels derived from mammalian tissues (e.g., collagen) support robust cellular ingrowth in vivo; however, polymers such as alginate that lack specific cellular interactions and do not support cell adhesion may not [44]. Nevertheless, these hydrogels could be modified with peptides or proteins that support cellular interactions and cellular infiltration [44]. Additionally, hydrogels will be employed as vehicles for localized protein delivery to enhance cellular and vascular ingrowth. Protein growth factors can be added to solutions of the hydrophilic polymer prior to gelation. Entrapped factors are soluble within the hydrated gel and can diffuse through the pores and into the surrounding tissue [45]. The diffusivity through the gel may be controlled by the extent of crosslinking and the degradation rate of the hydrogel, which determines the average pore size. Typical times for release by diffusion from these hydrogels can range from days to weeks [46].

Conclusion

The merging of tissue engineering principles and reproductive biology offers novel interdisciplinary opportunities in oncofertility. With regard to the in vitro growth and maturation approach, the ovarian follicle is unlike other tissues in that it does not require vascularization, as nutrients and waste products are transported by diffusion. Thus, the development of an in vitro culture system is limited only by the ability to present the appropriate combination of stimuli (e.g., diffusible, insoluble, and mechanical) during maturation. In addition to the follicle having uncommon properties, the industry surrounding fertility preservation is unique. Few cell therapies for preserving fertility are currently available, with in vitro fertilization among the most common techniques used. Thus, the development and application of an in vitro follicle culture system would provide immediate clinical opportunities for patients. Although in vivo transplantation techniques have been successfully applied to produce pregnancies in two women, a significant challenge lies ahead in enhancing engraftment and survival of the transplanted tissue.

References

1. Langer R, Tirell DA. Designing materials for biology and medicine. Nature 2004; 428:487–492.
2. Kreeger PK, Fernandes NN, Woodruff TK, et al. Regulation of mouse follicle development by follicle-stimulating hormone in a three-dimensional *in vitro* culture system is dependent on follicle stage and dose. Biol Reprod 2005;73:942–950.
3. Kreeger PK, Deck JW, Woodruff TK, et al. The in vitro regulation of ovarian follicle development using alginate-extracellular matrix gels. Biomaterials 2006;27:714–723.
4. Pangas SA, Saudye H, Shea LD, et al. Novel approach for the three-dimensional culture of granulosa cell-oocyte complexes. Tissue Eng 2003;9:1013–1021.
5. West ER, Shea LD, Woodruff TK. Engineering the follicle microenvironment. Semin Reprod Med. 2007;25(4):287–299.
6. Xu M, West E, Shea LD, et al. Identification of a stage-specific permissive in vitro culture environment for follicle growth and oocyte development. Biol Reprod 2006;75:916–923.

7. Xu M, Kreeger PK, Shea LD, et al. Tissue-engineered follicles produce live, fertile offspring. Tissue Eng 2006;12:2739–2746.
8. Jang JH, Rives CB, Shea LD. Plasmid delivery in vivo from porous tissue-engineering scaffolds: transgene expression and cellular transfection. Mol Ther 2005;12:475–483.
9. Sheridan MH, Shea LD, Peters MC, et al. Bioabsorbable polymer scaffolds for tissue engineering capable of sustained growth factor delivery. J Control Release. 2000;64:91–102.
10. Salha O, Abusheikha N, Sharma V. Dynamics of human follicular growth and in-vitro oocyte maturation. Hum Reprod Update 1998;4:816–832.
11. Eppig JJ, O'Brien M, Wigglesworth K. Mammalian oocyte growth and development in vitro. Mol Reprod Dev 1996;44:260–273.
12. Gosden R, Krapez J, Briggs D. Growth and development of the mammalian oocyte. Bioessays 1997;19:875–882.
13. Thomas FH, Walters KA, Telfer EE. How to make a good oocyte: an update on in-vitro models to study follicle regulation. Hum Reprod Update 2003;9:541–555.
14. Demeestere I, Centner J, Gervy C, et al. Impact of various endocrine and paracrine factors on in vitro culture of preantral follicles in rodents. Reproduction 2005;130:147–156.
15. Juneja SC, Barr KJ, Enders GC, et al. Defects in the germ line and gonads of mice lacking connexin43. Biol Reprod 1999;60:1263–1270.
16. Herlands RL, Schultz RM. Regulation of mouse oocyte growth: probable nutritional role for intercellular communication between follicle cells and oocytes in oocyte growth. J Exp Zool 1984;229:317–325.
17. Spears N, Boland NI, Murray AA, et al. Mouse oocytes derived from in vitro grown primary ovarian follicles are fertile. Hum Reprod 1994;9:527–532.
18. Eppig JJ, Schroeder AC. Capacity of mouse oocytes from preantral follicles to undergo embryogenesis and development to live young after growth, maturation, and fertilization in vitro. Biol Reprod 1989;41:268–276.
19. Cortvrindt RG, Hu Y, Liu J, et al. Timed analysis of the nuclear maturation of oocytes in early preantral mouse follicle culture supplemented with recombinant gonadotropin. Fertil Steril 1998;70:1114–1125.
20. Eppig JJ, O'Brien MJ. Development in vitro of mouse oocytes from primordial follicles. Biol Reprod 1996;54:197–207.
21. dela Pena EC, Takahashi Y, Katagiri S, et al. Birth of pups after transfer of mouse embryos derived from vitrified preantral follicles. Reproduction 2002;123:593–600.
22. Liu J, Van der Elst J, Van den Broecke R, et al. Live offspring by in vitro fertilization of oocytes from cryopreserved primordial mouse follicles after sequential in vivo transplantation and in vitro maturation. Biol Reprod 2001;64:171–178.
23. Donnez J, Dolmans MM, Demylle D, et al. Restoration of ovarian function after orthotopic (intraovarian and periovarian) transplantation of cryopreserved ovarian tissue in a woman treated by bone marrow transplantation for sickle cell anaemia: case report. Hum Reprod 2006;21:183–188.
24. Meirow D, Levron J, Eldar-Geva T, et al. Pregnancy after transplantation of cryopreserved ovarian tissue in a patient with ovarian failure after chemotherapy. N Engl J Med 2005;353:318–321.
25. Silber SJ, Lenahan KM, Levine DJ, et al. Ovarian transplantation between monozygotic twins discordant for premature ovarian failure. N Engl J Med 2005;353:58–63.
26. O'Brien MJ, Pendola JK, Eppig JJ. A revised protocol for in vitro development of mouse oocytes from primordial follicles dramatically improves their developmental competence. Biol Reprod 2003;68:1682–1686.
27. Lenie S, Cortvrindt R, Adriaenssens T, et al. A reproducible two-step culture system for isolated primary mouse ovarian follicles as single functional units. Biol Reprod 2004;71:1730–1738.
28. Cortvrindt R, Smitz J, Van Steirteghem AC. In-vitro maturation, fertilization and embryo development of immature oocytes from early preantral follicles from prepuberal mice in a simplified culture system. Hum Reprod 1996;11:2656–2666.
29. Cortvrindt RG, Smitz JE. Follicle culture in reproductive toxicology: a tool for in-vitro testing of ovarian function? Hum Reprod Update 2002;8:243–254.

30. Gutierrez CG, Ralph JH, Telfer EE, et al. Growth and antrum formation of bovine preantral follicles in long-term culture in vitro. Biol Reprod 2000;62:1322–1328.
31. Tambe SS, Nandedkar TD. Steroidogenesis in sheep ovarian antral follicles in culture: time course study and supplementation with a precursor. Steroids 1993;58:379–383.
32. Abir R, Franks S, Mobberley MA, et al. Mechanical isolation and in vitro growth of preantral and small antral human follicles. Fertil Steril 1997;68:682–688.
33. Roy SK, Treacy BJ. Isolation and long-term culture of human preantral follicles. Fertil Steril 1993;59:783–790.
34. Nayudu PL, Osborn SM. Factors influencing the rate of preantral and antral growth of mouse ovarian follicles in vitro. J Reprod Fertil 1992;95:349–362.
35. Wycherley G, Downey D, Kane MT, et al. A novel follicle culture system markedly increases follicle volume, cell number and oestradiol secretion. Reproduction 2004;127:669–677.
36. Fehrenbach A, Nusse N, Nayudu PL. Patterns of growth, oestradiol and progesterone released by in vitro cultured mouse ovarian follicles indicate consecutive selective events during follicle development. J Reprod Fertil 1998;113:287–297.
37. Boland NI, Gosden RG. Effects of epidermal growth factor on the growth and differentiation of cultured mouse ovarian follicles. J Reprod Fertil 1994;101:369–374.
38. Hartshorne GM, Sargent IL, Barlow DH. Meiotic progression of mouse oocytes throughout follicle growth and ovulation in vitro. Hum Reprod 1994;9:352–359.
39. Rowghani NM, Heise MK, McKeel D, et al. Maintenance of morphology and growth of ovarian follicles in suspension culture. Tissue Eng 2004;10:545–552.
40. Kong HJ, Smith MK, Mooney DJ. Designing alginate hydrogels to maintain viability of immobilized cells. Biomaterials 2003;24:4023–4029.
41. West E, Woodruff TK, Shea LD. Oxidized and irradiated alginate for the culture of ovarian follicles. [submitted].
42. Anseth KS, Bowman CN, Brannon-Peppas L. Mechanical properties of hydrogels and their experimental determination. Biomaterials 1996;17:1647–1657.
43. Heise M, Koepsel R, Russell AJ, et al. Calcium alginate microencapsulation of ovarian follicles impacts FSH delivery and follicle morphology. Reprod Biol Endocrinol 2005;3:47.
44. Marler JJ, Guha A, Rowley J, et al. Soft-tissue augmentation with injectable alginate and syngeneic fibroblasts. Plast Reconstr Surg 2000;105:2049–2058.
45. Davis KA, Anseth KS. Controlled release from crosslinked degradable networks. Crit Rev Ther Drug Carrier Syst 2002;19:385–423.
46. Burdick JA, Mason MN, Hinman AD, et al. Delivery of osteoinductive growth factors from degradable PEG hydrogels influences osteoblast differentiation and mineralization. J Control Release 2002;83:53–63.

Chapter 7
The Science of Cryobiology

Steven F. Mullen, PhD and John K. Critser, PhD

Introduction

The demand for effective bio-preservation methods in the medical community continues to increase with advances in transplantation and transfusion medicine [1]. In reproductive medicine, pre-implantation embryo cryopreservation has become an integral component of overall patient care, increasing the success rate per oocyte retrieval cycle [2,3]. Oocyte cryopreservation is becoming increasingly important due to legal restrictions on the creation and transplantation of supernumerary pre-implantation embryos as well as ethical considerations surrounding the cryopreservation of pre-implantation embryos [4,5].

Early investigations into the effects of sub-physiologic temperatures on living cells have been reviewed in great detail [6]. The current chapter will attempt to provide a broad overview of cryobiology, and refer to the reproductive biology literature when appropriate. Readers interested in learning more details are directed at several excellent texts and reviews on the various subjects [7–20].

Anatomy of Cryopreservation

Cryopreservation is the successful preservation of the normal function of cells or tissues by a reduction in temperature below which biochemical reactions take place. It is not the long-term storage of cells at these temperatures that is damaging, but the progression to these temperatures and back to normothermia that results in cryoinjury. Cryopreservation nearly always entails the use of one or more compounds that confer protection to cells during freezing. These so-called cryoprotectants are typically very simple, low molecular weight molecules with high water solubility and low toxicity. One feature that is common among these compounds is their ability to interact with water via hydrogen bonding [21]. Application of cryoprotectants is done (in most cases) simply by incubating the cells in solutions into which these compounds have been dissolved. After this exposure, the cells are cooled to a low sub-zero temperature (specimens are typically held at the temperature

T.K. Woodruff and K.A. Snyder (eds.) *Oncofertility*.
© Springer 2007

of liquid nitrogen; −196°C). At the appropriate time, the specimen is warmed, washed free of the cryoprotectants, and used in whatever manner is deemed appropriate. While this seems like a relatively straightforward procedure, many types of injuries can result from any one of the steps; thus numerous lethal effects need to be avoided.

The Effects of Water Precipitation (as Ice) During Cooling

Ice Nucleation, Crystallization, Vitrification, and Devitrification

Figure 7.1 shows a supplemented phase diagram for a generic aqueous solution. The physical transitions of water in solution which occur as a result of cooling and warming are described with such a diagram. The temperature at which these transitions occur depends upon the concentration of solutes in the solution. The curve

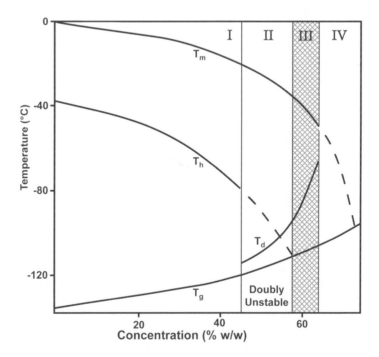

Fig. 7.1 A phase diagram for a hypothetical solution is shown. The concentration and temperature dependent physical transitions, including melting (T_m), homogenous nucleation (T_h), glass formation (T_g), and devitrification (T_d), are described by the respective curves. The use of such diagrams allows the calculation of variables which are important considerations for freezing injury [22]. Reprinted from Fahy et al. (1984) [7] with permission from Elsevier. See text for further details

labeled T_m describes the melting temperature of the solution (which is also the equilibrium freezing temperature). The dashed extensions of the curves represent extrapolations across hypothetical boundaries. As the solute concentration of the solution increases (moving along the X-axis from left to right), the melting temperature of the solution decreases. This is a well known result of the colligative effects of the solutes.

The curve labeled T_h characterizes the homogenous nucleation temperature. Homogenous nucleation is defined as the nucleation of ice crystals in the absence of nucleating agents. Aqueous solutions will usually crystallize at temperatures much higher than this due to impurities which act as effective ice nucleators. A solution containing pure water (i.e., free of heterogeneous nucleators) will remain liquid down to ~−39°C, at which point the entire solution will crystallize (the point where T_h intersects the Y-axis). The homogenous nucleation temperature decreases with increasing concentration of solutes.

The reason why water can remain liquid below its melting point is because the creation of a crystal entails the creation of a liquid–crystal interface with an associated interfacial free energy. The size of a thermodynamically-stable crystal (i.e., one that will continue to grow by the addition of water molecules) is dependent upon temperature (smaller crystals are more stable at lower temperatures). So as the temperature is lowered, the probability of formation of a stable crystal increases until T_h, where the probability is 1.

The curve labeled T_g represents the glass transition temperature. At this temperature, liquid solutions will transition to a stable glass (vitrify) and remain vitreous upon further cooling.

In region I of this chart (solutions with concentrations <= ~45 wt% (weight/weight) in this example), achieving true vitrification is nearly impossible. Nucleation (both homogenous and heterogeneous) is essentially unavoidable (at least with practical cooling rates). In region II, the difference between the T_h and T_g curves is small enough that vitrification can be achieved with practical cooling rates. However, a solution which does attain a vitreous state in this region is thermodynamically unstable. In the regions marked III and IV, vitrification is easily achievable. Notice that the T_h curve actually intersects T_g at the transition between regions II and III. Heterogeneous ice formation will not occur at temperatures below the glass-transition temperature.

If a sample with a composition described by regions II and III is cooled fast enough to vitrify, ice may still form during warming due to nucleation. The temperature at which this happens is described by T_d, the devitrification temperature. Essentially, between T_g and T_m, a solution free of ice is in a metastable state. Above T_g during warming, the solution is no longer a glass (the glass "melts" to form an unfrozen liquid with the molecules having translational mobility), and nucleation and ice growth can occur. Ice formation and crystal growth during warming is more likely than during cooling, all else being equal.

Why is this so? Consider the following two facts: (1) The probability of ice nucleation increases as temperature decreases (notice that as temperature decreases, the sample will get closer to T_h; (2) crystal growth, however, being a kinetic phenomenon, will be faster at higher temperatures. Now, imagine the following scenario. A sample with solutes at a concentration of 40% (w/w) is cooled very quickly so that nucleation occurs only at the temperature around T_h ($\sim$$-70°C$). However, at $-70°C$, ice crystal growth is very slow (at least relative to higher temperatures). Thus, crystal growth from the nucleation sites will be slow, especially considering that cooling is still taking place. However, during warming, once the sample gets above T_g ($\sim$$-120°C$), ice crystals can grow from the nucleation sites. However, it will still be slow at low temperatures, but the rate will increase as the sample warms. Because there were no ice nuclei above $-70°C$ during cooling in this example, ice growth at higher temperatures could not happen. However, ice nuclei are present during warming and crystal growth can occur until T_m. Therefore, if nucleation does occur during cooling, warming must be very fast to avoid crystal growth at temperatures below T_m. The striking differences between the critical cooling rate (defined as the cooling rate necessary to achieve vitrification) and the critical warming rate (defined as the warming rate necessary to avoid more than 0.2% crystallization during warming) are illustrated by the analysis of Baudot and Odagescu [23]. According to their calculations, for a 40% (w/w) solution of ethylene glycol in water, the critical cooling rate is 569°C/min, but the critical warming rate is $1.08 \times 10^{10}°C/min$.

Solute Concentration as a Result of Ice Crystallization, The Associated Osmotic Effects, and Cell Death at Supra-Optimal Cooling Rates

As ice forms during cooling, only water molecules comprise the ice crystals. As a result, all other components (salts, etc.) become concentrated in the remaining solution. As the solution concentration increases, the chemical potential of the water in the solution decreases. Water will continue to crystallize until the chemical potential of the water in the liquid phase equals the chemical potential of the water in the solid phase. In other words, the remaining solution will reach its equilibrium freezing point (the curve defined by T_m). Therefore, the concentration of the remaining liquid phase can also be determined from a phase diagram.

For example, assume that Fig. 7.1 represents the phase diagram of a sodium chloride–water binary solution. If you start with an isotonic saline solution (0.9 wt%) and cool it to $-20°C$, ice will form until the remaining solution is at its equilibrium freezing point. In this example, the remaining solution will attain a concentration of $\sim$45 wt% (note the point where the T_m curve reaches $-20°C$). In this hypothetical example, the unfrozen solution would be roughly 14 mol/L sodium chloride (compared to 0.15 mol/L initially). In reality, sodium chloride will only concentrate to $\sim$4 mol/L at $-20°C$ (the phase diagram for sodium chloride is markedly different than the one shown in Fig. 7.1).

When cells are frozen in suspension, the cells are sequestered in channels of concentrated unfrozen medium. The high concentration of this unfrozen solution establishes an osmotic gradient across the cell membrane, and as a result, water will flow out of the cell via exosmosis. Below a cell's equilibrium freezing point, the cytoplasm is in a supercooled state. If the sample is cooled slowly enough, exosmosis occurs to a sufficient degree to keep the cells in a near-equilibrium state with the extracellular solution. Such a situation will preclude intracellular ice formation. On the other hand, if the cooling rate is relatively rapid, water cannot leave the cell fast enough to maintain a near-equilibrium state with the extracellular solution, and at some point equilibrium will be re-established by intracellular ice formation (see Fig. 7.2).

This situation is described schematically in Fig. 7.3. The formation of intracellular ice is usually (but not necessarily) fatal to cells (see below for more details). Direct cryomicroscopic observation of intracellular ice formation in mouse oocytes (similar to that which is seen in Fig. 7.2) and the correlation to cell survival were some of the most convincing data to support the assertion that ice formation was the lethal cause of cell death at supra-optimal cooling rates [24,25].

The rate at which water flows out of a cell is dictated by the cell membrane water permeability. The permeability of cells to water is dependent upon several factors including temperature and the presence of cryoprotectants. For example, in the absence of cryoprotectant, human sperm water permeability is 1.84 μm/min/atm at 22°C, but is reduced to 1.23, 0.84, 0.77 and 0.74 μm/min/atm in the presence of propylene glycol, dimethylsulfoxide, glycerol, and ethylene glycol, respectively [26]. Furthermore, water permeability can vary greatly across cell types. For example, water permeability for human erythrocytes [27] is an order of magnitude higher than the value for human oocytes [28]. Because intracellular ice formation is

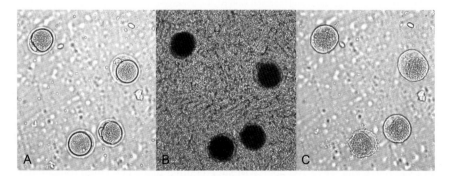

Fig. 7.2 Photomicrographs of intracellular ice formation in mouse oocytes cooled at 100 °C/min in an isotonic solution is shown. In Panel A, intact oocytes are shown prior to ice crystal formation; note the well-defined oolemma within the zona pellucida. As cooling proceeds, ice forms in the extracellular solution and eventually, the intracellular solution. The darker background in Panel B is due to ice, and the "blackening" of the oocytes indicates that intracellular ice formation has occurred. When the solution is warmed and the ice melts (Panel C), the cell membrane within the zona pellucida is no longer visible, indicating cell lysis. The speckled appearance of the background in Panels A and C is due to atmospheric water precipitation on the cold glass surface of the cell chamber, and not due to ice crystals

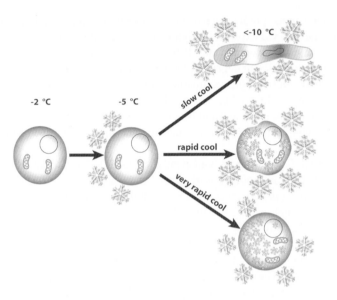

Fig.7.3 The cooling-rate-dependent fate of intracellular water resulting from extracellular ice formation is shown. As the temperature of the solution is cooled below the equilibrium freezing point, ice will form in the extracellular solution. As a result, water is driven out of the cell by an osmotic gradient across the cell membrane. If cooling is slow (upper cell, right side), sufficient water leaves the cell and intracellular ice formation does not occur. If the cooling rate is faster, ice will form inside the cell, and the amount of ice that forms and the size of the crystals will depend upon the cooling rate. Intermediate cooling rates (middle cell, right side) result in partial cell dehydration, larger crystals, and less intracellular ice. Very rapid cooling rates result in virtually no cell dehydration, a greater amount of ice formation, but smaller crystals. If cells are cooled very quickly (lower cell, right side) and warmed slowly, the average crystal size will increase (smaller crystals will tend to melt and larger crystals will tend to grow; a process known as recrystallization). This will be more damaging to the cell compared to very rapid warming. Figure adapted from Mazur, 1977 [29] with permission from Elsevier

dependent upon the degree of supercooling (hence the water content), the rate of cooling which results in intracellular ice formation differs widely across cell types. The theory of cell death due to intracellular ice formation resulting from the interaction of cooling rate and water loss outlined above was developed quantitatively by Peter Mazur [30] (see Mazur [19] for a recent review). The practical benefit of this theory comes from its potential to predict optimal cryopreservation procedures. For example, if one knew the degree of supercooling that a cell could tolerate during cooling and the membrane permeability, it would be possible to predict the cooling rate which would prevent intracellular ice formation and the temperature at which cooling could stop and the sample could safely be transferred to liquid nitrogen [31]. See the original description of mammalian embryo cryopreservation for a relevant example [32].

Ice formation in the cytoplasm of cells is not necessarily damaging. Studies over the years have investigated the correlation between the morphology of cytoplasmic ice, cooling and warming rates, and survival [33,34]. Results from such studies have shown that larger ice crystal size correlated positively with cell damage. As discussed above for bulk solutions, devitrification and re-crystallization can occur to cell water/ice during warming [35] resulting in the growth of large ice crystals [34]. Re-crystallization is the phenomenon whereby large ice crystals grow at the expense of small ice crystals due to the greater stability of large crystals at a given temperature. According to a more recent study, the formation of small ice crystals may actually be beneficial to cell survival [36]. Such a result is likely due to the reduced level of cell dehydration when water is trapped inside the cell in small ice crystals and the reduced level of osmotic stress and associated water flux during warming. However, the warming needs to be fast enough under such circumstances to avoid re-crystallization as just discussed.

Attempts have been made to explain the mechanism(s) which cause intracellular ice formation, and to date several theories have been put fourth. As explained in more detail by Mazur [19], theories of intracellular ice formation must account for several experimental facts: (1) in order for ice formation to occur in cells above $\sim-30°C$, extracellular ice must be present, and the proximity of the cells and ice is important; (2) extracellular ice is not a necessary precondition for intracellular ice below $\sim-30°C$; (3) intracellular ice formation usually happens immediately if the cells and the surroundings are supercooled -15 to $-20°C$ and extracellular ice is rapidly initiated; (4) if extracellular ice forms near the cell's equilibrium freezing point, intracellular ice usually does not form at slow cooling rates; and (5) the nucleation temperature decreases substantially if the extracellular solute concentration increases.

Several lines of evidence suggest that intracellular ice formation can be triggered by more than one mechanism. It is generally agreed that ice formation below $\sim-30°C$ in the absence of extracellular ice is due to the presence of intracellular nucleators (or as a result of homogenous nucleation at lower temperatures). The fact that intracellular ice formation above this temperature requires the presence of extracellular ice strongly suggests that the extracellular ice is acting to nucleate the intracellular ice. As extracellular ice does not nucleate intracellular ice at low degrees of supercooling, an intact plasma membrane effectively blocks the passage of ice into the cell. However, the plasma membrane is implicated mechanistically in the major theories put fourth to explain the initiation of intracellular ice formation above $\sim-30°C$.

Mazur [37] hypothesized that ice crystals can grow through membranes via protein pores like aquaporins. While evidence exists that ice can grow through channels which connect cells (i.e., gap junctions [38–40]), the pore size in these channels is much larger than those in aquaporins, making ice growth more likely. Mazur and colleagues are currently using genetic engineering techniques in oocytes as a means to test this hypothesis directly (see [41–43] for results from initial experiments). Toner and colleagues [44,45] have suggested that ice interaction with the plasma membrane causes a structural change to the inner membrane surface, resulting in an increase in the efficiency of ice nucleation. Muldrew and McGann [46,47] have put fourth a different mechanism altogether which suggests that ice grows through the membrane after the formation of a lesion as a result of the osmotic pressure gradient and resultant water efflux. A similar argument regarding

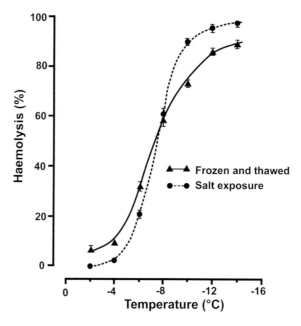

Fig. 7.5 The correlation between hemolysis and salt concentration for cells frozen or only exposed to salt is shown. The striking correlation lead Lovelock [54,57] to conclude that the concentration of salt resulting from ice formation was a primary mechanism of cryodamage. Others have argued that the effect of the salt concentration on cell volume was the true cause of cell damage [60]. Figure reproduced from Pegg 1987 [55] with permission from The Company of Biologists. See text for more details

   Cryoprotectants have also been shown to either directly interact with or be preferentially excluded from biosurfaces (e.g., the surface of lipid bilayers or proteins) [61–64]. The apparent opposite nature of these modes of interaction seems to suggest opposite effects. However, each mode of interaction can be beneficial to the stability of these structures. In addition, Rudolph and Crowe [65] have shown that trehalose and proline can prevent freezing-induced fusion of lipid vesicles. For more details on these mechanisms, interested readers are directed to recent reviews [53,66–68] and references therein.

   Perhaps it is not surprising that many organisms living in climates where freezing temperatures are encountered have evolved to include the metabolic production of cryoprotectants as a survival strategy. As discussed by Erica Benson [69] and reviewed by Ken Diller [70], the cryoprotective properties of sugars and glycerol in plants were described by Nikolay Maximov in the early 20th century (following on the work of others). The farsighted nature of his conclusions is remarkable considering what has been learned about cryoprotectants and their mechanisms since that time.

   A great deal of research has been conducted to understand the response of various members of the animal kingdom to freezing temperatures. The metabolic production of cryoprotectants is also a common strategy in these organisms. Inhibition of freezing at high sub-zero temperatures is one strategy among arthropods and fish,

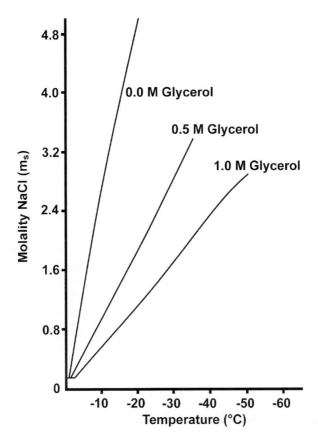

Fig. 7.6 The presence of cryoprotectants reduces the salt concentration at a given sub-zero temperature due to a colligative reduction in the freezing point of the solution (shown here for a glycerol and sodium chloride solution mixture). Notice that, as the concentration of glycerol increases, the salt concentration is significantly reduced. Figure reprinted from [71] with permission from The Biophysical Society

and is accomplished by regulative supercooling. In many instances the freezing point of physiological solutions is regulated by thermal hysteresis proteins [72]. The tertiary structure of these proteins allows them to directly interact with ice crystals due to polar residues along the protein backbone [73]. These proteins lower the freezing point of water without significantly altering the melting point. Thus, their mode of action is not colligative. According to a general model for their activity, these proteins bind to ice crystals and alter the radius of curvature of the growing crystal, which reduces the temperature at which it is thermodynamically favorable for additional water molecules to join the crystalline phase [74,75] (see Raymond et al. [76] for more detail on an early model of the mechanism of fish hysteresis proteins, and Kristiansen et al. [77] for a recent review on the mechanism of action). Overall, these proteins restrict ice growth when the environmental temperature is slightly below the equilibrium freezing temperature of the body fluids.

As an alternate strategy, organisms across many phylogenetic groups have developed mechanisms of regulating ice formation in situ. In naturally freeze-tolerant organisms, avoiding the formation of intracellular ice is managed by actively promoting and regulating the formation of extracellular ice. This allows freeze-induced dehydration of the cells and prevents ice from forming in the cytoplasm. As a coupled strategy, mechanisms to avoid the damaging consequences of cellular dehydration and ischemia that accompany freezing have also evolved.

Ken and Janet Storey, in a recent review on the subject [78], described four requirements for the successful freeze tolerance in animals: (1) ice must be confined to extracellular spaces and damage from ice crystals must be minimized; (2) the rate of freezing must be slow and controlled; (3) cell volume reduction beyond a minimum tolerable volume must be avoided; and (4) mechanisms must be present to prevent damage from resulting ischemia. These requirements are often met through both behavioral and physiological adaptations. For example, slow, controlled temperature change is often facilitated by the chosen hybernaculum of the organisms. Controlled ice nucleation can be performed by specific ice nucleating proteins in the blood [79,80]. Cryoprotectant synthesis (e.g., glucose production) in some organisms is initiated by freezing [81] (see the review by Storey and Storey [82] for more details). Membrane adaptations to cold have also been described [83]. As improved cryopreservation methods are sought, it is likely that attention paid to nature's laboratory will provide insights into appropriate means to avoid cryodamage.

Cryoprotectants: Detrimental Effects

As their name implies, cryoprotectants are beneficial during freezing. Their use, however, is not necessarily benign. Since the time of Lovelock's original work, it has been pointed out [84] and experimentally confirmed [55] that the correlation between the freezing damage in the presence of glycerol and the associated increase in salt concentration is strongest at low levels of hemolysis. In addition, as the concentration of glycerol is increased, the concentration of salt that causes a given degree of hemolysis decreases, suggesting that high concentrations of glycerol contribute to cell damage during freezing (Fig. 7.7). This suggests that high glycerol concentrations (particularly as a result of ice precipitation) contribute to the damage of cells frozen slowly. Similar results have also been shown for dimethylsulfoxide [85,86].

Injury from cryoprotectants is not limited to those which occur during freezing. Exposing cells to solutions containing cryoprotectants prior to cooling can be damaging due to an osmotic effect. Many of the commonly used permeating cryoprotectants have lower plasma membrane permeability coefficients compared to that of water. This relationship results in cells experiencing osmotically driven volume excursions during cryoprotectant addition to and removal from the cell during the

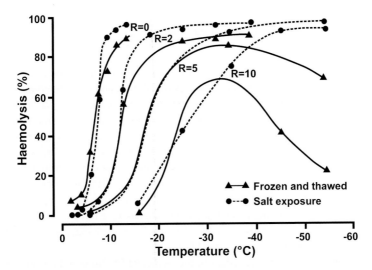

Fig. 7.7 The correlation between hemolysis and salt concentration is greatest at low levels of cell damage. As the ratio of glycerol to sodium chloride (R) increases, the correlation becomes weaker, particularly at high levels of hemolysis. Figure reproduced from Pegg 1987 [55] with permission from The Company of Biologists

course of a cryopreservation procedure. It has been shown in numerous cell types that damage to cells can occur as a result from volume excursions alone [87–106]. Furthermore, many studies have demonstrated a beneficial effect of prolonging the cryoprotectant addition and/or removal process which reduces the associated volume excursions [107–109].

The rate of water movement across the plasma membrane is determined by several factors and can be described by (7.1):

$$\frac{dV_w}{dt} = -L_p A R T \left(M_s^e + M_n^e - \frac{n_s^i}{V_w} - \frac{n_n^i}{V_w} \right)$$ (7.1)

where dV_w/dt represents the change in the cell water volume over time, L_p and A represent the cell membrane hydraulic conductivity and surface area, respectively, R and T represent the gas constant and temperature, M represents molal concentration, n represents the number of moles of solute (collectively, the terms in parentheses represent the concentration gradient across the cell membrane). The letters e, i, s, and n in the super- and subscripts represent the extra- and intracellular compartments, and permeating (s) and non-permeating (n) solutes respectively.

A concentration gradient of permeating cryoprotectants will also result in movement of these compounds across the cell membrane. The rate of change in intracellular cryoprotectant resulting from such a gradient can also be described by an ordinary differential equation (7.2):

$$\frac{dn_s^i}{dt} = P_s A \left(M_s^e - \frac{n_s^t}{V_w} \right)$$
(7.2)

where dn_s^i/dt represents the change in the number of moles of intracellular cryoprotectant over time, P_s represents the membrane permeability, and the remaining variables are equivalent to those in (1). Here we have shown the so-called two-parameter membrane transport model (L_p and P_s are the phenomenological parameters defining the permeability of the cell membrane to water and cryoprotectant). A three-parameter model incorporating an interaction coefficient (σ) was proposed on the basis of irreversible thermodynamics for membranes where water and solute move through a common pathway [110]. It has been argued that the interaction coefficient is not applicable to biological membranes as water and cryoprotectants usually travel through independent pathways. Furthermore, being phenomenological in nature, a three-parameter model is less parsimonious than a two-parameter model. Interested readers can find more details on this debate in a recent review [111].

Osmotic damage is often ascribed to the associated volume reductions [60, 93]. Cell volume response can be controlled during cryoprotectant addition and removal by modifying the procedures for loading and unloading these compounds [112]. As a result, cryoprotectant addition and removal can be accomplished in a manner that prevents injury due to excessive volume excursions. Because the volume response of cells can be modeled on a computer when the parameters in (1) and (2) for the cells are known, one can proactively predict optimal methods for this process (see Gao et al. [26] for a more thorough discussion).

True chemical toxicity is also a concern associated with the use of cryoprotectants [51,113]. This is particularly true for vitrification methods (see below) as very high concentrations of these compounds are necessary to achieve and maintain a vitreous state at practical cooling rates. The precise nature of the toxic effects of cryoprotectants remains, to a large degree, uncertain. Fahy and colleagues have concluded that protein denaturation is not a general effect of cryoprotectants [114]. They offered an argument that effects on membranes could provide an alternate explanation to a direct effect on proteins that would be consistent with some data and proposed models. Cryoprotectants have been shown to alter cytoskeletal components in mammalian oocytes, particularly the filamentous actin network and meiotic spindle [115–117]. Re-polymerization after treatments is common, but the particular organization of the polymers often does not resemble those of untreated oocytes. Frequently, toxicity is argued to be a significant cause of cell death in oocyte cryopreservation studies. However, rarely is the chemical effect isolated from the osmotic effect in such experiments. In a previously unpublished experiment in our laboratory, the osmotic effects associated with exposure to 2.5 mol/L 1,2-propanediol and ethylene glycol were controlled when assessing the effects of exposing mouse oocytes to these cryoprotectants by including a treatment simulating the volume excursions associated with cryoprotectant addition and removal. The results suggested that the damage associated from exposure to 1,2-propanediol was not a result of the osmotic effects, but a true chemical effect. Exposure to the same concentration of ethylene glycol was not detrimental to mouse oocyte survival (Fig. 7.8).

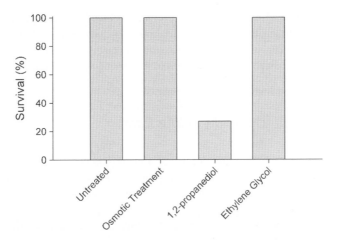

Fig. 7.8 The effect on cell viability of exposing mouse oocytes to 1,2-propanediol or ethylene glycol (2.5 M final with 0.3M sucrose) is shown. A solution containing 0.5 M sucrose which simulates the osmotically-driven volume excursions of the other treatments was included as a control. Neither osmotic stress or ethylene glycol exposure had an effect on oocyte viability after a 6-h incubation. Exposure to 1,2-propanediol resulted in a dramatic loss in cell viability (cell lysis)

It was mentioned earlier that most cryoprotectants have hydrogen bonding capability, and altering water structure is one of the mechanisms by which cryoprotectants are hypothesized to function. It is also recognized that the toxic concentration differs for different cryoprotectants. In a more recent report [118], Fahy and colleagues have determined that a compositional variable they call qv^* is directly associated with the toxic properties of a cryoprotectant when toxicity is non-specific. The proposal these authors make is that qv^* is related to the degree of hydration of a cryoprotectant. In their report, Fahy et al. show that the total concentration of cryoprotectants was not as strong of a predictor of toxicity as was the ratio of the molarity of water (M_W) in the solution to the molarity of polar groups in the solution (M_{PG}; i.e., $qv^* = M_W/M_{PG}$). Polar groups were defined as hydroxyl groups (−OH), sulfoxide groups (−S=O), carbonyl groups (−C=O), and amino groups (−NH$_2$) on the cryoprotectant. In their experiment, they initially tested the toxicity of various cryoprotectants with differing qv^* indices using rabbit renal cortical slices and examined the K$^+$/Na$^+$ ratio after exposure. As qv^* increased in the range from 2 to 6, the K$^+$/Na$^+$ ratio decreased from ~80% to ~10% relative to the controls.

The significance of the polar groups is such that they account for the interaction with water molecules, and compounds with a lower qv^* can interact with fewer water molecules. Such compounds are poorer glass formers compared to those with a higher qv^*. Hence, weak glass forming cryoprotectants are less toxic. Using this new information, the investigators were able to predict and confirm that substitution of 1,2-propanediol (a very good glass former) with ethylene glycol (a very poor glass former) in a previously developed vitrification solution (VS41A) would be a superior vitrification solution using rabbit renal cortical slices and mouse oocytes. Others have also shown that the protective potential of cryoprotectants was correlated to the molarity of potential hydrogen bonding groups [119]; (see the review by Mazur [120] for a more complete discussion). As discussed below, reducing cryoprotectant toxicity is one approach to improving vitrification methods.

Cell Death at Sub-Optimal Cooling Rates

Many of the factors which might contribute to cell damage as a result of freezing are interdependent. For example, ice crystal formation may have deleterious mechanical effects on cells in suspension or in tissues [46,55,71,121] and the amount of ice formed and the crystal structure is dependent upon cooling rate, warming rate, and the presence of cryoprotectants. Not surprisingly, the idea of a single optimal cooling rate for a cell is an oversimplification. The cooling rate at which cell survival is highest is dependent upon other factors such as cryoprotectant concentration and warming rate [50,122].

Intracellular cryoprotectants have noticeable effects on intracellular ice formation [50,41,42,123–125]. In general, in the presence of a permeable cryoprotectant, cell water will crystallize at a slower cooling rate compared to the cooling rate resulting in crystallization in the absence of an intracellular cryoprotectant [126]. This effect is likely a result of several factors. One includes the reduction in the water permeability of cell membranes in the presence of cryoprotectant as mentioned above. A second is likely a result of lowering the freezing point of the cytoplasm which causes a general reduction in the temperature at which a given driving force for water efflux is present. Because of the temperature dependence of water permeability, less water can move out of the cell in a given amount of time under such circumstances [124,127]; as discussed in Mazur [19].

The generic term "solution effects" has been coined to collectively describe the various forms of injury to cells cooled slowly enough to preclude damaging intracellular ice formation [128]. This term reflects a notion that the damage results from the solution conditions created by ice formation as described above. Meryman and colleagues suggested that damage was a physical and not a biological event [128], resulting either from the osmotic dehydration of the cells and the resulting stress placed upon the cell membrane due to cell volume reduction, or a direct osmotic effect on the membrane itself. In earlier work, Meryman described a hypothesis of cryoinjury based upon the cell reaching a minimum critical volume [129]. This later work supports this theory.

Another interesting hypothesis has been put fourth to explain solution effects damage in relation to the formation of ice. In a series of studies, Mazur and colleagues investigated the effects of the fraction of the solution which remained unfrozen on cell damage [71,130–132]. Their data showed a strong correlation between survival and the unfrozen fraction when the unfrozen fraction was low (5–15%). They proposed that as the unfrozen fraction was reduced, the cells were damaged by mechanical effects of the ice and/or close apposition with other cells.

When the unfrozen fraction is increased, damage was less strongly dependent on that variable and more on the salt concentration until the effects of the unfrozen fraction were lost. When the unfrozen fraction is not a damaging mechanism, the loss was attributed to the osmotic effect of the solute (both during exposure and dilution) [133].

The interpretation of these data came under scrutiny as Pegg and Diaper [134] pointed out that the unfrozen fraction variable was confounded by the treatments used to change the unfrozen fraction (changing the initial osmolality of the solution). Such treatments would systematically alter the volume excursions which the cells would undergo during the experiment, and this difference could also result in the outcome seen. Mazur [19] goes into greater detail about this debate and adds additional evidence for the unfrozen fraction hypothesis.

Perhaps the most important message to get from this particular debate is the difficulty in designing experiments to isolate the effect of a single variable on cell damage during freezing when numerous potential variables are interdependent (see [55,134] for an elaboration). Another good example of this is the challenge to the explanation for slow-cooling injury resulting from increased salt concentration. As discussed above, concentrated solutes cause exosmosis and result in a reduction in cell volume. Thus, either high salt concentration or volume reduction could explain the damage (it could also be an interaction of the two factors). The minimum volume hypothesis was strongly supported by the results of Williams and Shaw with erythrocytes [93] following up on earlier work by Meryman [60].

In more recent years, the molecular mechanisms of cryodamage, particularly the induction of apoptosis, have been investigated [135]. John Baust and colleagues have suggested that the trigger for apoptosis is not necessarily an immediate effect of the cryopreservation stresses, but can be delayed for several hours as the cells try to recover from these stresses [136]. Clearly, at the present time we are far from understanding all of the mechanisms which result in cryodamage.

Cooling and Cooling Injury/Cold Shock

Even in the absence of ice, cold temperatures have profound effects upon cells. Injury from cooling is often differentiated by the degree to which the rate of cooling causes the specific event. Injuries from rapid cooling are usually categorized as cold shock injuries. These types of injuries occur quickly after cooling, and are generally independent of the warming rate. In the context of cryopreservation, a significant body of literature has been produced which describes the effects of cold shock on cell membranes, particularly for spermatozoa [18,137].

A description of the liquid crystalline model of cell membranes can be found in a standard cell biology text [138]. In general, amphipathic lipid molecules form a bilayer structure with various proteins being integrated throughout. At physiologic temperatures, the membrane is fluid such that molecular mobility is high and many of the proteins and lipids are free to diffuse laterally within the bilayer (however, opposite faces of the bilayer are not identical, and moving from one face of the bilayer to the other is energetically unfavorable). The structure that lipids can take in solution is more diverse than just a simple bilayer configuration. A lamellar (i.e., bilayer) structure is common, but micelles, inverted micelles (micelles within the bilayer), hexagonal-II, and cubic-phase structures can occur (see Fig.1 in the review by Quinn [139]). The particular arrangements lipids take is dependent upon factors such as water activity, temperature, pH, salt concentration, and interactions with other molecules (e.g., proteins).

When membranes are cooled, they exhibit thermotropic behavior; that is to say they tend to undergo phase transitions. As membranes are cooled, the lipids tend to transition from a liquid-like state to a gel-like state, with the molecules being arranged in an orderly, crystalline fashion with a characteristic hexagonal arrange-ment [140]. Due to the complexity of biological membranes, a transition is not like a crystallization event in a simple solution (i.e., a rapid precipitation), but more like a (relatively) slow lateral separation of membrane lipids into distinct domains (see Fig. 7.9). Nevertheless, this transition is a distinct change from the usual lipid arrangement, and can have significant effects on membrane function.

The temperature at which this transition occurs is dependent upon several factors, including the length of the hydrocarbon chain in the lipid group, the presence and location of *cis*-unsaturated bonds (transition temperatures decrease as the position

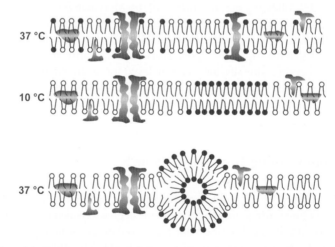

Fig. 7.9 A model of temperature-induced phase changes to membranes is described in this figure. In the upper portion of the figure, a typical biomembrane is shown, with various integral membrane proteins and lipid species. As the temperature is reduced from physiologic to hypothermic (10 °C in this instance), lateral redistribution of the various molecules occurs, with lamellar-forming lipid species (represented with white polar groups) and hexagonal-II-forming lipid species (represented with black polar groups) separating into distinct domains. Upon warming, an inverted micelle structure is created by the hexagonal-II-forming lipids. Such a configuration could result in a significant disruption of the membrane selective permeability, and the possibility of membrane failure and cell death. Figure adapted from Parks, 1997 [141], which was adapted from Quinn 1985 [139]

of the bond moves away from the polar group and toward the middle of the chain), and the concentration and valence of cations in the solution. An increase in the concentration of polyvalent cations increases the phase transition temperature, whereas monovalent cations increase lipid fluidity and decrease the phase transition temperature. The presence of cholesterol in a membrane can also affect phase transition behavior by (1) altering the ability of lipid species to transition to a gel-like configuration; and (2) increasing the disorder of the gel phase.

The propensity to develop a lamellar or hexagonal-II structure varies across lipid species. Different species tend to aggregate into domains during the phase change, and the creation of inverted micelles (hexagonal-II structures) within a bilayer can occur as a result (Fig. 7.9) [142]. Rearrangements such as these can alter the selective permeability of membranes, resulting in the loss of cell homeostasis.

Changes in the biochemistry of spermatozoa as a result of cold shock have been examined. A reduction in anaerobic glycolysis and respiration, ATP levels, Cytochrome *C* loss from the mitochondria, and release of numerous intracellular enzymes have all been described (reviewed in [18,143]). Furthermore, changes in the distribution of intracellular ions have also been noted.

Numerous compounds have been shown to confer protection to spermatozoa from cold shock. Protective agents include glycerol, phosphatidylserine, egg yolk, lecithin, milk, and albumin. The low density lipoprotein fraction of egg yolk is particularly effective at preventing cold shock injury [144], with phosphatidylcholine being a particularly active component [145]. The results from Quinn and colleagues [145] suggest that the effect is a result of interactions with the surface of the membrane, and not as a result of components intercalating within the lipid bilayer. The mechanisms of these compounds are not fully understood, but one model for the effect of adhering cryoprotectants on phase separations of membranes has been put fourth [4] and is shown schematically in Fig. 7.10.

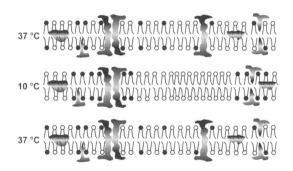

Fig. 7.10 A model of the effect of cryoprotectants on preserving biomembrane stability as described in Quinn 1985 [139] is shown. In the presence of cryoprotectants (not shown schematically), the hexagonal-II –forming lipid species preferentially associate with membrane proteins during cooling (compare middle panel to middle panel in Figure 7.9) and only lamellar-forming lipid species segregate into distinct domains. When the cell is warmed, the hexagonal-II-lipid – protein interactions prevent a non-lamellar transition, promoting the return to a normal bilayer configuration

16. Karow AM, Critser JK, eds. Reproductive Tissue Banking. San Diego: Academic Press; 1997.
17. Walters EM, Benson JD, Woods EJ, Critser JK. History of Sperm Cryopreservation. In: Pacey A, Tomlinson MJ, eds. Practical Guide for Sperm Banking. Cambridge: Cambridge University Press (In Press).
18. Watson PF, Morris GJ. Cold shock injury in animal cells. In: Bowler K, Fuller BJ, eds. Temperature and animal cells. Cambridge: The Company of Biologist Limited; 1987:311–340.
19. Mazur P. Principles of Cryobiology. In: Fuller BJ, Lane N, Benson EE, eds. Life in the Frozen State. Boca Raton: CRC Press; 2004:3–65.
20. Muldrew K, Acker JP, Elliott JAW, McGann LE. The water to ice transition: implications for living cells. In: Fuller BJ, Lane N, Benson EE, eds. Life in the Frozen State. Boca Raton: CRC Press; 2004:67–108.
21. Ashwood-Smith MJ. Mechanism of cryoprotectant action. In: Bowler K, Fuller BJ, eds. Temperature and Animal Cells. Cambridge: The Company of Biologists, Ltd.; 1987:395–406.
22. Cocks FH, Brower WE. Phase diagram relationships in cryobiology. Cryobiology 1974;11(4): 340–358.
23. Baudot A, Odagescu V. Thermal properties of ethylene glycol aqueous solutions. Cryobiology 2004;48(3):283–294.
24. Leibo SP, McGrath JJ, Cravalho EG. Microscopic observation of intracellular ice formation in unfertilized mouse ova as a function of cooling rate. Cryobiology 1978;15(3):257–271.
25. Toner M, Cravalho EG, Karel M, Armant DR. Cryomicroscopic analysis of intracellular ice formation during freezing of mouse oocytes without cryoadditives. Cryobiology 1991;28(1):55–71.
26. Gao D, Mazur P, Critser JK. Fundamental Cryobiology of Mammalian Spermatozoa. In: Karow AM, Critser JK, eds. Reproductive Tissue Banking, Scientific Principles. San Diego: Academic Press; 1997:263–328.
27. Terwilliger TC, Solomon AK. Osmotic water permeability of human red cells. J Gen Physiol 1981;77(5):549–570.
28. Hunter J, Bernard A, Fuller B, McGrath J, Shaw RW. Plasma membrane water permeabilities of human oocytes: the temperature dependence of water movement in individual cells. J Cell Physiol 1992;150(1):175–179.
29. Mazur P. The role of intracellular freezing in the death of cells cooled at supraoptimal rates. Cryobiology 1977;14(3):251–272.
30. Mazur P. Kinetics of water loss from cells at subzero temperatures and the likelihood of intracellular freezing. J Gen Physiol 1963;47:47–69.
31. Karlsson JO, Cravalho EG, Borel Rinkes IH, Tompkins RG, Yarmush ML, Toner M. Nucleation and growth of ice crystals inside cultured hepatocytes during freezing in the presence of dimethyl sulfoxide. Biophys J 1993;65(6):2524–2536.
32. Whittingham DG, Leibo SP, Mazur P. Survival of mouse embryos frozen to –196 degrees and –269 degrees C. Science 1972;178(59):411–414.
33. Shimada K, Asahina E. Visualization of intracellular ice crystals formed in very rapidly frozen cells at –27 degree C. Cryobiology 1975;12(3):209–218.
34. Bank H. Visualization of freezing damage. II. Structural alterations during warming. Cryobiology 1973;10(2):157–170.
35. Karlsson JO. A theoretical model of intracellular devitrification. Cryobiology 2001;42(3): 154–169.
36. Acker JP, McGann LE. Protective effect of intracellular ice during freezing? Cryobiology 2003;46(2):197–202.
37. Mazur P. The role of cell membranes in the freezing of yeast and other single cells. Ann N Y Acad Sci 1965;125:658–676.
38. Acker JP, Elliott JA, McGann LE. Intercellular ice propagation: experimental evidence for ice growth through membrane pores. Biophys J 2001;81(3):1389–1397.
39. Acker JP, Larese A, Yang H, Petrenko A, McGann LE. Intracellular ice formation is affected by cell interactions. Cryobiology 1999;38(4):363–371.

40. Irimia D, Karlsson JO. Kinetics of intracellular ice formation in one-dimensional arrays of interacting biological cells. Biophys J 2005;88(1):647–660.
41. Mazur P, Pinn IL, Seki S, Kleinhans FW, Edashige K. Effects of hold time after extracellular ice formation on intracellular freezing of mouse oocytes. Cryobiology 2005;51(2):235–239.
42. Mazur P, Seki S, Pinn IL, Kleinhans FW, Edashige K. Extra- and intracellular ice formation in mouse oocytes. Cryobiology 2005;51(1):29–53.
43. Guenther JF, Seki S, Kleinhans FW, Edashige K, Roberts DM, Mazur P. Extra- and intra-cellular ice formation in Stage I and II *Xenopus laevis* oocytes. Cryobiology 2006;52(3):401–416.
44. Toner M, Cravalho EG, Huggins CE. Thermodynamics and kinetics of intracellular ice formation during freezing of biological cells. J Appl Physiol 1990;69:1582–1593.
45. Toner M, Cravalho EG, Stachecki J, et al. Nonequilibrium freezing of one-cell mouse embryos. Membrane integrity and developmental potential. Biophys J 1993;64(6):1908–1921.
46. Muldrew K, McGann LE. Mechanisms of intracellular ice formation. Biophys J 1990;57(3):525–532.
47. Muldrew K, McGann LE. The osmotic rupture hypothesis of intracellular freezing injury. Biophys J 1994;66(2 Pt 1):532–541.
48. Dowgert MF, Steponkus PL. Effect of Cold Acclimation on Intracellular Ice Formation in Isolated Protoplasts. Plant Physiol 1983;72(4):978–988.
49. Steponkus PL, Dowgert MF, Gordon-Kamm WJ. Destabilization of the plasma membrane of isolated plant protoplasts during a freeze-thaw cycle: the influence of cold acclimation. Cryobiology 1983;20(4):448–465.
50. Mazur P, Leibo SP, Farrant J, Chu EHY, Hanna Jr MG, Smith LH. Interactions of cooling rate, warming rate and protective additive on the survival of frozen mammalian cells. In: Wolstenholme GEW, O'Connor M, eds. The Frozen Cell. London: J and A Churchill; 1970:69–58.
51. Fahy GM. The relevance of cryoprotectant "toxicity" to cryobiology. Cryobiology 1986;23(1):1–13.
52. Karow AM, Jr. Cryoprotectants – a new class of drugs. J Pharm Pharmacol 1969;21(4):209–223.
53. Acker JP. The use of intracellular protectants in cell biopreservation. In: Baust JG, Baust JM, eds. Advances in Biopreservation. Boca Raton, FL: Taylor & Francis; 2007:299–320.
54. Lovelock JE. The haemolysis of human red blood cells by freezing and thawing. Biochim Biophys Acta 1953;10:414–426.
55. Pegg DE. Mechanisms of freezing damage. In: Bowler K, Fuller BJ, eds. Temperature and Animal Cells. Cambridge: The Company of Biologists, Ltd.; 1987:363–378.
56. Pegg DE, Diaper MP. On the mechanism of injury to slowly frozen erythrocytes. Biophys J 1988;54(3):471–488.
57. Lovelock JE. The mechanism of the protective action of glycerol against haemolysis by freezing and thawing. Biochim Biophys Acta 1953;11:28–36.
58. Nash T. Chemical constitution and physical properties of compounds able to protect living cells against damage due to freezing and thawing. In: Meryman HT, ed. Cryobiology. New York: Academic Press; 1966:179–211.
59. Korber C, Scheiwe MW, Boutron P, Rau G. The influence of hydroxyethyl starch on ice formation in aqueous solutions. Cryobiology 1982;l9(5):478–492.
60. Meryman HT. Osmotic stress as a mechanism of freezing injury. Cryobiology 1971;8(5):489–500.
61. Anchordoguy TJ, Cecchini CA, Crowe JH, Crowe LM. Insights into the cryoprotective mechanism of dimethyl sulfoxide for phospholipid bilayers. Cryobiology 1991;28(5):467–473.
62. Xie G, Timasheff SN. The thermodynamic mechanism of protein stabilization by trehalose. Biophys Chem 1997;64(1–3):25–43.
63. Carpenter JF, Crowe JH. The mechanism of cryoprotection of proteins by solutes. Cryobiology 1988;25(3):244–255.

64. Anchordoguy TJ, Carpenter JF, Cecchini CA, Crowe JH, Crowe LM. Effects of protein perturbants on phospholipid bilayers. Arch Biochem Biophys 1990;283(2):356–361.
65. Rudolph AS, Crowe JH. Membrane stabilization during freezing: the role of two natural cryoprotectants, trehalose and proline. Cryobiology 1985;22(4):367–377.
66. Crowe JH, Crowe LM, Tablin F, Wolkers W, Oliver AE. Stabilization of cells diring freeze-drying: the trehalose myth. In: Fuller BJ, Lane N, Benson EE, eds. Life in the Frozen State. Boca Raton: CRC Press; 2004:581–601.
67. Crowe JH, Crowe LM, Carpenter JF, et al. Interactions of sugars with membranes. Biochim Biophys Acta 1988;947(2):367–384.
68. Crowe JH, Carpenter JF, Crowe LM. The role of vitrification in anhydrobiosis. Annu Rev Physiol 1998;60:73–103.
69. Benson EE. Cryoconserving algal and plant diversity: historical perspectives and future challenges. In: Fuller BJ, Lane N, Benson EE, eds. Life in the Frozen State. Boca Raton: CRC Press; 2004:299–328.
70. Diller KR. Pioneers in cryobiology: Nikolay Aleksandrovich Maximov (1890–1952). Cryo-Letters 1997;18:81–92.
71. Mazur P, Rall WF, Rigopoulos N. Relative contributions of the fraction of unfrozen water and of salt concentration to the survival of slowly frozen human erythrocytes. Biophys J 1981;36(3):653–675.
72. Barrett J. Thermal hysteresis proteins. Int J Biochem Cell Biol 2001;33(2):105–117.
73. Knight CA, DeVries AL, Oolman LD. Fish antifreeze protein and the freezing and re-crystallization of ice. Nature 1984;308(5956):295–296.
74. Hew CL, Yang DS. Protein interaction with ice. Eur J Biochem 1992;203(1–2):33–42.
75. Wilson PW. A model for thermal hysteresis utilizing the anisotropic interfacial energy of ice crystals. Cryobiology 1994;31:406–412.
76. Raymond JA, Wilson P, DeVries AL. Inhibition of growth of nonbasal planes in ice by fish antifreezes. Proc Natl Acad Sci USA 1989;86(3):881–885.
77. Kristiansen E, Zachariassen KE. The mechanism by which fish antifreeze proteins cause thermal hysteresis. Cryobiology 2005;51(3):262–280.
78. Storey KB, Storey JM. Freeze tolerance in animals. Physiol Rev 1988;68(1):27–84.
79. Storey KB, Baust JG, Wolanczyk JP. Biochemical modification of plasma ice nucleating activity in a freeze-tolerant frog. Cryobiology 1992;29(3):374–384.
80. Wolanczyk JP, Storey KB, Baust JG. Ice nucleating activity in the blood of the freeze-tolerant frog, *Rana sylvatica*. Cryobiology 1990;27(3):328–335.
81. Vazquez Illanes MD, Storey KB. 6–Phosphofructo-2-kinase and control of cryoprotectant synthesis in freeze tolerant frogs. Biochim Biophys Acta 1993;1158(1):29–32.
82. Storey KB, Storey JM. Natural freeze tolerance in ectothermic vertebrates. Annu Rev Physiol 1992;54:619–637.
83. Hazel JR. Effects of temperature on the structure and metabolism of cell membranes in fish. Am J Physiol 1984;246(4 Pt 2):R460–R470.
84. Fahy GM, Karow AM, Jr. Ultrastructure-function correlative studies for cardiac cryopreservation. V. Absence of a correlation between electrolyte toxicity and cryoinjury in the slowly frozen, cryoprotected rat heart. Cryobiology 1977;14(4):418–427.
85. Kahn RA. Biochemical changes in frozen platelets. In: Greenwalt TJ, Jamieson GA, eds. The blood platelet in transfusion therapy. New York: Alan R. Liss; 1978:167–180.
86. Fahy GM. Analysis of "solution effects" injury: rabbit renal cortex frozen in the presence of dimethyl sulfoxide. Cryobiology 1980;17(4):371–388.
87. Armitage WJ, Mazur P. Osmotic tolerance of human granulocytes. Am J Physiol 1984;247 (5 Pt 1):C373–C381.
88. Armitage WJ, Parmar N, Hunt CJ. The effects of osmotic stress on human platelets. J Cell Physiol 1985;123(2):241–248.
89. Agca Y, Liu J, Rutledge JJ, Critser ES, Critser JK. Effect of osmotic stress on the developmental competence of germinal vesicle and metaphase II stage bovine cumulus oocyte complexes and its relevance to cryopreservation. Mol Reprod Dev 2000;55(2):212–219.

90. Pukazhenthi B, Noiles E, Pelican K, Donoghue A, Wildt D, Howard J. Osmotic effects on feline spermatozoa from normospermic versus teratospermic donors. Cryobiology 2000;40(2):139–150.

91. Blanco JM, Gee G, Wildt DE, Donoghue AM. Species variation in osmotic, cryoprotectant, and cooling rate tolerance in poultry, eagle, and peregrine falcon spermatozoa. Biol Reprod 2000;63(4):1164–1171.

92. Mazur P, Schneider U. Osmotic responses of preimplantation mouse and bovine embryos and their cryobiological implications. Cell Biophys 1986;8(4):259–285.

93. Williams RJ, Shaw SK. The relationship between cell injury and osmotic volume reduction: II. Red cell lysis correlates with cell volume rather than intracellular salt concentration. Cryobiology 1980;17(6):530–539.

94. Zieger MA, Woods EJ, Lakey JR, Liu J, Critser JK. Osmotic tolerance limits of canine pancreatic islets. Cell Transplant 1999;8(3):277–284.

95. Gao DY, Chang Q, Liu C, et al. Fundamental cryobiology of human hematopoietic progenitor cells. I: Osmotic characteristics and volume distribution. Cryobiology 1998;36(1):40–48.

96. Men H, Agca Y, Mullen SF, Critser ES, Critser JK. Osmotic stress on the cellular actin filament organization of in vitro produced porcine embryos. Reproduction, Fertility, and Development 2004;12(1,2):177.

97. Koshimoto C, Gamliel E, Mazur P. Effect of osmolality and oxygen tension on the survival of mouse sperm frozen to various temperatures in various concentrations of glycerol and raffinose. Cryobiology 2000;41(3):204–231.

98. Songsasen N, Yu I, Murton S, et al. Osmotic sensitivity of canine spermatozoa. Cryobiology 2002;44(1):79–90.

99. Mullen SF, Agca Y, Broermann DC, Jenkins CL, Johnson CA, Critser JK. The effect of osmotic stress on the metaphase II spindle of human oocytes, and the relevance to cryopreservation. Hum Reprod 2004;19(5):1148–1154.

100. Agca Y, Liu J, Mullen S, et al. Osmotic tolerance and membrane permeability characteristics of Rhesus (*Macaca mulatta*) spermatozoa. Cryobiology 2004;49(3):316–317.

101. Walters E, Men H, Agca Y, Mullen S, Critser E, Critser J. Osmotic tolerance of mouse spermatozoa from various genetic backgrounds. Cryobiology 2004;49(3):344.

102. Walters EM, Men H, Agca Y, Mullen SF, Critser ES, Critser JK. Osmotic tolerance of mouse spermatozoa from various genetic backgrounds: Acrosome integrity, membrane integrity, and maintenance of motility. Cryobiology 2005;50(2):193–205.

103. De Loecker R, Penninckx F. Osmotic effects of rapid dilution of cryoprotectants II. Effects on human erythrocyte hemolysis. Cryo-Letters 1987;8:140–145.

104. Agca Y, Mullen S, Liu J, et al. Osmotic tolerance and membrane permeability characteristics of rhesus monkey (*Macaca mulatta*) spermatozoa. Cryobiology 2005;51(1):1–14.

105. Men H, Agca Y, Mullen SF, Critser ES, Critser JK. Osmotic tolerance of in vitro produced porcine blastocysts assessed by their morphological integrity and cellular actin filament organization. Cryobiology 2005;51(2):119–129.

106. Adams SL, Kleinhans FW, Mladenov PV, Hessian PA. Membrane permeability characteristics and osmotic tolerance limits of sea urchin (*Evechinus chloroticus*) eggs. Cryobiology 2003;47(1):1–13.

107. Shaw PW, Fuller BJ, Bernard A, Shaw RW. Vitrification of mouse oocytes: improved rates of survival, fertilization, and development to blastocysts. Mol Reprod Dev 1991;29(4):373–378.

108. Isachenko V, Montag M, Isachenko E, Nawroth F, Dessole S, van der Ven H. Developmental rate and ultrastructure of vitrified human pronuclear oocytes after step-wise versus direct rehydration. Hum Reprod 2004;19(3):660–665.

109. Fiéni F, Beckers JP, Buggin M, et al. Evaluation of cryopreservation techniques for goat embryos. Reproduction, Nutrition, Development 1995;35(4):367–373.

110. Kedem O, Katchalsky A. Thermodynamic analysis of the permeability of biological membranes to non-electrolytes. Biochim. Biophys. Acta 1958;27:229–246.

111. Kleinhans FW. Membrane permeability modeling: Kedem–Katchalsky vs a two-parameter formalism. Cryobiology 1998;37(4):271–289.
112. Gao DY, Liu J, Liu C, et al. Prevention of osmotic injury to human spermatozoa during addition and removal of glycerol. Hum Reprod 1995;10(5):1109–1122.
113. Baxter SJ, Lathe GH. Biochemical effects of kidney of exposure to high concentrations of dimethyl sulphoxide. Biochem Pharmacol 1971;20(6):1079–1091.
114. Fahy GM, Lilley TH, Linsdell H, Douglas MS, Meryman HT. Cryoprotectant toxicity and cryoprotectant toxicity reduction: in search of molecular mechanisms. Cryobiology 1990;27(3):247–268.
115. Johnson MH, Pickering SJ. The effect of dimethylsulphoxide on the microtubular system of the mouse oocyte. Development 1987;100(2):313–324.
116. Vincent C, Johnson MH. Cooling, cryoprotectants, and the cytoskeleton of the mammalian oocyte. Oxf Rev Reprod Biol 1992;14:73–100.
117. Vincent C, Pickering SJ, Johnson MH, Quick SJ. Dimethylsulphoxide affects the organisation of microfilaments in the mouse oocyte. Mol Reprod Dev 1990;26(3):227–235.
118. Fahy GM, Wowk B, Wu J, Paynter S. Improved vitrification solutions based on the predictability of vitrification solution toxicity. Cryobiology 2004;48(1):22–35.
119. Doebbler GF, Rinfret AP. The influence of protective compounds and cooling and warming conditions on hemolysis of erythrocytes by freezing and thawing. Biochim Biophys Acta 1962;58:449–458.
120. Mazur P. Cryobiology: the freezing of biological systems. Science 1970;168(934):939–949.
121. Sjostrom M. Ice crystal growth in skeletal muscle fibres. J Microsc 1975;105(1):67–80.
122. Mazur P, Schmidt JJ. Interactions of cooling velocity, temperature, and warming velocity on the survival of frozen and thawed yeast. Cryobiology 1968;5(1):1–17.
123. Rall WF, Mazur P, McGrath JJ. Depression of the ice-nucleation temperature of rapidly cooled mouse embryos by glycerol and dimethyl sulfoxide. Biophys J 1983; 41(1):1–12.
124. Myers SP, Pitt RE, Lynch DV, Steponkus PL. Characterization of intracellular ice formation in Drosophila melanogaster embryos. Cryobiology 1989;26(5):472–484.
125. Harris CL, Toner M, Hubel A, Cravalho EG, Yarmush ML, Tompkins RG. Cryopreservation of isolated hepatocytes: intracellular ice formation under various chemical and physical conditions. Cryobiology 1991;28(5):436–444.
126. Diller KR. Intracellular freezing of glycerolized red cells. Cryobiology 1979;16(2):125–131.
127. Karlsson JO, Cravalho EG, Toner M. A model of diffusion-limited ice growth inside biological cells during freezing. J Appl Physiol 1994;75:4442–4450.
128. Meryman HT, Williams RJ, Douglas MS. Freezing injury from "solution effects" and its prevention by natural or artificial cryoprotection. Cryobiology 1977;14(3):287–302.
129. Meryman HT. The exceeding of a minimum tolerable cell volume in hypertonic suspensions as a cause of freezing injury. In: Wolstenholme GEW, O'Connor M, eds. The Frozen Cell. London: J and A Churchill; 1970:51–64.
130. Mazur P, Cole KW. Influence of cell concentration on the contribution of unfrozen fraction and salt concentration to the survival of slowly frozen human erythrocytes. Cryobiology 1985;22(6):509–536.
131. Mazur P, Cole KW. Roles of unfrozen fraction, salt concentration, and changes in cell volume in the survival of frozen human erythrocytes. Cryobiology 1989;26(1):1–29.
132. Mazur P, Rigopoulos N. Contributions of unfrozen fraction and of salt concentration to the survival of slowly frozen human erythrocytes: influence of warming rate. Cryobiology 1983;20(3):274–289.
133. Zade-Oppen AM. Posthypertonic hemolysis in sodium chloride systems. Acta Physiol Scand 1968;73(3):341–364.
134. Pegg DE, Diaper MP. The effect of initial tonicity on freeze/thaw injury to human red cells suspended in solutions of sodium chloride. Cryobiology 1991;28(1):18–35.

135. Baust JM, Van B, Baust JG. Cell viability improves following inhibition of cryopreservation – induced apoptosis. In Vitro Cell Dev Biol Anim 2000;36(4):262–270.
136. Baust JM, Vogel MJ, Van Buskirk R, Baust JG. A molecular basis of cryopreservation failure and its modulation to improve cell survival. Cell Transplant 2001;10(7):561–571.
137. Morris GJ, Watson PF. Cold-Shock injury – a comprehensive bibliography. Cryo-Letters 1984;5:352–372.
138. Alberts B, Johnson A, Lewis J, Raff M, Roberts K, Walter P. Molecular biology of the cell. 4th ed. New York: Garland Science; 2002.
139. Quinn PJ. A lipid-phase separation model of low-temperature damage to biological membranes. Cryobiology 1985;22(2):128–146.
140. Chapman D. Phase transitions and fluidity characteristics of lipids and cell membranes. Q Rev Biophys 1975;8(2):185–235.
141. Parks JE. Hypothermia and Mammalian Gametes. In: Karow AM, Critser JK, eds. Reproductive Tissue Banking, Scientific Principles. San Diego: Academic Press; 1997:229–261.
142. Sen A, Brain AP, Quinn PJ, Williams WP. Formation of inverted lipid micelles in aqueous dispersions of mixed sn-3–galactosyldiacylglycerols induced by heat and ethylene glycol. Biochim Biophys Acta 1982;686(2):215–224.
143. Watson PF. The effects of cold shock on sperm cell membranes. In: Morris GJ, Clarke A, eds. Effects of low temperatures on biological membranes. New York: Academic Press; 1981:189–218.
144. Pace MM, Graham EF. Components in egg yolk which protect bovine spermatozoa during freezing. J Anim Sci 1974;39(6):1444–1449.
145. Quinn PJ, Chow PY, White IG. Evidence that phospholipid protects ram spermatozoa from cold shock at a plasma membrane site. J Reprod Fertil 1980;60(2):403–407.
146. Phadtare S, Alsina J, Inouye M. Cold-shock response and cold-shock proteins. Curr Opin Microbiol 1999;2(2):175–180.
147. Rieder CL, Cole RW. Cold-shock and the Mammalian cell cycle. Cell Cycle 2002;1(3):169–175.
148. Fujita J. Cold shock response in mammalian cells. J Mol Microbiol Biotechnol 1999;1(2):243–255.
149. Al-Fageeh MB, Marchant RJ, Carden MJ, Smales CM. The cold-shock response in cultured mammalian cells: harnessing the response for the improvement of recombinant protein production. Biotechnol Bioeng 2006;93(5):829–835.
150. Al-Fageeh MB, Smales CM. Control and regulation of the cellular responses to cold shock: the responses in yeast and mammalian systems. Biochem J 2006;397(2):247–259.
151. Inouye M, Phadtare S. Cold shock response and adaptation at near-freezing temperature in microorganisms. Sci STKE 2004;2004(237):pe26.
152. Phadtare S, Inouye M. Genome-wide transcriptional analysis of the cold shock response in wild-type and cold-sensitive, quadruple-csp-deletion strains of *Escherichia coli*. J Bacteriol 2004;186(20):7007–7014.
153. Rall WF, Fahy GM. Ice-free cryopreservation of mouse embryos at −196 degrees C by vitrification. Nature 1985;313(6003):573–575.
154. Kuwayama M, Vajta G, Kato O, Leibo SP. Highly efficient vitrification method for cryopreservation of human oocytes. Reprod Biomed Online 2005;11(3):300–308.
155. Lane M, Gardner DK. Vitrification of mouse oocytes using a nylon loop. Mol Reprod Dev 2001;58(3):342–347.
156. Martino A, Songsasen N, Leibo SP. Development into blastocysts of bovine oocytes cryopreserved by ultra-rapid cooling. Biol Reprod 1996;54(5):1059–1069.
157. Otoi T, Yamamoto K, Koyama N, Tachikawa S, Suzuki T. Cryopreservation of mature bovine oocytes by vitrification in straws. Cryobiology 1998;37(1):77–85.
158. Woods EJ, Benson JD, Agca Y, Critser JK. Fundamental cryobiology of reproductive cells and tissues. Cryobiology 2004;48(2):146–156.

Chapter 8
Ovarian Tissue Cryopreservation and Transplantation: Banking Reproductive Potential for the Future

David Lee, MD

Transplantation of cryopreserved ovarian tissue is a technology that holds promise for preserving reproductive potential for the future. It may be apropos for cancer survivors who will undergo treatment with sterility-inducing chemotherapy or radiation. Although there is some evidence suggesting cellular and molecular injury with the freezing and thawing process, there are examples in both animals and humans that transplantation of cryopreserved ovarian tissue can lead to successful restoration of fertility. Currently, cryopreservation of ovarian tissue is the only option available to preserve fertility in prepubertal girls or women who cannot delay their cancer treatment. For this patient population, ovarian tissue banking and subsequent transplantation is the only fertility-preserving method that has resulted in live-born pregnancies. The technology of ovarian tissue banking is currently at the forefront of the emerging field of oncofertilty.

Indications for Ovarian Tissue Banking

Scope of the Clinical Problem and Incidence of Ovarian Failure

There are more than 9 million cancer survivors living in the United States today. Furthermore, it is estimated that by 2010, 1 in every 250 people will be a survivor of cancer [1]. The prognosis for patients with childhood cancers is excellent, with greater than 70% surviving, and therefore, attention can be focused on patients' quality of life rather than just survival. Unfortunately for many young women, the chemotherapy or radiation therapy used to treat them is toxic to their ovaries and renders them infertile and dependent upon hormone replacement therapy. The incidence of ovarian failure may approach over 90% in patients undergoing high-dose chemotherapy [2]. Given that 1 in 52 females between birth and age 39 are diagnosed with cancer [3], many people are potentially affected.

One potential solution is to remove, freeze, and bank ovarian tissue before a patient undergoes gonadotoxic treatment, thereby removing the ovaries from harm, and then transplant the tissue back after completing treatment (autografting). Alternatively, ovarian tissue could be transplanted to an immunocompromised

T.K. Woodruff and K.A. Snyder (eds.) *Oncofertility.*
© Springer 2007

mouse host in order to minimize the risk of cancer transmission within the grafted ovarian tissue (xenografting), or oocytes isolated from the tissue could be matured in culture (in vitro maturation). Clinical decisions must always weigh the potential risks and benefits. Since there has been limited success with the aforementioned strategies, and since ovarian tissue banking requires removal of ovarian tissue, it is necessary to have a clear idea of the risk of ovarian failure from chemotherapy and/or radiation therapy. If the risk of ovarian failure is inevitable, it is reasonable to undertake these fertility-preserving strategies.

Gonadotoxicity of Chemotherapy

Chemotherapy can cause sterility in 38–56% of Hodgkin's lymphoma patients and the majority of bone marrow transplant patients [2]. The clinical course can be unpredictable. Oligomenorrhea can be followed by normal menses or premature ovarian failure (POF). Treatment with alkylating agents is particularly harmful (Table 8.1) [4,5]. The incidence of ovarian failure is dependent on the agent, dose, and age of the patient. Younger patients are more resistant to the gonadotoxic effects of the chemotherapy (Table 8.2) [6–9]. Offspring born to women who have received prior chemotherapy do not appear to be at increased risk for birth defects.

Table 8.1 The gonadotoxicity of chemotherapeutic agents

In 168 patients who received combination chemotherapy, the overall ovarian failure rate was 34%, representing an odds ratio of 1.0. The odds ratio of ovarian failure was calculated in exposed and non-exposed patients.

Group	Mechanism	Agents	Odds ratio for ovarian failure
Alkylating agents	Crosslinks DNA strands	Cyclophosphamide (Cytoxan)	4.0
	Inhibits RNA formation	Cholorambucil Mustine Melphalan Busulfan Carmustine Lomustine	
Platinum derivatives	Crosslinks DNA strands	Cisplatin Carboplatin	1.77
Vinca alkaloids	Disrupts microtubules and spindle	Vincristine Vinblastine	1.0
Antimetabolites	Inhibits pyrimidine or purine synthesis or incorporation into DNA	Cytarabine Methotrexate	0.3
Antibiotics	Multiple (transcription inhibition, DNA intercalation)	Adriamycin Bleomycin	0.25
Others	Unknown	Procarbazine	Unknown

Table 8.2 The gonadotoxicity of cyclophosphamide is dose and age dependent

Dose of cyclophosphamide before amenorrhea	Age of patient (years)
5,200 mg (5 g)	40
9,300 mg (10 g)	30
20,400 mg (20 g)	20
>50,000 mg (50 g)	Prepubertal

Table 8.3 Dose estimated to cause ovarian failure in 97.5% of patients as a function of age

Age (years)	Ovarian dose (cGy)
Birth	20.3 Gy (2,030 cGy)
10	18.4 Gy (1,840 cGy)
20	16.5 Gy (1,650 cGy)
30	14.3 Gy (1,430 cGy)

Gonadotoxicity of Radiation Therapy

Radiation therapy can adversely affect the ovaries, uterus, and hypothalamic-pituitary-ovarian axis such that future fertility is severely compromised.

Ovary

Radiation is harmful to the oocytes within the ovary. The LD50 of irradiation to the oocyte is 4 Gy [10], and some estimate that 5–10 Gy of radiation to the ovary causes ovarian failure in 97% of women. Younger patients are more resilient to radiation. Wallace et al. estimated that 18–20 Gy of ovarian radiation are necessary to induce ovarian failure in 97.5% of patients (Table 8.3) [11]. More conservative estimates by Chiarelli et al. showed that childhood cancer survivors receiving 20 Gy of abdominal irradiation had a relative risk of ovarian failure of only 1.02 [8]. Doses of 20–35 Gy caused infertility in 22% of patients, and doses greater than 35 Gy caused infertility in 32% of patients.

Uterus

High doses of abdominal irradiation (20–30 Gy) [12] and lower doses used in total body irradiation (14.4 Gy) [13] can adversely affect the growth and blood flow of the uterus. If subsequent pregnancy occurs, there is a statistically significant risk of preterm labor, low birth weight babies, and miscarriage.

Hypothalamic-Pituitary-Ovarian Axis

Cranial radiation to treat brain tumors can adversely affect the hypothalamic-pituitary-ovarian axis. Doses greater than 24–50 Gy are associated with delayed puberty [14,15], while lower does of cranial irradiation are associated with precocious puberty [14,16].

Limitations of Fertility: Preserving Techniques

Potential approaches to preserving fertility in women surviving cancer include ovarian suppression with gonadotropin releasing hormone (GnRH), pexying the ovaries outside the field of radiation, embryo freezing, oocyte freezing, and ovarian tissue banking with subsequent in vitro oocyte and follicle maturation. Each of these options has unique problems as summarized in Table 8.4.

Ovarian pexying involves surgically moving the ovaries medially behind the uterus, which is subsequently shielded, or laterally, outside the field of radiation. The ovaries can be sutured to prevent subsequent migration. The surgery can compromise the blood supply to the ovary, however, and transposition of the ovary does not always remove it from the field of radiation. Kwon reported that ovarian failure can still occur in 30–80% of cervical cancer patients undergoing pelvic irradiation after ovarian transposition. In addition, pexying does not protect the ovary from chemotherapeutic agents [17].

Gonadotropin releasing hormone agonist treatment may reduce the risk of POF; however, equivocal results indicate additional controlled trials are needed [18,19]. The observation was made that prepubertal girls had lower rates of ovarian failure after chemotherapy and radiation therapy than post-pubertal patients. With this in mind, some postulate that continuous GnRH exposure leads to downregulation of the pituitary and induction of a prepubertal state. This ovarian quiescence during cancer treatment might decrease susceptibility to gonadotoxic treatments. While some data in monkeys [20,21] and in small, non-randomized clinical studies [18,22] show benefit with GnRH therapy, one prospective randomized trial [23] showed no benefit. Primordial follicles in humans do not have follicle-stimulating hormone (FSH) receptors, so suppression of FSH with a GnRH agonist theoretically would not be protective. Younger patients may be less susceptible to chemotherapy because they have a greater number of oocytes, not because their ovaries are quiescent during chemotherapy.

In vitro fertilization (IVF) with embryo cryopreservation can be performed with pregnancy rates of 20–30% per frozen embryo transfer, but this approach requires ovarian stimulation and a male partner. Consequently, it is not applicable to children and can also create "orphan embryos" should the patient not survive. In addition, 2–6 weeks are required for ovarian stimulation and egg retrieval, which often delays initiation of cancer therapy.

Table 8.4 Summary of treatment options to preserve fertility

Method	Description	Advantages	Disadvantages	Efficacy	Cost
GnRH agonist	• Monthly injection to induce prepubertal state	• May decrease damage by chemotherapy	• Of no benefit in prepubertal girls or with radiation	• May decrease oocyte loss by 40%	$600–$900/month
Ovarian pexy	• Laparoscopically moving the ovaries outside the field of irradiation	• Minor surgical procedure	• Requires surgery • Not effective with chemotherapy • Ovary may migrate • Blood supply for ovary may decrease	• May decrease the dose of radiation to the ovary to 10% • Ovarian failure rate of 30–80%	$5,000
Ovarian tissue banking	• Laparoscopically remove ovarian tissue or ovaries and freeze • Maturation of eggs in the future by trans-plantation or in vitro methods	• Many oocytes preserved • Does not require stimulation • Does not delay cancer treatment • Appropriate for prepubertal girls	• Requires surgery • Eggs within the ovarian tissue need maturation before use • Limited efficacy	• Four human pregnancies to date	$5,000
Oocyte freezing	• Stimulation of ovaries with gonadotropins • Egg retrieval • Freeze mature unfertilized eggs	• Clinical efficiency improving • Appropriate for single young women • Not appropriate for prepubertal girls	• Requires 2–6 weeks for stimulation and retrieval • Only 20 oocytes banked per cycle	• 200 pregnancies worldwide • 1–3% pregnancy/oocyte frozen	$8,000–$18,000
Embryo freezing	• Stimulation of ovaries with gonadotropins • Retrieve eggs • Fertilize with partner's or donor sperm	• Proven technique	• Requires 2–6 weeks for stimulation • Not appropriate for prepubertal girls • Requires sperm • Limited number of embryos can be banked	• 20–30% pregnancy/embryo transfer	$8,000–$18,000

Cryopreservation of mature oocytes eliminates the need for a male partner and prevents creation of orphan embryos. To date, there have been 148 pregnancies in the world via oocyte freezing [24]. However, it too requires time and resources for ovarian stimulation. Second, ovarian stimulation is inappropriate in prepubertal girls because it initiates pubertal changes. Third, monitoring the growth of follicles and extraction of oocytes requires transvaginal ultrasound, which can be problematic in virginal or young patients. Fourth, a limited number of oocytes (15–20) are typically obtained at retrieval. Fifth, mature oocytes are challenging to freeze. The spindle is temperature sensitive, the zona pellucida hardens, and their relatively large size predisposes them to intracellular ice formation. Finally, the success rates are less than 2% per frozen oocyte [24–27].

Cryopreservation of immature oocytes with subsequent short-term in vitro maturation is another alternative and has been demonstrated in the mouse [28]; however, it has not yet yielded human embryos [29]. To date, there is no clear solution to this overwhelming clinical problem.

The Promise of Ovarian Tissue Banking

One potential solution is to freeze and bank ovarian tissue before patients undergo gonadotoxic treatment. Ovarian tissue banking involves surgically removing and cryopreserving ovarian tissue prior to the patient undergoing gonadotoxic cancer therapy, thereby removing the oocytes from harms way. The technology involves freezing immature primordial follicles in situ within the ovarian cortex or whole ovaries. Once the ovarian tissue is frozen, there are several options available for its future utilization, including autografting, xenografting, and in vitro maturation.

Ovarian tissue banking has several theoretical advantages over other fertility-preserving strategies. First, a 1-mm^3 piece of ovarian cortex may contain hundreds of oocytes [4]. Thus, cryopreservation of ovarian tissue is a potentially more efficient method of storing reproductive potential. Second, unlike collection of oocytes and production of embryos, which require time-consuming hormonal stimulation, oophorectomy does not delay cancer treatment. Oophorectomy or ovarian biopsy can usually be performed laparoscopically in less than an hour on an emergency basis. Third, primordial follicles consist of immature oocytes surrounded by a single layer of flattened pre-granulosa cells. These oocytes are much smaller, metabolically less active, and are not arrested at a stage where the spindle is present. All of these characteristics may make them better suited for cryopreservation than mature metaphase II oocytes. Finally, the immature oocytes within the ovarian tissue would be matured much later in life, thereby obviating the need for exogenous gonadotropin stimulation. Thus, ovarian tissue banking is appropriate for prepubertal girls.

Ovarian tissue banking has its disadvantages as well. First, surgery is required to obtain the ovarian tissue. Second, ovarian cortex is theoretically difficult to freeze because of its heterogeneity. Each cell type that comprises ovarian tissue (oocytes, granulosa cells, interstitial cells) has unique biological characteristics that require different freezing protocols. Finally, oocytes within ovarian tissue are immature, and require maturation before fertilization can occur. Follicles within ovarian tissue are arrested in early meiosis and cannot be fertilized. The process of follicular maturation is complex and requires multiple steps. The primordial to primary follicle transition involves numerous factors, primarily of the transforming growth factor (TGF) and platelet-derived growth factor families [30–35]. The formation of a fluid filled cavity, the antrum, within the layers of granulosa cells signifies the next stage of follicle growth and development, and is dependent on increased follicular vascularization and permeability of the blood vessels. As the follicle continues to grow, it resumes meiosis. In the primate, it is estimated that 150 days are required for growth from the primordial to the large preantral stage, followed by up to 70 days to reach the preovulatory stage [36,37]. Hence, with ovarian tissue banking, transplantation or extensive culture are needed before the harvested oocytes can be fertilized. Emerging technology utilizing three-dimensional follicle culture systems have led to successful in vitro maturation of mouse follicles [38–41]; IVF performed with these cultured oocytes has led to the birth of live, viable offspring [42]. These developments hold promise for the future use of banked, cryopreserved ovarian tissue for in vitro maturation and IVF. The current status of how these disadvantages have been overcome will be discussed below.

Cryopreservation of Ovarian Tissue has been Successful

Ovarian tissue banking is a two-step process. First, ovarian tissue must be cryopreserved with viable oocytes recovered upon thawing. Second, the primordial follicles within the frozen/thawed tissue must be matured. The freezing and thawing process can damage cells by both the formation of intracellular ice as well as the toxicity of the cryoprotectants. Cryoprotectants are molecules that help to prevent intracellular ice formation (see Mullen and Critser, this volume). The majority of pregnancies from banked oocytes have come after slow-rate freezing. Slow-rate (or equilibrium) freezing involves low, non-toxic concentrations of cryoprotectants and dehydration during cooling. Slow cooling involves the precipitation of water as ice, resulting in the separation of water from the solution. In contrast, vitrification involves very rapid freezing where solutions go directly from the aqueous phase to the glass state (amorphous solid) without going through the crystalline solid state in which damage can occur. Much higher concentrations of cryoprotectant are needed for this technique.

Oktay et al. [43] showed that ovarian tissue could be cryopreserved employing 1.5 M ethylene glycol and 0.1 M sucrose [44] and a slow-rate freezing process. A high percentage of primordial follicles survived the freezing/thawing process [43]. Our lab developed a novel system for vitrifying ovarian tissue (Fig. 8.1) [45]. We demonstrated that follicle viability was equivalent with vitrification (70.4 % ± 4.8%, $n = 1,705$) and slow-rate freezing (67.3% ± 4.7%, $n = 1,895$). Thus, this first step in ovarian tissue banking has been successful.

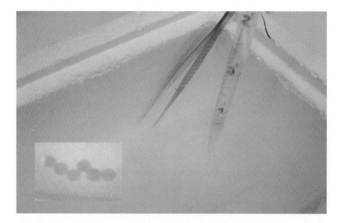

Fig. 8.1 A novel containerless system for vitrifying ovarian tissue developed by the authors. Pieces of ovarian cortex were placed into cryoprotectant and drops of the solution containing tissue were added directly to liquid nitrogen. Frozen droplets were then transferred into cryovials filled with liquid nitrogen for storage

Autotransplantation of Ovarian Tissue has been Successful

The second step in ovarian tissue banking involves maturation of immature follicles. Primordial follicles are immature eggs, arrested in the dictyotene stage of prophase I, and are surrounded by a single layer of flattened, pre-granulosa cells. Oocytes within primordial follicles cannot be fertilized before undergoing maturation. The maturation process is thought to take about 200 days, and the initial stages of growth are not dependent on FSH [36].

Autografting involves transplanting the ovarian tissue back into the donor from whom it was obtained. With autografting, the thawed, transplanted, immature oocytes would mature in vivo, thereby obviating the need for exogenous gonadotropin stimulation. Autografting of ovarian tissue would theoretically preserve a woman's endocrinologic function, unlike IVF and oocyte cryopreservation, which only address fertility.

History of Ovarian Transplantation

Ovarian transplantation is not new; it has a long history dating back to the early 1900s. People believed that waning sex steroids resulted in somatic cell aging, and that transplantation held the key to rejuvenation and eternal youth. However, it was not until the turn of the twentieth century that widespread interest was generated in reproductive organ transplantation. Despite many attempts of allogeneic ovarian transplantation in the 1900s, no clear clinical benefit was realized, primarily due to immune reactions. A breakthrough occurred in 1948 when the first cryoprotectant, glycerol, was discovered. The development of freezing methods using cryoprotectants led to work on the transplantation of cryopreserved gonadal tissue in the 1950s [46,47], eventually leading to viable offspring in mice [48]. In the 1990s, investigators begun to realize the potential clinical applications of cryopreservation, and research began again using new cryoprotectants.

Cortical Strips

Most recent experience with ovarian transplantation has utilized strips of ovarian cortex. Most of the primordial follicles in ovarian tissue lie in the "outer skin", just beneath the tunica albuginea (see Fig. 8.2). After the ovary is removed, it can be bi-valved, and the inner medullary tissue dissected away, leaving a thin "rind" of ovarian tissue that contains most of the eggs. Thinness (1 mm) of the cortical tissue is important to allow adequate exposure to and diffusion of cryoprotectants into the ovarian tissue prior to cryopreservation. In addition, since ovarian cortical strips are transplanted without vascular anastamoses, thinness of the tissue is important since the graft must initially survive via simple diffusion until neovascularization can occur.

Heterotopic vs. Orthotopic Grafts

The ideal location for transplantation of ovarian tissue has not yet been defined. Orthotopic transplantation is grafting tissue back to its native site. For ovarian tissue, this would include transplantation of cortical tissue back to the ovarian hilum or a nearby location such as the pelvic sidewall [49]. Orthotopic transplantation provides the potential for spontaneous pregnancy without IVF (i.e., the oocyte can ovulate from the transplanted ovarian tissue, be picked up by the tube, fertilized, and implant in the uterus) [50,51].

Heterotopic transplantation involves grafting tissue back to a non-native, ectopic site. Ovarian tissue has been transplanted into the arm and abdomen [52,53]. Heterotopic transplantation allows for easier monitoring of follicular development

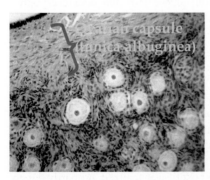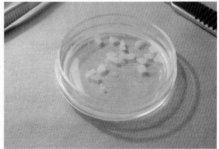

Fig. 8.2 (**A**) The density of primordial follicles is greatest just under the tunica albuginea. (**B**) The outer ovarian cortex has been cut in preparation for transplantation

and retrieval of oocytes. It also allows for easier monitoring of cancer growth within the transplanted ovarian tissue.

Animal Data

To date, successful cryopreservation and transplantation of ovarian tissue has been achieved in various animals. Cryopreservation of mouse ovarian tissue was found to produce good results with restoration of fertility after transplantation [48,54,55]. Fertility has also been restored using autografts stored at −196°C in ovariectomized sheep, whose ovaries more closely resemble those of humans [44]. Schnorr et al. transplanted autologous ovarian tissue into the upper arm of cynomolgus monkeys [56]. Menstrual cyclicity resumed in 5/6 (83%) fresh transplants and in 2/4 (50%) of thawed transplants.

Our lab [53] performed laparoscopic bilateral oophorectomies on seven rhesus macaques, and subsequently autologously transplanted fresh ovarian cortical tissue to the arm, abdomen, and kidney. Ovarian cortex was cut into 1×3×4 mm pieces ($n = 219$) in 4°C Leibovitz medium and transplanted immediately to the animal of origin in subcutaneous pockets or flaps juxtaposed to muscle or kidney (Fig. 8.3A, B). Four monkeys had transplants to both the arm and abdomen ($n = 23$–54), two to the kidney and abdomen ($n = 18$–42), and one to the arm only ($n = 26$). When 4 mm follicles developed, oocytes were collected via follicle excision 26–30 h after injecting 1,000 IU of human chorionic gonadotropin (hCG). Mature oocytes were fertilized via intracytoplasmic sperm injection (ICSI). All monkeys demonstrated estradiol (E2) levels greater than 50 pg/ml within 70–150 days post-transplantation. Estradiol and progesterone (P4) levels were higher in the local venous drainage of an arm transplant than in systemic venous blood, indicating the presence of functional grafted ovarian tissue (Fig. 8.3C). One monkey with renal and abdominal grafts showed repeated increases in P4 levels greater than 3 ng/ml approximately every 60 days, which is longer than the normal 28-day cycle (Fig. 8.4). FSH rose in this animal to 10.5 mIU/ml 84 days post-transplantation, but then declined to 2.79 mIU/ml by day 169, indicating adequate estrogen production. Several animals developed multiple follicles without exogenous gonadotropin stimulation; abdominal subcutaneous grafts showed the best follicular development (50%, Table 8.5). Follicles were excised ($n = 23$) from 4 hCG-treated monkeys; 16 oocytes were obtained. Eight were mature; six were fertilized via ICSI and cleaved in vitro. A five-cell, an eight-cell, and two morula-stage embryos were transferred laparoscopically to the oviducts of three recipient monkeys. A normal singleton gestation resulted from the transfer of the morulas, and ended in the birth of a healthy, 500-gram female in 2003 (Fig. 8.3D). She is named BRENDA for Bilateral oophorectomy, Resumption of ENDocrine function and Abdominal follicle pregnancy.

From the BRENDA data, several important conclusions can be drawn. First, transplantation into subcutaneous sites resulted in endocrine function and follicular development. Second, the abdomen appeared to be the best transplant site. Third, the resumption of endocrine function after about 130–150 days post-transplant is consistent with the time frame required for progression of primordial to antral

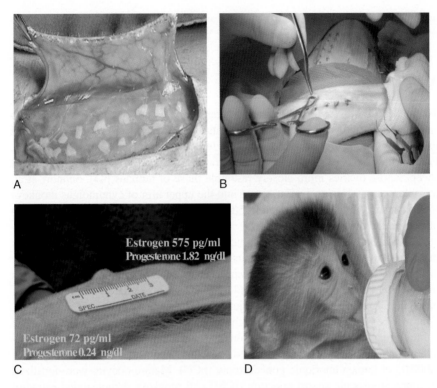

Fig. 8.3 (**A**) Ovarian tissue transplanted to the abdomen in flaps (**B**) and to subcutaneous pockets in the arm and abdomen (**C**) An ovarian follicle developing in the arm shows high local estrogen and progesterone secretion. Estradiol increased from 72 to 575 pg/ml in venous blood from the transplanted tissue. (**D**) Oocytes retrieved from heterotopic grafts were fertilized resulting in a healthy, term live-born monkey. From Lee DM et al. Nature 2004;428:137–138

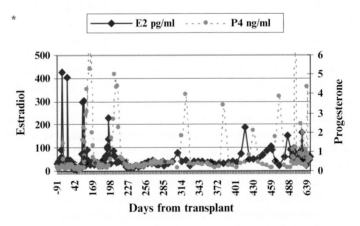

Fig. 8.4 Estradiol and progesterone are secreted cyclically after transplantation of ovarian tissue to the kidney and abdomen

Table 8.5 Of 219 ovarian tissue transplants, 49 developed follicles, and 23 were retrieved. Of 16 oocytes, 8 were mature, 6 were fertilized, and 3 embryos were transferred, resulting in 1 pregnancy

Site	#Graft	#Foll US	#Foll Ret	#Egg	#MII	#Fert	#Cleav	#ET	#Preg
L Arm	46	7	3	2	1	1	1	1	0
L Abd	54	27	15	11	6	5	5	2	1
L Kid	15	7	0	0	0	0	0	0	0
R Arm	44	5	4	3	1	0	0	0	0
R Abd	46	4	1	0	0	0	0	0	0
R Kid	14	1	0	0	0	0	0	0	0
Total	**219**	**49**	**23**	**16**	**8**	**6**	**6**	**3**	**1**
		22%	47%	70%		75%	100%		

Abd=abdomen; Cleav=cleaved; ET=embryo transfer; Fert=fertilized; Graf=grafted; Kid=kidney; L=left; MII=resumed meiosis; R=right; Ret=retrieved; US=ultrasound

follicle development [36,57,58]. Therefore, most likely, antral follicles are lost in the tissue preparation and transplantation process, and subsequent antral follicles represent in vivo maturation of the remaining primordial follicles.

Human Data

Oktay and colleagues first reported that ovulation occurred in autografted human ovarian tissue after gonadotropin stimulation [49,59]. A 29-year-old woman had undergone bilateral oophorectomy for benign indications. The ovarian tissue was cryopreserved in 1.5 M propanediol, thawed, and transplanted laparoscopically to the pelvic sidewall. The patient had follicular development documented by ultrasound with high doses of gonadotropins. In another case [52], ovarian tissue was transplanted to the forearm, and E2 measurements showed a gradient between the hand and cubital fossa, demonstrating functionality of the graft.

Radford et al. reported successful orthotopic transplantation of ovarian cortical tissue from a patient treated with chemotherapy for Hodgkin's lymphoma [60]. Seven months after transplanting ovarian cortical strips to the ovaries, she had resolution of hot flashes, E2 in the serum, a 10-mm endometrial lining, and a 2-cm diameter follicular structure seen by ultrasound.

Oktay et al. reported the first embryo derived from cryopreserved ovarian tissue that was heterotopically transplanted to the abdomen of a 30-year-old breast cancer patient [61]. Since then, four human pregnancies have been reported using both fresh and cryopreserved orthotopic ovarian tissue [50,51,62,63]. Donnez et al. [50] reported a 25-year-old patient with Hodgkin's lymphoma who underwent laparoscopic left ovarian cortical biopsies prior to MOPP/ABV chemotherapy and 38 Gy of radiation. She became amenorrheic with an FSH level of 91 mIU/ml. She then underwent laparoscopic peritoneal excision to promote vessel formation prior to ovarian tissue transplantation, followed by laparoscopic ovarian tissue transplantation to the pelvic sidewall 7 days later. A second laparoscopic transplant was also performed. She developed a follicle and became spontaneously pregnant. Although this is the first reported human pregnancy after ovarian tissue transplantation, it is possible that the pregnancy may have originated from an oocyte released from the ovary left in situ, and not from the transplanted ovarian tissue.

Silber et al. [51] subsequently reported a pregnancy from orthotopic transplantation of fresh ovarian tissue between monozygotic twins discordant for POF. One of two 24-year-old twins developed POF at age 13. The other twin went on to conceive three children spontaneously. After unsuccessful donor egg IVF, the sterile twin received a transplant of ovarian cortical tissue (fresh) from her sister via a mini-laparotomy. Within 3 months, the recipient's cycles resumed, and she conceived on the second cycle.

Meirow et al. [62] reported a definitive pregnancy from orthotopic transplantation of frozen/thawed ovarian tissue after chemotherapy-induced ovarian failure. The patient was a 28-year-old non-Hodgkin's lymphoma patient who had ovarian tissue harvested after first-line chemotherapy but before high-dose chemotherapy. Her FSH levels were consistently elevated (40–104 mIU/ml). Ovarian cortical tissue was transplanted via strips onto one ovary and via injection of a tissue slurry into the other ovary (Fig. 8.5). FSH levels decreased; Müllerian inhibiting substance and inhibin B increased. She conceived after natural cycle IVF.

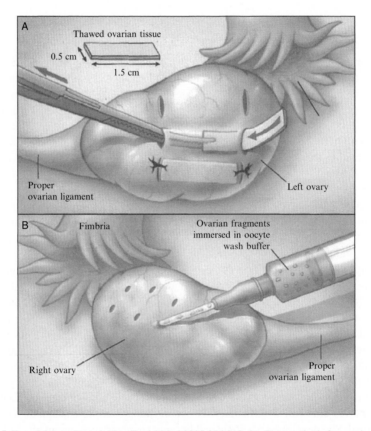

Fig. 8.5 From Meirow D et al. New Engl J Med 2005;355:318–21. Two methods for ovarian tissue transplantation: (**A**) Cortical strips, (**B**) Injection of ovarian tissue "slurry"

Demeestere et al. [63] performed simultaneous orthotopic and heterotopic transplantation of ovarian tissue. Follicles developed at the ovary, peritoneum, and abdomen. A spontaneous pregnancy ensued, but unfortunately ended in a miscarriage secondary to aneuploidy.

Whole Ovary Transplantation by Vascular Anastomosis

Transplanted ovarian cortical pieces rely upon simple diffusion for survival until new blood vessels form. Initially, the grafts are subject to ischemia. As an alternative approach, some have examined whether the intact ovary can be cryopreserved and subsequently transplanted via vascular anastomosis [64–67]. Wang et al. cryopreserved and then transplanted the upper uterus, fallopian tubes, and ovaries in mice, with a subsequent pregnancy [65]. Leporrier et al. performed heterotopic transplantation of an ovary to the arm using vascular anastomosis with extraction of a post-mature egg [64]. Bedaiwy et al. performed whole ovary transplantation in sheep, but in 8 of 11 animals, the vascular anastomosis had occluded completely [66]. Recently, Imhof et al. reported a live-born sheep from transplantation of a whole, frozen/thawed ovary [67]. One ovary was removed and the vessels cannulated so that the entire ovary could be perfused with cryoprotectant. After freezing and thawing, the contralateral ovary was surgically removed, and the thawed ovary transplanted back to the vascular pedicle. One of nine sheep became pregnant.

Problems with Ovarian Transplantation: Re-Introduction of Cancer

Although autografting seems promising, it is not without potential risks. Theoretically, ovarian tissue could carry micro-metastases that could "re-infect" a patient who had been previously cured of her cancer. Ovarian transplantation might be particularly concerning with blood-born malignancies, such as leukemia, where the cancer cells are already in the blood, and therefore presumably within the cryopreserved ovarian tissue. Shaw et al. showed that fresh and cryopreserved ovarian tissue samples taken from donors with lymphoma transmitted the cancer into previously healthy graft recipients [68]. This may bode poorly for the future of autografting, particularly for hematogenous malignancies like leukemia, or for patients with cancers known to metastasize to the ovary.

On the other hand, another study utilizing human tissue suggests that autologous ovarian transplantation is safe [69]. In this study, ovarian tissue from lymphoma patients was xenografted into immunodeficient mice. None of the mice developed lymphoma. However, when lymph nodes from the lymphoma patients were xenografted, mice transplanted with lymph nodes from the Hodgkin's disease patients did develop lymphoma (positive control).

Table 8.6 Risk of cancer metastases within the ovary [70]

Low risk of ovarian involvement	Squamous cell, cervix
	Ewing's sarcoma
	Breast cancer
	Stage I–III
	Infiltrative ductal
	Wilms' tumor
	Non-Hodgkin's lymphoma
	Hodgkin's lymphoma
	Osteogenic sarcoma
	Non-genital rhabdomyosarcoma
Moderate risk of ovarian involvement	Breast cancer
	Stage IV
	Infiltrative lobular
	Colon cancer (including tumors of rectum and appendix)
	Adeno/adenosquamous, cervix
	Upper gastrointestinal system
Cancers with high risk of ovarian involvement	Leukemia
	Burkitt's lymphoma
	Neuroblastoma
	Genital rhabdomyosarcoma

Hence, it is necessary to develop screening methods to detect minimal residual disease in ovarian tissue to eliminate the risk of cancer cell transmission with transplantation, or to consider xenografting or in vitro maturation, which would minimize re-introduction of cancer cells. A recent review attempts to stratify the risk of ovarian metastases (Table 8.6) [70].

Xenografting as a Potential Solution

Xenografting is another option for maturation of oocytes within cryopreserved ovarian tissue. Xenografting involves transplantation of ovarian tissue from one species (human) to another [severe combined immunodeficient (SCID) mice]. Because of the concern about re-introduction of cancer into patients via transplanted ovarian tissue, investigators have explored transplanting frozen-thawed ovarian tissue into an animal host that would serve as a biological incubator. With this technique, the possibility of cancer transmission and relapse can be minimized since maturation of the primordial follicles occurs in the animal host. When the follicle has matured in the mouse, a single egg can be isolated and fertilized, thereby theoretically eliminating exposure of the patient to cancer cells. However, xenografting may raise some ethical considerations; the concept of maturing human oocytes within another species is distasteful to some. Furthermore, xenografting raises the possibility of transmitting infectious agents or potentially altering the human genome.

Animal Data

Xenografting of cryopreserved ovarian tissue from non-human primates is feasible. Ovarian tissue from marmoset monkeys, which had been frozen and grafted into immunodeficient mice, developed viable, estrogen-producing follicles. Our lab [71] showed that rhesus ovarian tissue could be xenografted to SCID mice and that pre-antral and antral development could occur upon prolonged gonadotropin stimulation. The kidney capsule was a better site than subcutaneous sites for the grafts. There have already been live births reported from xenografting cyropreserved mouse ovarian tissue [72,73].

Human Data

Transplantation of frozen-thawed ovarian tissue into an animal host with subsequent gonadotropin stimulation and oocyte retrieval may offer considerable advantages to cancer survivors. Several groups have shown that human ovarian tissue can survive and grow to large antral stages in immunodeficient mice when transplanted subcutaneously, over the peritoneum, or under the kidney capsule [74–77]. Revascularization is critical for graft survival, and these sites are well vascularized, especially the subcapsular region of the kidney. Finally, Cha's group demonstrated that human fetal ovarian tissue could be vitrified in ethylene glycol and xenografted into NOD-SCID mice with resumption of follicular growth [78].

While these results are promising, a recent study raised the question of whether oocytes derived from xenografted ovarian tissue are ultrastructurally and

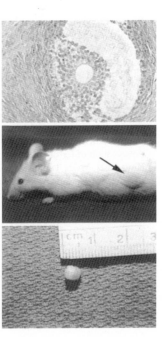

Fig. 8.6 Xenografted human ovarian cortex transplanted into a male NOD-SCID mouse following gonadotropin stimulation produces antral follicles [74]

reproductively competent [79]. When these oocytes were analyzed immunocyto-chemically, the microtubule organization and chromatin configuration were abnormal. It is possible that xenografting of human ovarian tissue will be more valuable as a research tool than as a clinical treatment. Xenografts could be used to examine which conditions might optimize autologous transplant conditions. Numerous factors, including anti-apoptotic agents [71], antioxidants like vitamin E or ascorbic acid, and angiogenic factors like vascular endothelial growth factor (VEGF), TGF, and FSH have been postulated to be beneficial. Further research is necessary to maximize the efficiency of ovarian tissue transplantation.

Conclusion

Ovarian tissue cryopreservation and transplantation is currently the most effective fertility-preserving treatment for prepubertal girls undergoing gonadotoxic cancer treatment and for women whose chemotherapy or radiation therapy must start immediately. Although there have been human pregnancies reported utilizing these methods, the underlying principles of cryobiology and transplantation biology must be further refined within the new field of oncofertility before widespread clinical application is possible.

References

1. Blatt J. Pregnancy outcome in long-term survivors of childhood cancer. Med Pediatr Oncol 1999;33:29–33.
2. Meirow D, Nugent D. The effects of radiotherapy and chemotherapy on female reproduction. Hum Reprod Update 2001;7:535–543.
3. Greenlee RT, Murray T, Bolden S, et al. Cancer statistics, 2000. CA Cancer J Clin 2000;50:7–33.
4. Meirow D. Ovarian injury and modern options to preserve fertility in female cancer patients treated with high dose radio-chemotherapy for hemato-oncological neoplasias and other cancer. Leuk Lymphoma 1999:33:65–76.
5. Meirow D. Epidemiology and infertility in cancer patients. In: Gosden R, Tulandi T, editors. Preservation of fertility. London: Taylor and Francis, 2004:21–38.
6. Koyama H, Wada T, Nishizawa Y, et al. Cyclophosphamide-induced ovarian failure and its therapeutic significance in patients with breast cancer. Cancer 1977;39:1403–1409.
7. Goldhirsch A, Gelber RD, Castiglione M. The magnitude of endocrine effects of adjuvant chemotherapy for premenopausal breast cancer patients. The International Breast Cancer Study Group. Ann Oncol 1990;1:183–188.
8. Chiarelli AM, Marrett LD, Darlington G. Early menopause and infertility in females after treatment for childhood cancer diagnosed in 1964–1988 in Ontario, Canada. Am J Epidemiol 1999;150:245–254.
9. Falcone T, Attaran M, Bedaiwy M, et al. Ovarian function preservation in the cancer patient. Fertil Steril 2004;81:243–257.
10. Wallace WH, Shalet SM, Hendry JH, et al. Ovarian failure following ovarian irradiation in childhood: the radiosensitivity of the human oocyte. Br J Radiol 1989;62:995–998.

4. Deansley R. Egg survival in immature rat ovaries grafted after freezing and thawing. Proc R Soc Lond B Biol Sci 1957;147:412–421.

5. Newton H, Aubard Y, Rutherford A, et al. Low temperature storage and grafting of human ovarian tissue. Hum Reprod 1996;11:1487–1491.

6. Whittingham DG, Leibo SP, Mazur P. Survival of mouse embryos frozen to –196 degrees and –269 degrees C. Science 1972;178:411–414.

7. Willadsen SM. Factors affecting the survival of sheep embryos during-freezing and thawing. Ciba Found Symp 1977;52:175–201.

8. Gosden RG, Boulton MI, Grant K, et al. Follicular development from ovarian xenografts in SCID mice. J Reprod Fertil 1994;101:619–623.

9. Harp R, Leibach J, Black J, et al. Cryopreservation of murine ovarian tissue. Cryobiology 1994;31:336–343.

10. Cox SL, Shaw J, Jenkin G. Transplantation of cryopreserved fetal ovarian tissue to adult recipients in mice. J Reprod Fertil 1996;107:315–322.

11. Sztein J, Sweet H, Farley J, et al. Cryopreservation and orthotopic transplantation of mouse ovaries: new approach in gamete banking. Biol Reprod 1998;58:1071–1074.

12. Shaw JM, Cox SL, Trounson AO, et al. Evaluation of the long-term function of cryopreserved ovarian grafts in the mouse, implications for human applications. Mol Cell Endocrinol 2000;161:103–110.

13. Gosden RG, Mullan J, Picton HM, et al. Current perspective on primordial follicle cryopreservation and culture for reproductive medicine. Hum Reprod Update 2002;8:105–110.

14. Baird DT, Webb R, Campbell BK, et al. Long-term ovarian function in sheep after ovariectomy and transplantation of autografts stored at –196°C. Endocrinology 1999;140: 462–471.

15. Arav A, Revel A, Nathan Y, et al. Oocyte recovery, embryo development and ovarian function after cryopreservation and transplantation of whole sheep ovary. Hum Reprod 2005;20:3554–3559.

16. Lee DM, Yeoman RR, Battaglia DE, et al. Live birth after ovarian tissue transplant. Nature 2004;428:137–138.

17. Aubard Y, Piver P, Cogni Y, et al. Orthotopic and heterotopic autografts of frozen-thawed ovarian cortex in sheep. Hum Reprod 1999;14:2149–2154.

18. Radford JA, Lieberman BA, Brison DR, et al. Orthotopic reimplantation of cryopreserved ovarian cortical strips after high-dose chemotherapy for Hodgkin's lymphoma. Lancet 2001;357:1172–1175.

19. Oktay K, Aydin BA, Karlikaya G. A technique for laparoscopic transplantation of frozen-banked ovarian tissue. Fertil Steril 2001;75:1212–1216.

20. Donnez J, Dolmans MM, Demylle D, et al. Livebirth after orthotopic transplantation of cryopreserved ovarian tissue. Lancet 2004;364:1405–1410.

21. Oktay K, Tilly J. Livebirth after cryopreserved ovarian tissue autotransplantation. Lancet 2004;364:2091–2092; author reply 2092–3.

22. Wallace WH, Pritchard J. Livebirth after cryopreserved ovarian tissue autotransplantation. Lancet 2004;364:2093–2094.

23. Meirow D, Levron J, Eldar-Geva T, et al. Pregnancy after transplantation of cryopreserved ovarian tissue in a patient with ovarian failure after chemotherapy. N Engl J Med 2005;353:318–321.

24. Leporrier M, von Theobald P, Roffe JL, et al. A new technique to protect ovarian function before pelvic irradiation. Heterotopic ovarian autotransplantation. Cancer 1987;60:2201–2204.

25. Leporrier M, Roffe JL, Von Theobald P, et al. Autologous transplantation of whole ovaries vs ovarian cortical strips. JAMA 2002;287:44–45.

26. Marconi G, Quintana R, Rueda-Leverone NG, et al. Accidental ovarian autograft after a laparoscopic surgery: case report. Fertil Steril 1997;68:364–366.

27. Oktay K, Economos K, Kan M, et al. Endocrine function and oocyte retrieval after autologous transplantation of ovarian cortical strips to the forearm. JAMA 2001;286:1490–1493.

28. Oktay K, Buyuk E, Rosenwaks Z, et al. A technique for transplantation of ovarian cortical strips to the forearm. Fertil Steril 2003;80:193–198.

29. Oktay K, Buyuk E, Veeck L, et al. Embryo development after heterotopic transplantation of cryopreserved ovarian tissue. Lancet 2004;363:837–840.
30. Oktay K, Oktem O. Sustained endocrine function and spontaneous pregnancies after subcutaneous transplantation of cryopreserved ovarian tissue in stem cell transplant recipients. Fertil Steril 2005; 84(Suppl 1):S68.
31. Johnson J, Canning J, Kaneko T, et al. Germline stem cells and follicular renewal in the postnatal mammalian ovary. Nature 2004;428:145–150.
32. Oktay K. Spontaneous conceptions and live birth after heterotopic ovarian transplantation: is there a germline stem cell connection? Hum Reprod 2006;21:1345–1348.
33. Shaw JM, Bowles J, Koopman P, et al. Fresh and cryopreserved ovarian tissue samples from donors with lymphoma transmit the cancer to graft recipients. Hum Reprod 1996;11: 1668–1673.
34. Spears N, Boland NI, Murray AA, et al. Mouse oocytes derived from in vitro grown primary ovarian follicles are fertile. Hum Reprod 1994;9:527–532.
35. Eppig JJ, O'Brien MJ. Development in vitro of mouse oocytes from primordial follicles. Biol Reprod 1996;54:197–207.
36. Xu M, Kreeger PK, Shea LD, et al. Tissue-Engineered Follicles Produce Live, Fertile Offspring. Tissue Eng 2006; [Epub ahead of print].
37. Reaman GH. Pediatric oncology: current views and outcomes. Pediatr Clin North Am 2002;49:1305–1318, vii.
38. Poirot C, Vacher-Lavenu MC, Helardot P, Guibert J, Brugieres L, Jouannet P. Related Articles, Links et al. Human ovarian tissue cryopreservation: indications and feasibility. Hum Reprod 2002;17:1447–1452.
39. Poirot CJ, Martelli H, Genestie C, et al. Feasibility of ovarian tissue cryopreservation for prepubertal females with cancer. Pediatr Blood Cancer 2006; [Epub ahead of print].

Part IV
Health Care Decision-Making

Chapter 10
Oncofertility and the Social Sciences

Karrie Ann Snyder, PhD

Due to breakthroughs in medical technology and more aggressive forms of cancer treatment, today most people diagnosed with cancer survive. In 2000, over 2.5 million adults of childbearing age were survivors of cancer [1,2]. And by 2010, it is estimated that one out of every 250 adults will be a survivor of childhood cancer [3,4]. The more aggressive forms of treatment that have made it possible for more people, particularly those diagnosed at younger ages, to survive cancer, however, also often impair an individual's fertility. The field of oncofertility has emerged as a way to address lost or impaired fertility in those with a history of cancer. Biomedical research in this area is active in developing new ways to help those afflicted preserve their ability to have biological children. Oncofertility is also an interdisciplinary field that bridges biomedical and social sciences and examines issues regarding an individual's fertility concerns, options, and choices in light of cancer diagnosis, treatment, and survivorship. Although the potential effects of cancer treatment on an individual's fertility are well documented, the rate and extent of fertility impairment among those who have undergone cancer treatment are not fully known. Similarly, within the social sciences, how cancer patients are affected by infertility in their day-to-day lives and the impact on their sense of self have been largely overlooked. Improved survivorship rates over the last several decades, however, mean that cancer-related infertility is an issue that will become a concern for an increasing portion of the population along with their partners and families.

Biomedical and social science research have largely been separate areas of scholarship with little discussion or inquiry across fields. However, a recent issue of *Science* implored that "the successful application of new knowledge and breakthrough technologies, which are likely to occur with ever-increasing frequency, will require an entirely new interdisciplinary approach" (p. 1847) [5]. Similarly, the interdisciplinary nature of oncofertility recognizes that understanding the social dynamics, institutional behaviors, and structural factors that envelop emerging technologies are not secondary research issues but require careful empirical inquiry as technologies are developed because the surrounding social environment influences and is affected by how those technologies are integrated into society and used by individuals and institutions. Including social science research as a constitutive part of oncofertility will help to broaden understanding within the

137

T.K. Woodruff and K.A. Snyder (eds.) *Oncofertility*.
© Springer 2007

health care community regarding cancer patients' concerns about their fertility and future family plans. Specifically, social science can help to uncover how cancer patients, along with their families and physicians, make health care decisions that are cognizant of fertility concerns and how these decisions are couched in specific social, legal, economic, and cultural contexts. Social science insight will be vital to the field of oncofertility as it grows. The intent of this chapter is to highlight some important first steps that build upon existing scholarship within the social sciences, including medical sociology, gender studies, racial/ethnic studies, communications research, and stratification.

Studying Cancer Within the Social Sciences

There are few health issues that have received as much attention within biomedical sciences, the political arena, and the media as cancer. As a leading cause of death, cancer receives much in the way of government-sponsored and private research monies, volunteer efforts, political advocacy, and public interest. Social scientists have well considered many aspects of health and illness, including the stigma associated with illness (particularly mental illness); disparities in health care prevention, treatment, and outcomes; the organization and access to health care systems; and issues of professionalization and expert knowledge within the health care community. Curiously, less attention has been paid to cancer as a realm of inquiry. Tritter, in fact, calls for a distinct "sociology of cancer" because cancer challenges how we think of disease and illness [6]. For one, it is a diffuse category that includes over 200 variants recognized by histopathologists and its treatment cuts across many medical disciplines, including surgery, oncology, palliative care, and occupational therapy, resulting in a highly complex and blurred network of caregivers and health care institutions treating a single patient [6]. It is not always clear which medical professional is in "charge" of a particular issue, particularly who should advise cancer patients regarding potential fertility impairment.

Cancer also challenges how we think of a "sick" person [6]. Many cancer patients do not exhibit feelings of illness upon diagnosis (although this varies with the form). It is often the treatment, including chemotherapy and radiation therapies, that results in sickness. Moreover, a cancer diagnosis itself is often a transformative experience in a person's life akin to other major illness (such as mental illness, HIV/AIDS, or muscular sclerosis) whereby the illness becomes a master status. But unlike most other illnesses and disorders, cancer becomes a prominent part of an individual's biography, even after someone is successfully "cured." People who have overcome cancer are forever viewed as "survivors."

Cancer is a transformative experience in an individual's life not only because of the survivorship status it confers, but because of the secondary health issues that can be caused by the cancer or its subsequent treatment, including impaired fertility. As a broad discipline, oncofertility intends to look at reasons leading to fertility impairment and to develop ways to safeguard a cancer patient's fertility. The aim of oncofertility is also to explore how infertility impacts those with cancer, their families, and their future family goals and plans. The perspective of oncofertility is that fertility and cancer combine to create a unique set of issues to be researched. It is not simply that cancer patients have a different set of options than non-cancer patients in terms of becoming a parent, but rather having cancer qualitatively alters how one makes choices regarding family planning and goals. Undoubtedly, there is a host of issues that social scientists can tackle within the realm of oncofertility, but important first steps would be to look at health care decision making regarding cancer and fertility preserving treatment choices because of the impact of cancer and related infertility has on the lives of those with cancer and their families. Moreover, social science inquiry within oncofertility should be particularly attuned to issues of gender and race/ethnic diversity because of the implications for disparities in the experiences of cancer survivors in terms of reaching family and parenting goals.

Gender and Oncofertility

An important avenue for research within oncofertility would be to look at gender differences in the fertility concerns of male and female cancer patients, differences in the health care decisions men and women make regarding whether or not to take steps to pursue fertility-conserving treatment options (such as sperm banking or emergency IVF), and the impact of infertility on men's and women's survivorship experiences. Historically, men with cancer have had more effective options in terms of safeguarding their fertility. Men who have reached puberty have long had the option of cryopreserving sperm for later use (as was done by Lance Armstrong when diagnosed with advanced testicular cancer). Women have had far less successful options (see Appendix, this volume, for overview of options). For those with cancer of non-reproductive organs, shielding ovaries during radiation treatment or emergency in vitro fertilization (IVF) are the most common options. However, shielding only has a limited effect and emergency IVF delays cancer treatment and can only be performed on those who have reached puberty. Because emergency IVF requires fertilization and results in an embryo, the decision is also fraught with ethical issues (e.g., What happens to fertilized embryos if the woman does not survive? What if a married couple divorces prior to the embryos being used? What about women who do not have a partner?). Although women who have been diagnosed with cancer have much improved chances of being able to bear children today, the chances of post-diagnosis parenthood is still far greater among male cancer patients [7]. The field of oncofertility emerged as a way to address this gender inequity by developing more options for women. Yet, there is little insight into "what survivors know about their own fertility status, how and when they obtain information regarding the impact of cancer treatment on their fertility, and how they respond to that information" (p. 869) [8]. Research could look at differences in the fertility concerns of men and women at the time of diagnosis as well as a comparison of the health care decisions that men and women regarding fertility-conserving treatments.

Gender and Patient-Physician Interactions

One major question that remains unanswered is how cancer patients learn about possible fertility impairment and fertility-conserving treatment options, particularly in the context of the doctor-patient relationship, and how this may differ by gender. While those facing cancer may turn to the Internet or other sources for information, most still rely on their doctors as their primary information source [9,10]. The small body of research on patient-physician interaction regarding cancer and fertility (most of which exists outside of the social sciences) points to rather worrisome findings. In several studies, many, if not most, respondents did not recall having discussions with their physicians regarding the possible impact of cancer treatment on their fertility. Less than 60% of young adults who have survived cancer could recall discussions of possible infertility due to cancer treatment [11–14]. Although studies of adult survivors of childhood cancer often rely on recollections of conversations held years earlier, results for those diagnosed as adults are similar. Only 72% of younger women with breast cancer discussed fertility with their doctor in one study [15], and half of physicians in another study reported "rarely" or "never" addressing sperm banking or infertility issues with male cancer patients at risk for infertility [16]. Also, cancer patients who want fertility information do not always get adequate information. Younger women dealing with breast cancer have reported receiving insufficient information on the impact of cancer treatment on their fertility or what could be done [17].

So while a lack of information regarding fertility seems to be a common feature of most cancer patients' diagnostic and treatment experiences, what is not known is how men and women facing fertility-threatening cancer treatment interact with health care staff, if this differs by gender, and how these potential gender differences affect the flow of fertility-related information. In particular, there are almost no direct comparisons of men and women in terms of the likelihood of discussing fertility or treatment options with a doctor. Research has shown that the gender of the physician can alter what topics or issues are brought up with male and female patients [18]. Further, one study of proactive fertility-related behaviors of men who have undergone treatment for testicular cancer suggests that some behaviors (i.e., fertility testing) were more likely to occur among the higher educated, suggesting "that physicians identify more closely with the men with whom they share status characteristics and, therefore offer them more encouragement or information" (p. 353) [19]. This may indicate that when doctor and patient share status similarities (such as gender), physicians may be more likely to discuss such sensitive issues. Because men still outnumber women among doctors, women may be disadvantaged in discussing fertility with a physician because men are more likely to have a physician of their same gender. Understanding how fertility information is shared between physician and patient and how this may differ by gender is vital because it has been found that concerns over infertility can alter treatment decisions [13,15], and the biggest barrier to undergoing fertility-conserving treatment is a lack of information (even for relatively simple procedures such as sperm banking) [20].

Gender and the Experience of Infertility

A key part of oncofertility involves looking at the post-treatment fertility of cancer survivors and its impact on their lives. Those who have investigated the impact of infertility on the concerns of cancer survivors from a social science perspective tend to focus on a group of cancer survivors (e.g., breast or childhood cancer survivors), which is often limited to a particular gender and with most focusing on women. This research has shown that for some women infertility can be as distressing as cancer itself [1,21,22]. Very few studies exist that compare men's and women's experiences with infertility directly (for exception, see [1]), leading to a lack of understanding within the social sciences of how men and women experience infertility post-cancer.

More generally, research has looked at the emotional distress that often accompanies infertility (see [23] for review) and suggests that women and men do in fact experience infertility differently. Women's infertility tends to challenge their status or self-image as a "complete" woman, which for many involves being a good wife and mother, whereas male infertility calls into question sexual potency and masculinity [23].[1] In one study of infertile couples, Clarke et al. found that both men and women saw parenthood as a mark of adulthood and that infertility called into question their gendered self-image. However, men were more concerned with how infertility called into question their masculinity and sexual prowess, whereas women placed greater emphasis on their bodies in needing of repair, which stemmed from the fact that medical interventions are often aimed at women in infertile couples.

As a field, oncofertility recognizes that cancer and fertility combine to create a new set of issues to be addressed, such as infertility having a unique impact on individuals because of their cancer diagnosis. Most research on infertility has been on "healthy" individuals and couples. For example, those who are infertile commonly desire to feel "normal" when compared with their peers who can conceive [23]. But for those who have survived cancer, having a child may take on an even greater importance because it allows them to feel not only normal, but healthy as well [8]. Further, cancer may alter the experience of infertility differently for men and women. For example, Clarke et al., who studied otherwise healthy couples, concluded that "Infertility shatters previously held perceptions of the body and the self as healthy, whole, and normal" (p. 110) [23]. For cancer patients, their bodies have already "let them down." Men with cancer are placed in a unique position compared with men who have infertility issues in that they may be more likely to be targeted for medical treatments or take the "blame" for a couple's infertility, an experience more akin to those of women in studies of infertility.

---

[1] There are many conceptions of masculinity and feminity available to men and women that may not rely so heavily on fertility and parenthood, but those that are more socially validated tend to be premised on more traditional notions of women as caregivers (including mothers) and men as sexually potent providers (see Clarke et al. 2006).

Moreover, for cancer patients, infertility may interplay with concerns over sexual identity and performance in a unique way from those who are infertile. Clarke et al. found that men's sense of sexual identity was more compromised than a woman's because men equated infertility with sexual dysfunction whereas women's desirability as a sexual partner was not called into question. Depending the form of cancer, issues of sexual dysfunction or desirability may take on a different meaning for those with cancer. Testicular cancer can lead to sexual difficulties in men, so issues of infertility may be even more closely tied to issues of sexual performance and virility. Women, such as those with breast cancer, must contend with infertility in addition to changes in body image related to cancer treatment (such as a mastectomy or hair loss), which can alter their feelings of sexual desirability, and other bodily changes that may alter one's desire or ability to engage in sexual activity, including hormonal changes and fatigue [24,25]. Those with or who have had cancer must confront possible infertility in a context where one's entire sexual being has been impacted by having cancer.

Beyond one's perceived status as a sexual partner, cancer survivors have reported that infertility, or its possibility, can cause tension in relationships, particularly ones viewed as "serious" or "committed" [8,25]. In fact, in looking at testicular cancer, an important determinate of "good health-related quality of life" 3–13 years post-treatment is associated with having intact fertility, having children, and living with a partner (p. 1597 [26], also see [27,28]). Those who are infertile may also be troubled over their ability to maintain or begin a partner relationship, and for cancer patients, this issue is further complicated by their own concerns of reoccurrence and survivorship. Many women who have had cancer are concerned that becoming pregnant will make the reoccurrence of cancer more likely or that their children will be more susceptible to illness.[2] Infertility and having children may be markedly distinct experiences for those with or who have survived cancer, which makes parenthood and infertility among cancer survivors an interesting topic for social scientists interested in family studies. It also presents an intriguing gender comparison because of the potential differences in the long-term impact of infertility on the survivorship experiences of men and women.

Race/Ethnicity and Oncofertility

The above discussion highlights the importance of building on the long tradition in gender comparative research to better understand how cancer patients deal with possible infertility, associated health care decisions, and the long-term impact of infertility on their lives. The experience of cancer and fertility, however, may differ along other social statuses as well. An important area of inquiry would be

---

[2] Despite these common fears among those who have had cancer, there is little scientific evidence. For complete discussion, see fertilehope.org.

comparative analyses looking at the fertility concerns and related health care decisions by race/ethnicity. Research within the social sciences has well-documented inequities across racial and ethnic groups in terms of infant mortality, life expectancy, exposure to health insurance, and the quality of medical care available. This inequity extends to cancer as well. Overall, cancer rates vary by racial and ethnic background. For example, African–American men and women in general have a higher overall incidence of cancer, including higher rates of prostate, cervix, and lung cancers [29]. There are also disparities in when cancer is diagnosed and mortality rates. For example, although Caucasian women have the highest overall incidence rate of breast cancer, they are diagnosed at earlier stages and have lower mortality rates than African–American women [29,30]. These disparities in terms of cancer diagnosis, treatment, and morbidity have been linked to a host of interlocking economic, social, cultural, and environmental factors including health insurance coverage, access to quality health care, and the availability of economic resources, as well as differences in risk-behaviors (e.g., smoking rates), cancer screening behaviors (e.g., mammographies), and underlying risk factors for some cancers (e.g., obesity and history of infectious disease within a group) [29].

Research within oncofertility could build upon this firm foundation of looking at health care inequalities by race/ethnicity and associated differences in socioeconomic status. This area of research is important because whether or not a woman or man takes steps to help maintain fertility functioning (or is made aware of potential options) will impact his or her later ability to bear children. Hence, systematic variation in the options and information accessed by various groups (such as poorer women or racial/ethnic minorities) and their subsequent health care decisions may lead to later disparities in terms of which survivors are able to preserve fertility through the latest and emerging reproductive technologies. Down the road, those who have impaired fertility will also have different access to resources (e.g., financial resources and health insurance) to take advantage of costly fertility treatments (e.g., IVF) in order to conceive and bear biological children. Similarly, those with impaired fertility will differ in their ability to pursue other avenues to become parents, including adoption and surrogacy, due to financial constraints, legal issues (e.g., bans on adoption for single or homosexual women), and cultural or ethical concerns (e.g., cultural proscriptions against surrogacy).

Race/Ethnicity and Patient–Physician Interactions

In particular, research should consider racial/ethnic differences in patient–physician communication and their impact on health care decision-making regarding fertility and fertility preservation options. This emphasis will help to uncover possible inequities in terms of cancer patients' access to information, their ability to pursue fertility preservation treatments, and ultimately, differences in terms of which groups of survivors are able to become parents. Today, racial and ethnic minority groups make up 25% of the United States, but by 2,050 these groups will constitute the majority of the population [31]. Increasingly, doctor and patient interactions will take place in a setting of cultural dissimilarity, which may influence how information and concerns are shared, how fertility preservation options are considered, and how health care decisions are made [31]. Research would be advised to understand how such sensitive health care decisions regarding fertility are made in the context of racial/ethnic (along with socio-economic) dissimilarity that will continue to become more commonplace. An important part of this research would be to understand how gender further influences the discussion of infertility between cancer patient and doctor. Depending on religious or cultural backgrounds, women and men with cancer may be more willing to share concerns regarding sensitive topics like loss of fertility or sexual performance with a physician when they share a common cultural background or language skills as their doctor.

How doctors approach fertility may differ based on the patient they are advising. For example, research has shown that doctors with different patient populations can vary in how they convey medical information. Doctors with largely minority populations, as compared with those with a Caucasian client base, are less likely to suggest preventative care (e.g., mammographies) and these differences have been attributed to physician education, time spent with patients, and the socioeconomic status of patients [32]. As stated above, doctors may share more fertility-related information with cancer patients when they share a similar status or cultural background.

Examining issues of racial and ethnic variation in doctor–patient relationships and its impact on infertility-cancer related treatment choices is vital because of the varied histories of racial and ethnic groups within the United States health care system, particularly the legacy of distrust for some groups. A patient may distrust the medical system based on their personal experiences with overcrowded or outdated health care facilities (which are undoubtedly linked to economic resources), and also from historical antecedents. Culturally, many racial and ethnic groups may avoid of medical treatment because of "deeply embedded distrust of the medical system" [33] stemming from a negative racial or ethnic history with the medical community (e.g., Tuskegee experiments) and perceived cultural insensitivity among doctors [34]. Tense interactions between health care staffs and patient may differ by gender as well. For example, the gendered nature of the traditional doctor (male)–patient (female) relationship has resulted in women's health being compromised based on the history of forced sterilization for many minority groups [35]. This history may make minority women particularly wary of discussions regarding fertility with physicians, who tend to be Caucasian males.

Race/Ethnicity and Family and Community Involvement

While health care decisions are commonly thought of in terms of a patient–physician dyad, exploring the role of family, and even the larger community, will be particularly important for understanding fertility-related concerns and decisions across racial/ethnic groups. For example, research on African–Americans with cancer has shown a reliance on family as a source of information (along with misinformation) [34]. The role of the larger community in the experience of illness can also differ by race/ethnicity as well as gender. One study found that Japanese–American men and European–American women facing cancer were "able to draw on their social support networks more readily and accept the dependent role more easily" whereas European–American men and Japanese–American women were more distressed in facing cancer (p. 579, [31]). Further, an individual's fertility treatment decision may be influenced by their family through larger community, cultural, and religious traditions and values. Many treatment options, such as emergency IVF or alternative routes to parenthood, such as surrogacy or adoption, are not seen as acceptable within some cultural or religious groups. Understanding the nature of cultural differences between patient and doctor, the roles of families and communities in health care decisions, and how these impact fertility treatment decisions and concerns is important because of the increasing relevance of post-cancer infertility for many families and the increasing diversity of the United States.

The Digitial Divide and Race/Ethnicity

Finally, an increasingly important area of research within oncofertility would be to look at racial/ethnic differences and disparities in terms of access to health care information beyond health care practitioners, including Internet- and Web-based resources. In general, "e-health" refers to information and communication technologies, most notably the Internet, as sources of health-related information for individuals and as mechanisms that can promote health-related behaviors. Although patients still rely heavily on practitioners for health care advice, other sources of health-related information, including e-health Web sites (e.g., cancer information sites and online support groups) have become increasingly important avenues for information related to prevention behaviors, treatment options, and even emotional support [36–38]. Generally, it has been well documented that a "digital divide" exists along socio-economic, education, and racial/ethnic lines with regard to access to the Internet (although this gap has somewhat narrowed from the late 1990s) [36]. Being newer sources of information and intervention, e-health Web sites and programs have not been widely evaluated, but early research shows positive results in the potential of e-health sources to contribute to better health outcomes, including promising findings on shared decision-making and healthy behavioral changes (for overview, see [38]).

In terms of those with cancer, comparative research is needed on differences in access to computers and the World Wide Web, but also on how racial/ethnic groups use online sources (e.g., entertainment or health-related purposes) and the accessibility and relevancy of information on the Web that meets "the cultural, language, or literacy needs of the individual user" [37]. Improved communication technologies will undoubtedly have consequences for a range of cancer-related issues, including the use of preventative screening procedures (e.g., self-exams for testicular and breast cancer) and healthy lifestyle behaviors (e.g., smoking cessation). Studying access to electronic forms of information is, however, particularly relevant for oncofertility because of the rapidity with which health care decisions regarding fertility preservation need to be made. Procedures often need to occur prior to cancer treatment. The Web may provide a source of not only quick information, but also the most up-to-date information because new and experimental options may not be familiar to all doctors. Also, since doctors do not often prioritize issues of infertility or treatment options when treating patients with cancer, online sources and even support group sites may provide much needed information regarding infertility and treatment options for patients. Looking at access to e-health sources is vital because differences in the availability of e-health information across racial/ethnic and socioeconomic groups may have long-term consequences on cancer survivorship experiences with regard to parenthood and family formation.

Conclusion

The above discussion highlights some of the important issues that need to be addressed within the social sciences and oncofertility. I focused on individual level experiences and decision-making processes because so little is known about the fertility concerns of those with cancer, how they make fertility-conserving treatment choices, and their survivorship experiences regarding parenthood and family planning. An understanding of how these issues may differ by key social status, particularly gender and race/ethnicity (along with socioeconomic status or religious affiliation), is important because of the possibility of disparities in terms of fertility and parenthood for cancer survivors.

As oncofertility as a field of scholarship grows and as its biomedical techniques become mainstreamed into medical practice, there will be ample opportunity for research focusing on meso- and macro-levels of analysis. How do scholars come together and build an interdisciplinary field? How do norms concerning research and scholarship develop when actors come from a variety of fields and backgrounds? Oncofertility social researchers can also examine how emerging technologies become integrated into cancer care. How do hospitals and medical education programs integrate new standards into practice? How are such reforms institution-alized and is there ever resistance to new technologies? Research could also look at how biomedical technology affects the social perception of illness. Cancer is increasingly a survivable condition with most patients returning to the trajectories of their lives, but what is the cultural image of the cancer patient? Will expanding awareness that cancer patients often can and do become parents post-cancer help to change the societal image of cancer from one of a devastating illness to that of a manageable disease? These are just some of the ways that social scientists can expand on the initial scholarship advanced here. The ideas put forth here are just some important first steps in developing robust scholarship that will draw together scholars from a range of fields to ask new questions and develop new concepts and ways of looking at the important and growing concern of infertility among cancer survivors.

References

1. Schover LR. Motivation for parenthood after cancer: a review. J Natl Cancer Inst Monogr 2005;34:2–5.
2. Bureau. USC. US Summary 2000: 2000 Census Profile. Washington, DC: Government Publication C2KPROF00US, 2002.
3. Ries L, Harkins D, Krapcho M, editors. SEER cancer statistics review, 1975–2003. Bethesda, MD: National Cancer Institute.
4. Bleyer W. The impact of childhood cancer on the United States and the world. Cancer 1990;40:355–367.
5. Lane N. Alarm bells should help us refocus. Science 2006;312:1847.
6. Tritter J. The sociology of cancer. Research advances in medical sociology. Presented at: XV World Congress of Sociology. July 12, 2002, Brisbane, Australia.
7. Fossa S, Magelssen H, Melve K, et al. Parenthood in survivors after adulthood cancer and perinatal health in their offspring: a preliminary report. J Natl Cancer Inst Monogr 2005;34:77–82.
8. Zebrack B, Casillas J, Nohr L, et al. Fertility issues for young adult survivors of childhood cancer. Psycho-oncology 2004;13:689–699.
9. Nelson DE, Kreps GL, Hesse BW, et al. The Health Information National Trends Survey (HINTS): development, design, and dissemination. J Health Commun 2004;5:443–460.
10. Shaw B, Gustafson D, Hawkins R, et al. How underserved breast cancer patients use and benefit from eHealth programs. Am Behav Sci 2006;49:823–834.
11. Schover L. Psychosocial aspects of infertility and decisions about reproduction in young cancer survivors: a review. Med Pediatr Oncol 1999;33:53–59.
12. Schover L, Rybicki L, Martin B, et al. Having children after cancer: a pilot survey of survivor's attitudes and experiences. Cancer 1999;86:697–709.
13. Canada A, Schover L. Research promoting better patient education on reproductive health after cancer. J Natl Cancer Inst Monogr 2005;34:98–100.
14. Schover L, Brey K, Lichtin L, et al. Knowledge and experience regarding cancer, infertility, and sperm banking in younger male survivors. J Clin Oncol 2002;20:1880–1889.
15. Partridge A, Gelber S, Peppercorn J, et al. Web-based survey of fertility issues in young women with breast cancer. J Clin Oncol 2004;22:4174–4183.
16. Schover L, Brey K, Lichtin L, et al. Oncololgists' attitudes and practices regarding banking sperm before cancer treatment. J Clin Oncol 2002;20:1890–1897.
17. Thewes B, Butow P, Girgis A, et al. The psychosocial needs of breast cancer survivors: a qualitative study of the shared and unique needs of younger versus older survivors. Psyco-oncology 2004;13:177–189.
18. Tabenkin H, Goodwin M, Zyzanski S, et al. Gender differences in time spent during direct observation of doctor-patient encounters. J Women's Health. 2004;13:341–349.
19. Rieker P, Fitzgerald E, Kalish L. Adaptive behavioral responses to potential infertility among Survivors of testis cancer. J Clin Oncol 1990;8:347–355.
20. Statistics 2006. Available at: Fertilehope.org. Accessed November 13, 2006.
21. Dow K. Having children after breast cancer. Cancer Pract. 1994;2:407–413.
22. Surbone A, Petrek J. Childbearing issues in breast carcinoma survivors. Cancer 1997;79:1271–1278.

23. Clarke L, Martin-Matthews A, Matthews R. The continuity and discontinuity of the embodied self in infertility. Canadian review of sociology and anthropology. 2005;4:95–113.
24. Thaler-DeMers D. Intimacy issues: sexuality, fertility, and relationships. Sem Oncol Nurs 2001;17:255–262.
25. Takahashi M, Kai I. Sexuality after breast cancer treatment: changes and coping strategies among Japanese survivors. Soc Sci Med 2005;61:1278–1290.
26. Gurevich M, Bishop S, Bower J, et al. (Dis)embodying gender and sexuality in testicular cancer. Soc Sci Med 2004;58:1597–1607.
27. Rudberg L, Nilson S, Wikblad K. Health-related quality of life in survivors of testicular cancer. J Psychosoc Oncol 2000;18:19–31.
28. Wenzel L, Dogan-Ates A, Habbal R, et al. Psychosocial, ethical, and legal issues defining and measuring reproductive concerns of female cancer survivors. J Nat Cancer Inst Monogr 2005;34:94–98.
29. Ward E, Jemal A, Cokkinides V, et al. Cancer disparities by race/ethnicity and socioeconomic status. CA. 2004;54:78–93.
30. Ghafoor A, Jemal A, Ward E, et al. Trends in breast cancer by race and ethnicity. CA. 2003;53:342–355.
31. Kagawa-Singer M, Kassim-Lakha S. A strategy to reduce cross-cultural miscommunication and increase the likelihood of improving health outcomes. Acad Med. 2003;78:577–587.
32. Gemson DH, Elinson J, Messeri P. Differences in physician prevention patterns for white and minority patients. J Community Health 1988;13:53–64.
33. Gadson S. The health disparities question: will pay-for-performance measure up? Presented at: 2006 Leadership Summit on Health Disparities, AMA/National Minority Health Month Foundation. April 12, 2006, Washington, DC, 2006.
34. Matthews A, Sellergren S, Manfredi C, et al. Factors influencing medical information seeking among African American cancer patients. J Health Commun 2002;7:205–219.
35. Auerbach J, Fiert A. Women's health research: public policy and sociology. J Health Soc Behav 1995;35:115–131.
36. Gibbons MC. A historical overview of health disparities and the potential of eHealth Solutions. J Med Internet Res. 2005;7:e50.
37. Kreps G. Communication and racial inequities in health care. Am Behav Sci 2006;49:760–774.
38. Neuhauser L, Kreps G. Rethinking communication in the E-health era. J Health Psychol 2003;8:7–23.

Chapter 11
Shared Decision Making:
Fertility and Pediatric Cancers

Marla L. Clayman, PhD, MPH, Kathleen M. Galvin, PhD,
and Paul Arntson, PhD

> *We live our lives like chips in a kaleidoscope, always part of*
> *patterns that are larger than ourselves and somehow more*
> *than the sum of their parts.*
> — *Salvador Minuchin*

Childhood cancer is a familial disease; no family member escapes unscathed from the impact of a young person's cancer diagnosis, treatment, and follow-up procedures. As new treatment options unfold and more children survive, families are faced with multiple critical decisions at the time of diagnosis. This chapter will address one of the goals of oncofertility research – to improve the decision making competencies of family members confronting the news of a child's cancer diagnosis plus the additional information that the treatment may or will affect the child's future fertility. We will bring together key constructs and research from family systems theory and the shared decision making model in order to understand better how families whose children are newly diagnosed with cancer can make informed choices about the future fertility of their children while immediately confronting a potentially life-threatening illness.

To accomplish this purpose, the chapter will unfold in the following manner: first, we will briefly articulate the current state of childhood cancer and fertility preservation. Second, we will explicate a systems approach to family communication and decision making. Third, we will summarize the recent evolving work on shared decision making in health care. Fourth, the current state of childhood cancer and fertility preservation options will be described as a highly stressful context into which a family systems approach and shared decision making models must be integrated for immediate and long-range successful health care outcomes. In doing so, we will review the recent research that has investigated how families and health care professionals do and want to make decisions about fertility preservation when children are diagnosed with cancer. We will conclude by summarizing what we now know about shared decision making by families and health care professionals concerning fertility preservation for children with cancer and what we still need to know.

As family members and health professionals confront this situation together, the desired outcome is a shared decision-making process that involves parent(s),

T.K. Woodruff and K.A. Snyder (eds.) *Oncofertility*.
© Springer 2007

potentially the child, and relevant medical personnel. Few family members are prepared for such stressful experiences; even fewer are prepared to engage in decision making that is both informed and takes personal values into account about such critical topics in such limited time frames. Therefore, there is a growing need to prepare medical professionals with the knowledge and tools for managing these stressful circumstances and to develop information and strategies to empower family members faced with such a life crisis.

The Current State of Pediatric Oncofertility

In 2006, an estimated 9,500 new cases of pediatric cancer were diagnosed in the United States [1]. Over the last several decades, survival rates for children with cancer have increased tremendously, and most children who develop cancer can be expected to survive [1]. Concurrent with these advances in cancer treatment, interest in cancer survivorship for childhood and adult cancer survivors has grown in both the academic and lay communities. Although the survival rate for those with childhood cancer has risen to almost 80%, such a diagnosis sends families into a crisis mode that alters life as they know it. Parents must come to terms with the reality that their child has cancer, a life-threatening disease, at the same time they are confronted by numerous related decisions regarding treatment and clinical trials. This period after diagnosis involves a steep learning curve [2]. Such revelations are accompanied by an expectation on the part of the treatment team that treatment decisions will be made quickly. During this time, some parents learn that side effects of the recommended treatments will, or may, render the patients infertile.

Therefore, these parents, and perhaps the patients, are faced with considering fertility preservation options at the same time they are struggling with understanding the cancer diagnosis and immediate treatment possibilities. In general practice, only parents of pubescent males learn of fertility preservation options because highly developed techniques for partnerless patients exist only for post-pubescent males [3]. The fertility options for females, however, are more limited, as egg harvesting and preservation have low success rates with unfertilized mature oocytes and are not options for girls with immature oocytes [4,5]. Further, many pediatric oncology providers are not adequately informed about current standards in fertility preservation and may have difficulty finding and contacting fertility specialists in a timely manner [6]. Experimental options for women and young girls include harvesting and freezing immature ovarian tissue for later auto-transplantation (i.e., restoring the tissue to her body) when the patient is ready to have children or maturation of the ovarian tissue in vitro and then fertilizing the mature egg [5]. In other words, parents of girls and young women are likely to learn that the options for preserving fertility are few and unpredictable (see Agarwal and Chang, this volume, for further discussion of fertility preservation options).

Family Communication in Context

Systems theory provides a root metaphor for thinking about family interactions as well as language for talking about ongoing changing family interactions with other human systems [7]. In the case of a family member's cancer diagnosis, systems theory is particularly apt and useful. Family therapist Virginia Satir [8] used the image of a mobile to describe a family system because as circumstances impact one or more members of the family, the other members reverberate in response to the change in the affected members. When individuals form families they also create family systems through their interaction patterns. Such human systems reflect characteristics of interdependence, patterns, interactive complexity, mutual influence, equifinality,[1] and openness [9]. Human systems depend on interchange with the larger ecosystem in order to survive and thrive; these systems function within larger social systems such as friendship, religious, educational, and health networks.

As developmental changes and unpredictable stresses occur, the family system mobile moves as members work through the issues, often creating a slightly different mobile configuration as a result. Most changes send the mobile into limited motion from which recovery is reasonably swift and sure; based on discussion, careful decision making, and negotiations, family members assimilate the new information or situation and find a new sense of balance. On occasion, a family encounters an unpredictable stress that sends the mobile spinning out of control; the gravity, complexity, and uncertainty of the situation shatters the possibility of relying on previous knowledge or coping patterns. The announcement that a child has life-threatening cancer sends the family mobile into chaotic movement. In minutes, the family's world as they know it has changed forever. A further statement that the child may face fertility issues as a result of treatment only deepens the vortex in which members find themselves. No option for gradual assimilation exists.

The family system must interact continually with other systems, including those of medical personnel within health care institutions, as well as the family's established support systems. As the family system faces upheaval and stress, the parental figures, and potentially the patient, confront making multiple decisions regarding unfamiliar issues that are difficult to discuss. As medical personnel describe an array of concerns, procedures, and options, the family is drawn into a web of communication involving medical, psychological, and ethical issues that is challenging emotionally and intellectually. Family decision making is frequently described as a phased problem solving loop beginning with phase 1 (identifying the problem, formulating a goal, and assessing resources), phase 2 (generating and assessing alternatives), phase 3 (selecting the best option) and phase 4 (accepting a decision, putting it into effect, and evaluating the outcome) [10]. Such a model assumes decisions are made over a period of time and conclusions may be reached before the family assimilates the change and moves on. This is not the pattern if the

---

[1] Equifinality is a concept central to family systems theory. It supposes that there is more than one route or option that can lead to the same final outcome.

issue involves immediate decisions regarding life-threatening and quality-of-life-threatening concerns of a child.

Shared Decision Making in Theory and in Practice

The concept of shared decision making in the medical context refers to a process of creating a course of action that is acceptable to the parties involved. Central to this model is more than the requirement that patients be informed of their relevant options, but in addition, patient values and self-efficacy serve as important factors in what is the "right" decision for that patient at that time [11]. The idea of shared decision making was first put forth by the President's Commission for the Study of Ethical Problems in Medicine and Biomedical and Behavioral Research in 1982 [12]. It described shared decision making as a process (rather than a singular point in time) based on both mutual respect and partnership between the patient and the physician. This description represented a shift from paternalistic care, in which physicians make decisions on behalf of the patient, to a model in which patient preferences, values, and concerns are taken into account. Although the Commission was concerned chiefly with this process as a part of biomedical research, the shift away from paternalism has been endorsed as a model of clinical care as well.

Beginning in the 1990s, many researchers and clinicians have expanded upon and tried to operationalize shared decision making [13–17]. A summary of these and other models of shared decision making, as well as an integrative model, are presented in a recent article by Makoul and Clayman [11]. A fundamental aspect of shared decision making is the concept that patients should be informed of the relevant information, including both risks and benefits to the extent that they desire, combined with the authority to participate in the process of decision making to the extent that they wish. This does not mean that physicians and other health care providers have no role in decision making. Rather, the respect for patients as individuals, with particular and unique desires and values, is paramount. Even if patients choose to let the responsibility for the final decision rest with the physician, which may be appropriate in many cases, the goals of shared decision making may still be attained [11]. In a sense, the process of decision making and the point of making the "final" decision are two separate events [11].

Decision Making in Pediatrics and Cancer

Both the family systems approach and shared decision making models have particular complementary characteristics that are useful to the study of pediatric oncofertility. Two shortcomings of shared decision making research as applied to this context are that it has generally focused on interactions (1) within the medical visit with a single practitioner; and (2) with only dyadic (i.e., patient–provider) communication.

That is, information, such as that garnered from other sources, even other clinicians, and relationships relevant to decision making, including spouses or other family members, have not been well integrated into the empirical research on this topic. Similarly, family systems theory has seldom been applied explicitly to medical decision making, although many professionals intuitively exhibit thinking along the lines of this theory. These shortcomings may be remedied by combining the structure and logic of family systems theory with that of shared decision making.

Bioethicists insist that children whose parents are considering enrolling them in clinical trials be informed of their choices at a level that is consistent with their age and cognitive capacity. This process of informing and gaining the child's permission is referred to as "assent" [18,19]. This principle has been recommended and incorporated, with varying success, into clinical practice in non-research settings [18,19]. That is, although the parents have legal authority to make decisions regarding the child's care until he or she reaches 18 years of age, it is generally frowned upon in Western societies to keep medical information and the opportunity to participate in medical decisions from older children and adolescents [18,20]. Despite this, research into shared decision making in the pediatric context is limited, and tends to focus on parents as the decision makers rather than also including the role of the child [21]. Among adult cancer patients at various stages of disease and treatment, investigators consistently find that most want detailed information about their condition, even if they do not want control over decision making [22–26]. The type of information and how that information is presented can influence how patients view their disease, their treatment, and even the competence of their physicians [27]. Yet, the literature suggests that, although physicians are important sources of information for cancer patients, they may both underestimate the patients' information needs and overestimate the amount of information they provide [28]. Young cancer survivors have reported a lack of counseling and information regarding the impact their diagnosis and treatment may have on future fertility [29].

Understanding how families confront and communicate about such potential concerns is critical. The role of the patient in this process is poorly understood because little research exists on how affected children and adolescents come to understand general treatment alternatives and make reasoned decisions [2]. Even less is known about how they confront fertility issues. Moral and ethical objections render real-life decision making difficult to study and little is know about how well children are able to understand their medical realities or make rational decisions about their own treatment [2].

A study of 60 children and adolescents, ranging in age from 10 to 16 years, focused on a general population of children and their knowledge of infertility and related issues as well as options to preserve fertility [30]. Gender differences seem to appear quite early. Of 31 females in this study, only one did not have the concept of an inability to have children, while 10 of the 29 males in the group were unaware of infertility. The remaining 49 participants completed in-depth interviews, in which it became clear that many of them understood that illness or "bad luck" could cause someone to not be able to have children, although some respondents intertwined infertility with issues of sexuality. This same population of 60 respondents was also asked about their views on parenthood and their own goals for the future [31]. Themes that emerged included having children as a part of a loving relationship and wanting to watch them grow up. Again, gender differences emerged: only females stated that prior experience caring for and spending time with children influenced their desire to eventually become parents, whereas both girls and boys mentioned parenting as the fulfillment of other sociocultural expectations (e.g., everyone has children after reaching adulthood). This indicates that even young girls with cancer may view the prospect of losing their fertility differently and more concretely than has previously been recognized.

In their study designed to determine whether female adolescents with a diagnosis of cancer and their parents were interested in trying to preserve fertility, Burns et al. interviewed parents and female adolescents [32]. The latter were between the ages of 10 and 21 and had started or completed treatment; their fertility status was unknown. The discussion areas included: adolescents' thoughts about the future, whether someone had talked to them about how the treatment might affect fertility, their interest in pursuing research-based fertility preservation techniques, and their willingness to wait to start therapy. The researchers concluded that the respondents were willing to explore research options to preserve fertility as long as their health was not put in jeopardy in the attempt to preserve fertility.

In her study of child and adolescent involvement in decisions regarding their own medical treatment, McCabe [33] asserts, "We need to support minors' involvement in decision making, particularly for treatment decisions where the clarity of the 'right choice fades, where treatment preferences are based upon personal values and 'quality-of-life' issues" (pp. 505–506). She cites clinical issues, including child factors, family factors, and situational factors that facilitate or impede the child's use of developmental capacities. Although the wishes of patients over the age of 18 are considered in such decision making, those under the age of 18 are represented by parents who may or may not include them in the treatment decision-making process. Even among older adolescents, the complexity of dealing with the medical system may be more overwhelming than it would be for an adult who has more life experience. Additionally, some families and patients are never informed, or fully informed, about potential fertility concerns, leaving them ignorant of such concerns until after treatments have commenced or even later (see reference 34 and Nieman et al., this volume).

Sperm banking has been available for decades, but since the 1990s, advances in in vitro fertilization made it more effective [35]. This process is highly functional for most adolescent males because it can be completed quickly and through noninvasive procedures without delaying the cancer treatments. Therefore, adolescent and young adult males have a reasonable probability of preserving their fertility. According to Schover, "Teens as young as 12 have the physical capacity and emotional maturity to provide semen samples and should be informed routinely of this option" (p. 525). As such, research that has focused on the role of children in decision making about fertility often deals solely with males [3,36,37].

Young women have fewer viable options and often experience limited communication about the issues. The fertility implications are significant. Young women who undergo cancer treatment may lose functioning ovarian tissue both at the time of treatment (acute ovarian failure) and in the long term [38]. In their study of young women (average age at diagnosis was 32.9 years) who were treated for breast cancer, Partridge et al. [39] found that although 72% of women reported discussing fertility with their doctors, only 51% felt their concerns were addressed adequately. Women diagnosed more recently were better aware of the possible impact of chemotherapy on fertility. These authors report "concerns about fertility are present for the majority of young premenopausal women, regardless of their age and extent of the disease" (p. 4181). They conclude that "there may be a need for improved communication about fertility between young women with breast cancer and their health care providers" (p. 4182) regarding issues such as risk of infertility, premature menopause, and options to preserve fertility. Clearly this does not address issues of girls and young women under 18, but it does highlight a gap in the information provided to cancer patients about their future fertility. In their examination of discussions of reproductive health with young women with breast cancer, Duffy et al. [40] report the medical conversations centered on the patients' understanding of the impact of chemotherapy treatment on prognosis, alternative treatments, and risks and benefits of treatments, but the patients desired more discussion of reproductive health for those about to undergo chemotherapy. Yet, only 34% of women in this study reported discussing fertility issues with a health provider.

Many younger women report that, although fertility was not of great importance to them at the time of diagnosis, it became increasingly important as time passed [41]. A major concern was the lack of enough fertility-related information at the time of diagnosis. Many remained unclear about their fertility status. The group reported a series of current questions such as "Am I going to be fertile/able to conceive after treatment? If I am still fertile does that mean that I can still have children? How do treatments affect the reproductive system? By what mechanism?" (p. 505). These women reported receiving only verbal information about the impact of their treatment on fertility. Given the stress of the moment, they felt overwhelmed and found it difficult to recall the information. If young adult women report such responses, what might teens report who may know less about the issues and questions? To what extent are young women and/or their parents informed and prepared to raise this issue?

It is impossible to consider parent–child interactions on the topic of fertility without framing the issue within the larger, complicated topic of parent–child discussions about sex, given that the two are inextricably linked. Discomfort in the general area of discussing sexuality will impact the parental willingness and perception of competence in discussing fertility, especially at a moment of high stress. Maddock delineates three types of families according to their communication patterns regarding sexuality: (1) sexually neglectful, (2) sexually abusive, and (3) sexually healthy families [42]. Whereas sexually healthy families are characterized by effective and flexible communication patterns that support intimacy, sexually neglectful families exhibit an absence of discussion on the topic and sexually abusive families reflect a perpetrator-victim pattern with limited communication. The growing literature on parent–child discussions of sex reflects the tendency of mothers to discuss this topic more frequently with their children, particularly daughters; even when both parents are involved, they are more likely to talk about sex with daughters rather than sons [43]. Mothers are predominantly responsible for sexual communication with their children but their children report friends are the main source of sexual information, followed by their mothers. Some parents may have difficulty talking with their adolescents about sex because they are unsure about their own knowledge and skill and concerned that their children will not take them seriously [44]. Due to their insecurities, parents rate themselves low on the list of influences on children's sexual behaviors, whereas children rate their parents high on the list [45]. In addition, most parents seem too squeamish to get into the subtleties of instilling sexual ethics [46]. Thus, some parents facing a diagnosis of a child's cancer and potential infertility are communicatively challenged because of their past interaction patterns. How do parents who have not addressed sexual issues begin to deal with fertility concerns under severe health-threatening conditions? Families in which a mother is unwilling or unavailable to talk about sexuality and fertility may avoid such conversations in the stress of the moment. Young women may wish to involve friends in their consideration of the issues.

Very little is known about how children and/or parents may react to holding such difficult conversations. In one of the few studies of teenagers and young adults faced with possible or actual fertility impairment following cancer treatment, Crawshaw and Sloper interviewed 38 individuals diagnosed with cancer between the ages of 13 and 21 and who were aware of a risk that their fertility might have been affected [34]. The age at interview ranged from 16 to 30 years, allowing for information from both teenagers and young adults. Many did not understand their fertility concerns until some time after treatment. In keeping with the general findings of mother–daughter communication about sexuality, Crawshaw and Sloper found examples of open communication about fertility among all groups of respondents, although this was more often the case in families of females, especially mothers and daughters; in the latter case, there was some ambiguity as to whether the topic was limited to menstrual difficulties. Some respondents found it difficult to talk openly with any family members about fertility issues. The authors concluded that, "Pre-existing verbal patterns within families were maintained or strengthened in some families but altered in others. However, the pattern of communication around cancer matters tended to differ in most families to those around cancer-related fertility matters in that it was much more likely to be closed" (p. 113).

Some key findings from this study, with an emphasis on those that related to both genders or that related to females, included that both genders strongly supported telling patients about the potential impact of the treatment on the reproductive system at the time of diagnosis, and there was an emphasis on the need for professionals to raise the subject sooner, more frequently, in a low-key way and without ambiguity. Respondents wished professionals would treat them as partners, therefore prioritizing their input over their parents. Families were much less likely to talk about cancer-related fertility issues than cancer issues at any stage. In some cases, patients talked more to siblings and extended family members than parents and some patients were more likely to discuss cancer-related fertility matters with a small number of close friends. Females were more likely to find themselves managing conversations about parenthood plans (and actual pregnancies). Eventually, the uncertainty about fertility affected romantic relationships. Respondents experienced anticipated and actual concerns about when and how to tell a romantic partner. Essentially coping with the impact of cancer-related fertility concerns was a dynamic process with different aspects arising at different times, in different contexts, and in different life stages (pp. 5–9).

Whereas the previous study relied totally on in-depth interviews with the cancer survivors, another recent study addressed the experiences of mothers and daughters (see Nieman et al., this volume). Two focus groups were conducted with adult survivors of childhood cancer; four survivors and three parents participated in one group and six survivors and seven parents participated in the other group. Survivors who had been diagnosed between the ages of 13 and 21 and experienced fertility-threatening treatments remembered that their short-term concerns after diagnosis included appearance, missing activities at school, and how friends would treat them, whereas long-term concerns included dying, relapse, and infertility. Parents focused on their child's survival after diagnosis and some reported long-term concerns, including infertility. "Similar to survivors, some parents reported that their daughter's fertility was a concern at the time of diagnosis, while others, particularly fathers, state that it 'wasn't even on the radar screen'" (p. 206). Although all survivors felt included in the informational sessions regarding treatment, they did not see any option other than receiving the treatment. Parents viewed treatment decisions as the medical provider's role and their responsibility was to find the right provider. In essence, survival was the key goal at the time of diagnosis.

In addition, parents reported a need to educate themselves about cancer and cancer treatments although they felt overwhelmed by the enormity of information and found it difficult to consider long-term issues. Survivors felt that fertility was rarely discussed by the medical team prior to treatment. Some parents remembered discussing fertility, while others did not. "Some parents reported that they wished they knew more about the possibility of their child's infertility and what to do before the first treatment was initiated, but acknowledged that they may not have been able to think about it at the time of diagnosis" (p. 207).

The difficult conversations are not confined within the family boundaries. Medical personnel cross the family's boundary from the time the child is presented for diagnosis of a problem. Many families move from the familiar pediatrician to the specialist, while some encounter the medical system through emergency rooms without a traditional medical history. These families bring with them their attitudes toward, and familial history with, medical professionals. Their culture or religion may influence the types of decisions they are prepared to make [33]. Most also present with a history of discussing significant health issues with particular members of their support systems, such as extended family members, religious leaders, and close friends.

The science of fertility preservation is advancing; girls and young women with cancer and their parents will soon be asked about experimental methods of fertility preservation, including laparoscopic removal of ovarian tissue. These scientific advances may further complicate the process of decision making for parents, children, and their health care providers. It is vitally important that researchers understand how families come to make decisions about their ill children's fertility, who and what are important sources of information and support for families, and what information needs still exist for families as they make and reflect on their decisions. Longitudinal studies are particularly important when studying patient–provider communication and the patient and family experience because needs change, perspectives shift, and behaviors among the players in decision making may not be stable over time [28,47–49]. Further, as a child ages, her level of maturity, familiarity with the disease (including medical procedures, terminology, and providers), and cognitive capabilities change, sometimes quite radically. In addition, recent research has suggested that decision-making preferences among patients are malleable [50,51]. Moreover, since most studies of communication in the cancer context have been cross-sectional, patients' and their families' communication needs throughout the trajectory of cancer care and into survivorship are unclear.

This chapter has demonstrated a growing body of research that can be drawn on in the emerging field of pediatric oncofertility and decision making. Yet there are still many values-based criteria and medical options that need to be identified and investigated in order to generate valid and useful information. In a way, this entire volume is about building a clinically functional and relevant shared decision-making model for families, their children with cancer, their friends, and relevant professionals.

References

1. American Cancer Society. Cancer facts and figures 2006. Atlanta: American Cancer Society, 2006.
2. Eiser C. Children with cancer: the quality of life. Mahwah, NJ: Lawrence Erlbaum Association, 2004.
3. Schover L. Sexuality and fertility after cancer. Hematology 2005;523–527.
4. Nieman CL, Kazer R, Brannigan RE, et al. Cancer survivors and infertility: a review of a new problem and novel answers. J Support Oncol 2006;4:171–178.
5. Picton H. Fertility preservation methods and treatments for females. In: Balen R, Crawshaw M, editors. Sexuality and fertility issues in ill health and disability: from early adolescence to adulthood. London: Jessica Kingsley Publishers, 2006:85–98.
6. Goodwin T, Elizabeth Oosterhuis B, Kiernan M, et al. Attitudes and practices of pediatric oncology providers regarding fertility issues. Pediatr Blood Cancer 2007;48:80–85.
7. Galvin KM, Dickson FC, Marrow SR. Systems theory: patterns and (w)holes in family communication. In: Braithwaite D, Baxter L, editors. Engaging theories in family communication: multiple perspectives. Thousand Oaks, CA: Sage, 2006:309–324.
8. Satir V. The new peoplemaking. Mountain View, CA: Science and Behavior Books, 1988.

9. Galvin KM, Bylund C, Brommel B. Family communication: cohesion and change. 6th ed. Boston: Allyn & Bacon; 2006.
10. Kieren D, Maguirfe T, Hurblut N. A marker method to test a phasing hypothesis in family problem-solving interaction. J Marriage Family 1996;58:442–455.
11. Makoul G, Clayman ML. An integrative model of shared decision making in medical encounters. Patient Educ Couns 2006;60:301–312.
12. President's Commission for the Study of Ethical Problems in Medicine and Biomedical and Behavioral Research. Making health care decisions. The ethical and legal implications of informed consent in the patient–practitioner relationship. Washington, DC, 1982.
13. Towle A. Physician and patient communication skills: competencies for informed shared decision making. Vancouver, Canada: University of British Columbia, 1997.
14. Elwyn G, Edwards A, Wensing M, et al. Shared decision making observed in clinical practice: visual displays of communication sequence and patterns. J Eval Clin Pract 2001;7:211–221.
15. Elwyn G, Edwards A, Wensing M, et al. Shared decision making: developing the OPTION scale for measuring patient involvement. Qual Saf Health Care 2003;12:93–99.
16. Charles C, Gafni A, Whelan T. Shared decision-making in the medical encounter: what does it mean? (or it takes at least two to tango). Soc Sci Med 1997;44:681–692.
17. Charles C, Whelan T, Gafni A. What do we mean by partnership in making decisions about treatment? BMJ 1999;319:780–782.
18. Lee KJ, Havens PL, Sato TT, et al. Assent for treatment: clinician knowledge, attitudes, and practice. Pediatrics 2006;118:723–730.
19. Committee on Bioethics, American Academy of Pediatrics. Informed consent, parental permission, and assent in pediatric practice. Pediatrics 1995;95:314–317.
20. Parsons SK, Saiki-Craighill S, Mayer DK, et al. Telling children and adolescents about their cancer diagnosis: cross-cultural comparisons between pediatric oncologists in the US and Japan. Psycho-oncology 2007;16:60–68.
21. Merenstein D, Diener-West M, Krist A, et al. An assessment of the shared-decision model in parents of children with acute otitis media. Pediatrics 2005;116:1267–1275.
22. Blanchard CG, Labrecque MS, Ruckdeschel JC, et al. Information and decision-making preferences of hospitalized adult cancer patients. Soc Sci Med 1988;27:1139–1145.
23. Cassileth BR, Zupkis RV, Sutton-Smith K, et al. Information and participation preferences among cancer patients. Ann Intern Med 1980;92:832–836.
24. Henman MJ, Butow PN, Brown RF, et al. Lay constructions of decision-making in cancer. Psycho-oncology 2002;11:295–306.
25. Stewart DE, Wong F, Cheung AM, et al. Information needs and decisional preferences among women with ovarian cancer. Gynecol Oncol 2000;77:357–361.
26. Barnett MM. Does it hurt to know the worst?—psychological morbidity, information preferences and understanding of prognosis in patients with advanced cancer. Psycho-oncology 2006;15:44–55.
27. Ziebland S, Evans J, McPherson A. The choice is yours? How women with ovarian cancer make sense of treatment choices. Patient Educ Couns 2006;62:361–367.
28. Arora NK. Interacting with cancer patients: the significance of physicians' communication behavior. Soc Sci Med 2003;57:791–806.
29. Canada AL, Schover LR. Research promoting better patient education on reproductive health after cancer. J Natl Cancer Inst Monogr 2005:98–100.
30. Balen R, Fraser C, Fielding D. Children and young people's understanding of infertility. In: Balen R, Crawshaw M, editors. Sexuality and fertility issues in ill health and disability: from early adolescence to adulthood. London: Jessica Kingsley Publishers, 2006:49–64.
31. Fraser C, Balen R, Fielding D. The views of the next generation: an exploration of priorities for adulthood and the meaning of parenthood amongst 10–16-year-olds. In: Balen R, Crawshaw M, editors. Sexuality and fertility issues in ill health and disability: from early adolescence to adulthood. London: Jessica Kingsley Publishers, 2006:33–48.
32. Burns KC, Boudreau C, Panepinto JA. Attitudes regarding fertility preservation in female adolescent cancer patients. J Pediatr Hematol Oncol 2006;28:350–354.

33. McCabe MA. Involving children and adolescents in medical decision making: developmental and clinical considerations. J Pediatr Psychol 1996;21:505–516.
34. Crawshaw M, Sloper P. A qualitative study of the experiences of teenagers and young adults when faced with possible or actual fertility impairment following cancer treatment. 2006. Available at: http://www.york.ac.uk/inst/spru/pubs/pdf/fertility.pdf. Accessed December 28, 2006.
35. Schover LR. Sexuality and fertility after cancer. Hematology Am Soc Hematol Educ Program 2005;523–527.
36. Schover LR. Psychosocial aspects of infertility and decisions about reproduction in young cancer survivors: a review. Med Pediatr Oncol 1999;33:53–59.
37. Schover LR, Brey K, Lichtin A, et al. Knowledge and experience regarding cancer, infertility, and sperm banking in younger male survivors. J Clin Oncol 2002;20:1880–1889.
38. Chen WY, Manson JE. Premature ovarian failure in cancer survivors: new insights, looming concerns. J Natl Cancer Inst 2006;98:880–881.
39. Partridge AH, Gelber S, Peppercorn J, et al. Web-based survey of fertility issues in young women with breast cancer. J Clin Oncol 2004;22:4174–4183.
40. Duffy CM, Allen SM, Clark MA. Discussions regarding reproductive health for young women with breast cancer undergoing chemotherapy. J Clin Oncol 2005;23:766–773.
41. Thewes B, Meiser B, Rickard J, et al. The fertility- and menopause-related information needs of younger women with a diagnosis of breast cancer: a qualitative study. Psycho-oncology 2003;12:500–511.
42. Maddock J. Healthy family sexuality: positive principles for educators and clinicians. Family Relations. 1989;38:130–136.
43. Warren C. Communicating about sex with parents and partners. In: Galvin KM, Cooper P, editors. Making connections: readings in relational communication. 3rd ed. Los Angeles: Roxbury, 2003:317–324.
44. Jaccard J, Dittust P, Gordon V. Parent-adolescent communication about premarital sex: factors associated with the extent of communication. J Adoles Res 2000;15:187–208.
45. Wilson P. 1994: forming a partnership between parents and sexuality educators: reflections of a parent advocate. SIECUS Report. 2004;32:6–8.
46. Stodghill II R. Where'd you learn that? In: Davidson J Sr, Moore NB, editors. Speaking of sexuality. 2nd ed. Los Angeles: Roxbury, 2005:370–374.
47. Ford S, Fallowfield L, Lewis S. Doctor–patient interactions in oncology. Soc Sci Med 1996;42:1511–1519.
48. van Dulmen AM, Verhaak PF, Bilo HJ. Shifts in doctor-patient communication during a series of outpatient consultations in non-insulin-dependent diabetes mellitus. Patient Educ Couns 1997;30:227–237.
49. Graugaard PK, Holgersen K, Eide H, et al. Changes in physician–patient communication from initial to return visits: a prospective study in a haematology outpatient clinic. Patient Educ Couns 2005;57:22–29.
50. Arora NK, Ayanian JZ, Guadagnoli E. Examining the relationship of patients' attitudes and beliefs with their self-reported level of participation in medical decision-making. Med Care 2005;43:865–872.
51. Mallinger JB, Shields CG, Griggs JJ, et al. Stability of decisional role preference over the course of cancer therapy. Psycho-oncology 2006;4:297–305.

Part V
Ethical and Psychosocial Impact of Cancer-Related Infertility

healthy peers and family members enjoy. Yet some of these goals are simply unattainable, for side effects of the chemotherapy or radiation that saved their lives has often compromised or eliminated their fertility.

For children and adults faced with a sudden cancer diagnosis, the immediate priority is survival and support for the difficult time period surrounding treatment. But the coincident infertility created by advances in cancer treatment often paradoxically create a patient of a different sort—an infertility patient. At this juncture, the medical disciplines of oncology and infertility have become intertwined, and a new area of medicine, oncofertility, emerges.

With this new field comes new issues: complex dilemmas and ethical and practical issues that arise when discussing fertility preservation in the context of cancer are only the first horizon of our moral concern. The concerns around these topics deepen when the wider social implications of this work are considered. The medical breakthroughs created in oncofertility are a portal to a far wider prospect. Using the techniques described in this book, can gametes be preserved against a host of physical and social events that will compromise fertility, often with the same prospective statistical certainty as chemotherapy and radiation?

Finally, as basic research on human embryonic stem cells accelerates, a rate-limiting step is the acquisition of human eggs from women for research, especially for the creation of disease-specific cell lines for the study of early cellular reprogramming and for the creation of patient-specific histocompatible tissue. As the debate about how to obtain human oocytes for research and for potential cures intensifies, serious moral issues about the risk of multiple egg extraction emerge. It has not escaped our attention that the creation of a stable, renewable, and plentiful source of human ova has the potential to relocate and transform the entire debate about egg acquisition for research or therapy. Such an advance could solve several of the ethical complexities of stem cell research by ensuring the just, safe, and scalable acquisition of eggs.

The questions of fertility preservation have an obvious threshold consideration—they are strongly affected by the sex of the participant. For men, sperm can be safely retrieved, frozen, and stored once a boy begins to produce spermatocytes (see Brannigan, this volume, for further discussion). Unfortunately, options for women facing cancer treatment are less reliable. Mature human oocytes cannot be effectively frozen, stored, and thawed because of the fragility of the human egg cell [4,5]. For a woman facing fertility-impairing cancer treatment, a male partner or willingness to use donor sperm, the time to safely delay cancer therapy, and a cancer that will not grow in response to hormonal treatments makes her a candidate for ovarian hyperstimulation and emergency IVF. Ideally, this results in embryos for potential future use (see Agarwal and Chang, this volume, for further discussion). This option is currently the most widely used and proven method for preserving fertility, however, it has limitations, can be emotionally and physically difficult, is a viable option for only a fraction of patients, and carries some risk to the patient. Scientific expertise and technical advances have begun to overcome many of the obstacles of female fertility preservation in the face of cancer, with the goal of offering solutions that are feasible for a wider range of patients [5].

Expanding Options for Women – Follicle Preservation and Maturation

Should more be offered and attempted? Biomedical research in the field of oncofertility has begun to extend experimental research to explore this question. Could ovarian tissue containing immature ovarian follicles be frozen, stored, and then thawed, matured, fertilized, and result in successful pregnancy [6–8]? Was this idea both practical and ethical? Yet offering the procedure is itself an ethical problem: the techniques available are experimental, and participation in research protocols offers limited hope for the participants today, while holding the promise of developing options for future patients [8]. The complexity of the decisions for both patients and their families increases yet further in the case of childhood cancer, when the child's assent and parental consent for the child patient's participation in research come into play [9]. The best interest of the child now must simultaneously be held in balance with the best interest for the adult the child will hopefully become.

In this chapter, we uncover the core themes that have emerged and reflect on how the canonical literature on the topic is reinforced or altered by new work in oncofertility. First, we explore infertility as a disease state or disability. Why is it important to continue research on fertility preservation? Does the loss of fertility for any reason have a moral high priority and deserve allocation of resources and health care dollars? We then look at an instance whereby the technology of ovarian cryopreservation and maturation will have particular ethical considerations: the case of fertility preservation and research in children. What special considerations surround cancer, fertility, and research involving children? Is it appropriate to be concerned with a child's future reproduction or treatment-related infertility? How might the issue be approached to avoid discomfort with regarding children as future sexual beings? Lastly, these questions are used to frame the potential next uses of an emerging ability to cryopreserve ovarian tissue for future transplantation or maturation of primordial follicles in vitro. The potential of these techniques is far-reaching, not only because it may provide a new choice for fertility preservation for girls and women with cancer, but also because it has the potential to revolutionize fertility treatments for other reproductive-age women, change the nature of egg donation, reduce the number of unused embryos in infertility clinic freezers, and influence the acquisition of embryonic stem cells.

A Prairie Horizon: The Long View of Research on Fertility

The landscape of reproduction has shifted throughout history, both as an adaptation to circumstances and as a reaction to advances in technology. The scientific breakthrough of efficient ovarian tissue cryopreservation and in vitro maturation [7] of human female gametes will likely change the horizon of this landscape in the near future. The purpose of this chapter is to provide roots for the utilization of this technology. By reflecting on ethics literature, historical precedents, recommended medical practices, and desires of cancer survivors, we will frame some of the important questions about advancing fertility preservation treatments and anticipate future dilemmas.

The development of ovarian cryopreservation represents a significant step forward for fertility-preserving options for cancer patients who are either sexually immature, do not have a partner at the time of diagnosis and/or do not wish to use donor sperm, or who are not able to or choose not to delay treatment for emergency IVF [5–7]. In the scenario that this treatment becomes readily available for humans, a patient could elect to have one ovary removed by laparoscopic (minimally invasive) surgery and cryopreserved. If she chooses to start a family and is unable to do so without assistance, a piece of the ovarian tissue would be thawed, the follicles matured and fertilized in vitro, [10] and then introduced into her uterus as in current IVF protocols. Alternatively, the tissue could be transplanted into the patient and matured prior to IVF [11]. If the patient no longer has a uterus or is not able to carry a pregnancy, the embryos could be gestated by a surrogate.

Cryopreserving immature follicles would have several distinct advantages for cancer patients or any woman needing an oophorectomy. First, it allows her to bank her own gametes, allowing her to have her own genetic offspring in the future if she chooses. Second, if she is eligible for emergency IVF but does not have a partner, it gives her the opportunity to wait until she has a partner. She also can choose against the delay of her own cancer treatment and have an alternative to emergency IVF. Third, it will likely eliminate the risk of reintroduction of malignant cells back into the patient [5,12]. Fourth, it may decrease the number of embryos made with each cycle, thus eliminating the dilemma of what to do with unused embryos once a pregnancy has been achieved. Fifth, it allows her to delay childbearing until an age that approximates that of the normal population. Female survivors of cancer treatment may recover normal ovarian function early in their reproductive life, but they often experience premature ovarian failure by their thirties [13]. The subsequent pressure to reproduce may hasten her choice of a partner or restrict the other life choices of education and career that her peers enjoy.

Despite the medical breakthrough that this technology represents, let us ask a priori the questions: Is the premise of infertility research a just and prudent use of research resources and attention? Why is it important to focus research and offer new reproductive technologies (NRT)? Many would argue that IVF research is precisely the sort of highly technological medicine that drives up health care costs by focusing on desire instead of need. In a world that has significant infant mortality and orphans in need of homes, should medicine continue to refine this field? Let us turn to the defenses as mounted in the literature by Daniel Brock and John Robertson.

The right to reproduce is regarded as an important freedom within society that is seldom questioned or restricted. This reflects a long-standing sense of a procreative respect for the "right to reproduce" as a moral imperative, often defended as bearing on autonomy, identity, self-determination, and dignity [14]. Our cultural value of being able to have one's own genetic children is clearly displayed as the emotional reaction of an individual or couple to their own infertility.

When discussing the rights of individuals, it is customary to describe them in terms of negative and positive rights. The right to procreate is inherently regarded as a moral "negative right", which is to say that others have a duty to not interfere with this right unless there is sufficient and weighty moral ground to do so. For example, individuals and the government should not sterilize citizens against their will nor interfere with an individual's access to NRTs. The right to procreate has not, however, been afforded the status of a "positive right." This would propose that others must act in a way to secure this right and guarantee the right to NRTs to anyone who needs them regardless of cost. The designation of this claim is certainly a matter of current debate given the prevalence and emotional consequences of infertility. By recognizing the fact that reproductive technologies are not widely available or funded, however, we do not intend to make an argument against insurance coverage of reproductive technologies. It is beyond the scope of this chapter to discuss social injustices with regard to access to health care services for fertility, contraception, or other mechanisms of "procreative liberty" as described by John Robertson [15]. The fact that infertility treatments are covered by insurance in a minority of states in the U.S. or that citizens are not accustomed to expecting these services should not pave the way for this precedent to become ingrained in our social thinking [14].

If a moral right protects procreation by coital means, then one can extend this right to also protect non-coital reproduction [15]. The desire for an infertile person or couple to reproduce is rooted in the same desire to parent as it is for a couple that can coitally reproduce: to rear children that are genetically related to one or both of the parents. The fact that the individual or couple is infertile should not exclude them from an experience that is the norm for people in their lifetime [15]. In this case, the disability is an inability to coitally produce children, and to disqualify them from treatment would be tantamount to denying any medical treatments that aim to approximate normal life. If insurance will cover the diagnosis and treatment of the sequelae of chemotherapy or radiation, for example lung or heart problems, it follows that infertility as a consequence of treatment should also be covered. Furthermore, many medical conditions, such as hypertension, diabetes, arthritis, and cancer have associated genetic predispositions as well as behavioral influences. Why should other medical conditions that also have genetic or behavioral components, such as premature ovarian failure, immotile sperm, or delayed childbearing not be allocated the same status with regard to health care dollars? The direct consequences of infertility may not be life threatening, but many medical conditions that hinder quality of life are readily treated and covered [14]. Perhaps the limited allocation of health care dollars for this service is biased by the decision being made by a portion of the population that has already reproduced, thus they know they will not need these services [14].

As Daniel Brock notes:

"Norman Daniels has argued that the importance of health care for justice lies most fundamentally in its securing and protecting for individuals access to the normal range of opportunities in their society. Health care can often prevent, restore, or limit the loss of normal
function that is the typical mark of disease. While we tend to associate equality of
opportunity most commonly with education and work, it is not limited to those venues.
NRT's often represent the means by which the opportunity to bear and raise children can
be restored to infertile individuals. The moral importance—on grounds of equality of
opportunity and justice—of doing so depends largely on the relative importance of parenting within the normal life plans of most people. This suggests that infertility is a disability
whose alleviation by means such as NRT has a very high moral priority." [14]

For the authors of this chapter, the case for allowing women to have children after
cancer treatments presents a compelling case for research. In the case of cancer
when the cure may cause harm, we argue that there is a duty to prevent damage
or repair that which is damaged by treatment, when possible. Infertility is
understood as a disease of reproductive-age individuals that can often be
overcome by medical treatment, and it is just to allocate resources to its research
and treatments. There is yet another reason to actively pursue this research. It is
our contention that the growing search for oocytes for stem cell research presents
another, non-rights-based argument for continuation. Thus, we can focus on the
particular case of oncofertility, while understanding that the research has a
mutable future.

The Role of Oncologists and Infertility Specialists

In large part, the most profound ethical issues when a new treatment is developed
are the presentation of the advance without fictions or promises. The issue of
realistic consent is the second ethical problem in oncofertility. Cancer and its
aftermath present a difficult case, with a long history of invasive, risk-laden treatments. Patients depend on their physician to present to them their illness, educate
them about treatment, and expect to be warned about side effects of the treatment.
Developing a clear ethical interaction can be complicated by the swiftness of new
research as well as its uncertain application.

   As this technology goes forward, it is also imperative that appropriate patients
have access to information regarding experimental fertility-preserving techniques.
Oncologists who treat reproductive-age patients or patients who have not yet
reached sexual maturity need to not only be aware of the potentially gonadotoxic
effects of treatments in order to discuss treatment related infertility with patients, but
also should be aware of both established and experimental fertility preserving
options for both male and female patients [9,12]. Studies suggest that oncologists
either explain sub-optimally the potential of treatment-related infertility, or fail to do
so at all (see Snyder, this volume, and Clayman, Galvin, and Arntson, this volume,
for further discussion). This can be attributed to a number of factors, including an
appropriate focus on treatment and cure of the cancer, lack of physician knowledge

about available methods to preserve fertility, physician judgment about patient prognosis, or discomfort with broaching the subject with patients or their parents, as in the case of children. While oncologists may get the appropriate training in fellowship programs to discuss well established methods of fertility preservation such as sperm banking and oophoropexy, they may lack appropriate training and knowledge about newer techniques, particularly those that are experimental [9,12].

Ongoing training and effort on the part of the practitioner will ultimately be required to stay abreast of experimental techniques, particularly in the case of children and women without partners who will need to store gametes, not embryos. The American Society of Clinical Oncology (ASCO) recognizes the scope of this problem and has published "Recommendation on Fertility in Cancer Patients" that emphasizes the importance of early discussion and referral to appropriate resources for all patients of reproductive age. In the case of children or women who cannot or do not wish to freeze embryos, the patients should also be referred to appropriate specialists and centers capable of carrying out institutional review board (IRB)-approved protocols when established methods do not exist [12]. The process of patient education about fertility preservation prior to cancer treatment will ultimately require a combination of approaches that involve education by patient advocacy groups and also a sea change within the climate of oncology practice [12].

Unfortunately, the measure of damage and the need for restoration of function is often hard to quantify. It is often difficult to place a number on the risk of infertility for any given patient and the type of treatment he or she is to receive. The fertility status of the patient after treatment will vary greatly depending on sex, age, dose and duration of chemotherapy or radiation treatments, method of administration, field of radiation, and the pre-treatment fertility status of the individual [5–7,12] (see Gracia and Ginsberg, this volume). For experimental fertility-preserving techniques, it is impossible to quantify success as there is no current success rate to offer to the patient. The patient who is offered the opportunity to enroll in experimental trials must explicitly understand that the true benefit may not be available within his or her reproductive life span, yet may contribute to the development of an option for other patients in the future. Experimental techniques should only be undertaken at appropriate research centers under IRB-approved protocols. Oncologists must work closely with the reproductive endocrinologists and with psychosocial providers in order to be able to refer as needed and help to develop an appropriate treatment plan and refer patients to clinical trials [6,7,12,16].

Reproductive endocrinologists need to not only be aware of both established and experimental options, but also have an increased awareness of the patient that is facing the crisis of cancer simultaneously with the potential crisis of infertility. Full consideration of the cancer diagnosis, consultation with the patient's oncologist, the range of fertility preserving options, and the patient's desires for future fertility will inform the appropriate plan. Infertility training programs should work to increase exposure of training fellows and obstetrics and gynecology residents to oncology patients seeking fertility preservation in order to improve patient referral to appropriate trials and specialized centers in the future [6,7,12] (also see Kondopalli, this volume, for further discussion).

   From the beginning of the consent process, the patient must be presented with
any and all options available to either preserve fertility or pursue other means to
have children, including adoption, egg donation, and surrogacy. The distinction
between established and experimental options must be made clear and the patient
must consent for any research that will be done on their tissue. Patients must clearly
understand how long the tissue will be stored by the research team and made aware
of their options for storage after that time has expired. Although the current research
(including developments in the mouse) is promising [10,11], we must bear in mind
that in vitro maturation is still experimental and should be presented as such without
giving the patient false hope. Furthermore, the older the patient is, the less likely the
experimental technique will be available to her in her reproductive years. Directives
about how to handle the tissue posthumously in the event of the patient's death
should be included with the consent to obtain the tissue. These directives need to
specify if a partner or spouse may use the tissue for IVF after the death of the patient.
In the case of children, the age at which the patient will have access to use the tissue
to initiate a pregnancy and if parents have any right to the tissue needs to be established prior to obtaining the ovarian tissue [9,16,17].
   Ethical concerns regarding the theoretical increased risk of cancer in a child
born to a cancer survivor, due to a possible genetic predisposition, have been
discussed by other researchers [16,18]. A discussion of the estimated risk to
patient's offspring should be part of the informed consent process prior to ovarian
cryopreservation, but does not preclude the patient's access to these services.
Physicians have also questioned if it is ethical to allow a patient to reproduce when
they may have a reduced life-span, thus leaving a child with only one parent.
Although the loss of a parent is undeniably stressful for a child, the ethical analysis
provided in other works [19] argues that this burden does not exceed other stresses
children may experience in their lifetime and does not yield a convincing argument
to deny cancer survivors access to reproductive services.

Ethical Issues in the Case of Childhood Cancers

The Special Case of Young Girls

When faced with the diagnosis and treatment regimes for pediatric cancer, parents
face a particular burden of choice. They will be asked not only about the range of
treatment options for their child, but also about somewhat disquieting options regarding the theoretical adult that their child may become, if she survives. Such a complex
set of dilemmas is overwhelming. Parents must contemplate the problem of the best
interests of the child at two completely different times of life, one of which is entirely
abstract. They must negotiate the needs of a desperately (and suddenly) sick child in
need of urgent treatment and their desire to believe the treatment will be successful
and it will allow the child to live and grow. Parents then must hold a distant and often
conflicted vision about the child's future, where he or she is an adult who will make

choices about education, family, and career—indeed, as sexually active adult men and women desiring children of their own. The choice to engage in an utterly experimental intervention, minor surgery, and a set of complicated conversations about the future is a unique responsibility for parents of children with cancer.

It was because of these very difficulties that our research turned to this question. In understanding this ethical question, we turned to a logical cohort most likely to give thoughtful answers: women and their parents who had faced cancer in the past. Choosing families who had faced pediatric cancer, we asked whether such conversations and the experiment proposed—even if no hope for translation to clinical use was offered—would be warranted. The research strongly indicated that this difficult conversation is critical. The respondents indicated that careful consideration of even experimental fertility preservation ought to be presented (see Nieman et al., this volume).

For some physicians and parents, the concern about discussing a child's future fertility is unalterably a discussion that sexualizes a young child and attempts to predict her reproductive choices. While acknowledging this, we argue that an alterative view is possible, that of the preservation of organ function, in much the way other organs are protected and restored after cancer therapies damage them; the ovary, after all, is a reproductive organ. In the view of many, it is a morally distinction function, for an ovary contains gametes, whose special status has long been considered distinction and who cells are entities deserving of special concern and respect, a fact that cannot be ignored when ovarian tissue is stored or used.

The goal of cancer treatment is cure with the least amount of damage to the rest of the organs in the body. With this model, any discussion with parents and the child should include a discussion of the effort to minimize damage and the associated advantages and risks. In the case of ovaries, which are particularly susceptible to damage by chemotherapy and radiation, one option for preserving function is to remove ovarian tissue or an entire ovary for cryopreservation.

The risks and benefits of fertility-preserving surgery can be explained in an age-appropriate manner in order for her to give assent. The surgery is being done to protect the cells in an organ that may allow the child to have children in the future if she chooses. If the surgery is not done, then there is an estimated risk she will not have her own children, and she will need to choose from other options such as adoption, egg donation, or childlessness. We cannot guarantee she can have her own genetic children if the surgery is performed, nor can we guarantee she will or will not be able to bear her own genetic children if the surgery is not done. Preserving the ovary simply increases the chance that she will be able to have her own genetic children if she chooses to do so in the future.

Research in Children

The special problem of research in children is central to our ethical concern – both because research will have to be done long in advance of therapeutic use, as described above and that in all cases, the surgical intervention necessary will raise unique ethical questions of how any pediatric research is framed. Ethical guidelines for research in children must strike a balance between the need to improve treatments for children with protection of the individual child. IRBs are able to approve pediatric research in three risk and benefit categories under federal regulations: (1) studies that offer participating children a prospect of direct benefit, (2) studies that do not offer a prospect of direct benefit but pose only minimal risk, and (3) studies that do not offer a prospect of direct benefit and pose a minor increase over minimal risk [20].[1] As a result, the enrollment of children in clinical research is highly dependent on regulators at each institution and how they struggle to interpret risk and benefit guidelines [21].[2] While it is understood that it is important to protect children from excessive risks in research, it is also important to consider that an overestimation of the risks will prevent important advances in pediatric treatments [22].

Research with children requires their assent, which differs from the consent obtained from the patient's parents or an adult patient [9]. Informed consent has two main components: that the patient has comprehension or understanding of the treatment and that the consent is freely given [23]. Assent is "a child's affirmative agreement to participate in research." The process of assent from a child acknowledges both their legal status as a minor and also their decreased decision-making capacity or ability to comprehend a treatment [9].

The requirement of assent may be waived by the IRB only in cases when the research "offers a prospect of direct benefit that is important to the health or well-being of the children and is available only in the context of research" [21]. We fully understand that children many not have the capacity to understand the nature of rare but serious risks, and thus the consent to this intervention must be a parental decision for younger girls.

In the case of oophorectomy for fertility preservation in girls with cancer, the treatment may or may not provide direct benefit to the child, and will put the child at above minimal risk compared with that of daily life. The federal guidelines are vague in how to assess capacity for assent and how much information about risks should be given to children asked to assent. Based on the recommendation of the American Academy of Pediatrics (AAP) and the National Commission, it is appropriate to obtain assent[3] from children 7 years of age and older. Parental consent must also be given. As described above, the need for the surgery may be presented

---

[1] Minimal risk is defined as "ordinarily encountered in daily life or during the performance of routine physical or psychological test" (22).

[2] A recent study of how IRB chairpersons applied these guidelines yielded highly variable results, revealing either overestimation of tests that are considered routine, or underestimations of risks of daily life, such as riding in a car in rush-hour traffic (22).

[3] The components of competent assent are (1) rudimentary understanding of the procedures, that is, what subjects will be required to do, or what will be done to them, if they participate; (2) basic comprehension of the general purpose of the research; and (3) a preference to participate in the research. The result is a lower level of requirement of comprehension than consent and the expression of a preference to participate. As the age and development of the child advances, appropriate respect needs to be given to the child or adolescent assent for treatment (29).

as part of the treatment package and in an age-appropriate manner that describes the protection of organs involved in reproduction. Both assent and consent must be obtained in order for the surgery to be performed. For children under age 7, parental consent is sufficient if a reasonable person would agree that the potential benefit to the child justifies the potential risks [21,22]. Further guidelines need to be developed on the nature of explicit information that must be provided to children about risks in order to obtain assent.[4] The age at which a pediatric patient would have access to the tissue to initiate a pregnancy and if parents have any right to the tissue needs to be established prior to obtaining the ovarian tissue [16,24].

Why is it important to involve children in the decision about their treatment or research protocol at all? Although legal requirements may apply, the ethical analysis and psychological benefits to involvement of children in such decisions yield far more compelling arguments. Just as in the treatment of adults, it is important to respect the child's autonomy, dignity, individuality, and opportunity for self-determination. The psychological literature supports that children involved in their treatment decisions have the positive benefits of feeling effective, competent, and in control and may experience better self esteem, decreased anxiety, and decreased depression as a result. In cases where research may not directly benefit the patient but may benefit future patients in a similar situation, participation in research may allow the adolescents to feel altruistic and as if they are contributing to society and scientific knowledge. This may also be the first major decision, not only in the course of disease treatments, but in a long life of difficult decisions, and allowing the patient to make the decision in a supportive environment may have long-lasting benefits [25].

Assessing the Intervention: A Community Consent Process in Action

At the beginning of the project of ovarian preservation, the primary ethical concern was that a procedure that was not even entirely dependable in the murine model would be offered to young girls and their families who were already facing enormous and difficult decisions about cancer chemotherapy. Was such a request itself even ethical? Or would the very notion of the question be too difficult to bear? Reflecting on this, we decided to go to the people most directly involved – for the only expertise that actually mattered here was the expertise of patients and families.

---

[4] The recommendation from the National Commission and the AAP is that assent be obtained from children ages 7 and older, but a recent study found that only 20% of IRBs follow this recommendation. This study also found that approximately 25% of IRBs are not requiring investigators to inform children of serious, however rare, risks. This is a deviation from the normal analogous regulations for children developed from adult requirements, but the requirement of serious risks explained to children is not explicitly recommended in guidelines (21).

As new technologies emerge, it is important to have the experience of survivors and their families inform the approach taken with patients who may qualify for experimental fertility-preserving techniques. Literature on childhood cancer often focuses on the scientific, ethical, and legal considerations for fertility preservation [9,16,17], but rarely on the attitude and opinions of parents or survivors with fertility concerns or fertility-preserving options at the time of diagnosis [12]. One recent focus group study on female adult survivors of childhood cancer and their parents, however, has looked at parents' and survivor's concerns regarding cancer-related infertility (see Nieman et al., this volume). The study finds that although the parents acknowledged that they were overwhelmed with information at the time of their daughter's cancer diagnosis, they agreed that fertility preserving options, even if experimental, should be presented as part of the "treatment package" for all children with cancer, similar to how clinical trials are presented to parents. Survivors and parents said that they would have given serious consideration to participation in a fertility preserving study. Survivors also indicated that helping medical advancement, helping other women in the future, and the possibility that it might help them have a child were all potential benefits of participating in a study. Parents also raised concerns about exposing their daughter to another surgery that could be potentially emotionally and physically draining as well as harmful. But these parents also indicated that they would have like more information and believe that, in hindsight, they would have considered having their daughters participate in the study if it had been available at the time of diagnosis. This research indicates that patients and their families will likely be interested in information about fertility-preserving options at the time of diagnosis and prior to the initiation of chemotherapy and radiation, even if they are experimental, and that patients faced with similar fertility damaging therapy may choose to participate if presented with this option. (For further discussion of this focus-group study, see Kinahan, Didwania and Nieman, this volume and Nieman et al., this volume).

The Ethical Implications for a New Terrain: Therapy or Enhancement?

While we have argued that offering an experimental intervention and pursuing research in oncofertility is fully warranted when done under the norms and policies we suggest above, we are aware of the obvious implications of this research. Do our arguments apply to the use of cryopreservation of ovarian tissue for any cause that might imperil fertility? For any use of the matured eggs, including stem cell research? Let us address each question separately.

It is an understandable therapy to attempt to preserve the potential to have genetic children for a cancer patient, but should this therapeutic intervention be extended to women who may face infertility due to other causes? Must there be an immediate or iatrogenic threat to fertility in order for a woman to choose to preserve it? Although we acknowledge that this may be an infrequently requested service, the arguments in favor or against such a practice are important to consider as technologies to store female gametes improve. An extension of the risk/benefit analysis for fertility preservation surely must include other circumstances that threaten fertility or delay childbearing. In order to explore this idea, we discuss both the established method of banking embryos by cryopreservation, and then ask if the principles that apply to embryo storage would extend to male or female gametes.

For example, what if a woman knew that her ability to have children may be impacted by a need for extended professional training or graduate education, a duty to serve in the armed forces or foreign service, or engagement in precarious occupations such as space travel or radiation research? Her risk of infertility will be markedly increased either due to her age or her exposure to hazards, perhaps even approximating the risk of infertility presented to a patient being treated with chemotherapy or radiation. As a society we have clearly become comfortable with a woman's choice to use contraception to prevent pregnancy. The preservation of fertility could be argued as the extension of reproductive choices [15]. Perhaps few women would consider the risk, time commitment, and cost of ovarian hyperstimulation to retrieve eggs for IVF and storage of embryos without demonstrated infertility. But would the ability to store eggs instead of embryos, analogous to storage of sperm, make this option more tempting? Is a law student required to partner before she has children, or a Navy recruit with six years to serve actually "socially infertile" due to obstacles imposed by society?

By the criteria of effectiveness, safety, and ability to pay, IVF could be offered to anyone who requests it. The idea of 25-year-old women preserving fertility by freezing embryos would be disconcerting to many, but a 25-year-old woman undergoing hyperstimulation to help an infertile couple create embryos is current practice. Does the ethical dilemma lie in the storage of embryos that may not ever be used, or in preserving female fertility for "lifestyle" reasons? Who should make the distinction between "lifestyle" and the circumstances of an individual's life that threaten fertility or delay childbearing for any reason, such as finding a partner late in life, pursuing a challenging career, or recovering from an illness? That moral values undergird access to fertility treatments is a largely undescribed issue, yet single mothers and same-sex couples often are sometimes denied fertility services – are they also "socially infertile?"

The American Society for Reproductive Medicine (ASRM) currently recommends against offering ovarian and oocyte cryopreservation as a means to defer reproductive aging based on the current risk-to-benefit ratio and experimental status of the techniques [7]. It remains, however, that the body of work that represents oncofertility is striving to improve techniques to acquire and store gametes until they are established rather than experimental. The storage of gametes, unlike the creation and freezing of embryos, is less ethically problematic for practitioners and society. Sperm banking has been an established technique that is not currently met with much deliberation or protest. As techniques to bank gametes for women emerge, the practical advantages should be weighed against the risk of obtaining the ovarian material. Fertility specialists, women who seek the procedure, and ethicists will need to consider the risk-to-benefit ratio at which fertility preservation could be offered at the request of a healthy patient. We would add that a fair debate about the propriety of the storage of ovarian material would re-open a debate that must include storage of sperm. In light of new data linking conditions such as autism and schizophrenia to paternal age >40 [26], the request for sperm storage by healthy men in their thirties may increase in frequency.

Such a debate walks the familiar fence line of all enhancement debates – where does normal aging become a risk factor in the newly framed disease of infertility? The statistics are startling. Approximately 12% of U.S. women of childbearing age have received infertility services [2], and married women in their thirties who have not yet had a child have a 20–25% rate of infertility after 12 months of unprotected intercourse [27]. Assuming in vitro maturation would allow a woman to conceive by IVF in the future, there could be distinct advantages to a woman storing ovarian tissue in her twenties. It would literally stop the clock and the aging events that begin to increase rates of infertility in older women. The ovary is removed when she is sexually mature and in her reproductive prime, when she has more follicles than she will in her thirties, her ovary has not become resistant to the hormones that mature eggs each month, and the younger eggs are less likely to have chromosomal abnormalities. At what risk-to-benefit ratio, considering the risk of surgery, the success of the preservation, and risk of infertility, could she elect to have this surgery at age 25?

Since ovarian cryopreservation is experimental, it will first be offered to patients who have an iatrogenic threat to their fertility [6,7]. But once the method is no longer considered experimental and its success rate begins to approximate current IVF techniques and normal monthly fecundity, then it is reasonable that access be considered under guidelines similar to other ARTs. Furthermore, as hormonal and physical markers are improved to assess the potential of maturing follicles, only the best candidates will be fertilized, ideally leading to fewer embryos created each cycle. This could virtually eliminate the dilemma of what to do with unused embryos once a pregnancy has been achieved, and to the creation of a new source of eggs for stem cell research.

Recalling a Complex History

Nearly 30 years has passed since the birth of Louise Brown, a breakthrough in medicine and a startling change in the meaning and construction of fertility. Then an experimental technique of IVF, now a routine medical treatment for infertility, the disaggregation of the steps of ovulation, fertilization, implantation, and embryonic development allowed each step to be studied in the in vitro clarity of the lab. The remarkable success of the technique and its eventual commonality allow a certain level of complacency about the extraordinary difficulty of its technical and social achievement.

In their book *A Matter of Life*, Steptoe and Edwards record March 1968 as the first IVF procedure using eggs from a woman who needed her ovary removed for medical reasons. In the subsequent months, they worked with ovaries from 12 women who needed medically indicated oophorectomy, and performed 56 in vitro fertilizations for a paper published in *Nature* in 1969. It was only after several years of working out the details of acquiring in vivo matured oocytes and achieving fertilization that the first trial transfer of any embryo back to the mother was made (January 1972). The first pregnancy was not achieved until the summer of 1975 and was not carried to term. An unspecified number of patients and embryos, and trial and error, resulted in the pregnancy of Lesley Brown with Louise in December of 1977, and the historic birth in 1978 [28].

It is important to note that Steptoe and Edwards only briefly tried IVF in non-human primates and discovered that technical difficulties prevented the technique to be efficient or a good research model. Since the mouse model worked well, and as they had desperate couples willing to try their last hope at biological children, they moved straight to efficient fertilization and embryo transfer in humans. This is an important detail, for it set the precedent for all future IVF interventions, many of which would move directly into clinical use as a matter of practice guidelines rather than in controlled, double-blinded clinical trials. In a sense, the entire IVF enterprise has been an extended clinical trial, but without the standard guidelines, IRBs, and DSMBs. Much of the work was advanced in the private commercial sector. Yet IVF is now an established technique that has a monthly success rate, according to the CDC, that approximates, or even exceeds, normal human fecundity. We wish to note that such an advance did in fact rest on a certain degree of public trust, the willingness of women to be human subjects, and scientific risk.

As we gaze on the possibility of a radically new landscape in human reproduction, not only for cancer survivors, but for all women, we need to re-state the need for the clearest oversight and regulations. Can we turn to this complex history, and yet remain cautious about its shortcomings in this parallel case? We argued that this is the case, as in IVF, non-human primate trials may prove inconclusive or unsustainable. We argue that, as in IVF, other mammalian models may prove sufficient to allow a move to human trials, especially given that the proposed technique of in vitro maturation can be considered a scientifically logical extension of IVF techniques used with regularity today. For the research to proceed in humans will require IRB-approved trials, using standards of quality that current protocols for embryo transfer require in order to give the optimal chance for normal, healthy offspring. Initial patient selection would be limited to women who would not otherwise have the opportunity to have genetic offspring.

Regulatory norms are only a part of the picture. A remarkable advance in so basic a human activity requires a wide-ranging ethical debate about the nature, goal, and meaning of the science. The debate will concern the issues we have summarized here: cancer and its meaning, infertility and its construction, pediatric research, justice issues, iatrogenic harms, and resultant duties. Yet more will be required. This further disaggregation of human reproduction is, after all, about women, families, and how we bring children into the world. The complex negotiation of new roles and the complex and delicate new science offer unprecedented hope and unprecedented responsibilities.

Conclusion

This chapter discusses a subset of the ethical issues surrounding the expanding field of oncofertility. Fertility preservation will continue to be a concern of many adult oncology patients, but also of pediatric patients as they become adult survivors of their childhood cancer. We establish that work in both fertility preservation in the face of iatrogenic threat to fertility and infertility research hold a moral high priority. Fertility preservation procedures for both children and adults should be routinely discussed with patients whose disease treatment may impair fertility, but only be offered in the context of specialized research centers and IRB-approved protocols. Furthermore, patients should understand the limitations of what can be offered at the time of their treatment. Although current experimental fertility preservation protocols should be reserved for individuals who face iatrogenic threat to fertility, we acknowledge that these techniques may not be considered experimental in the near future and may be requested in the context of life circumstances that delay childbearing, to create stem cells, or in conjunction with alternative IVF protocols. We encourage an ongoing discussion between physicians, ethicists, and society at large that carefully weighs the risk-to-benefit ratio of the uses of these technologies in the context of other fertility protocols that are currently routinely offered, such as ovarian hyperstimulation, sperm donation, and embryo storage. As oncofertility grows as a multidisciplinary field, ethics will be a constitutive part of the discussion and research. In this chapter, our aim was to outline some of the more pressing issues regarding ovarian tissue preservation and maturation of oocytes in vitro, particularly with regard to cancer diagnosis and in children. As the techniques put forth in this volume become mainstreamed into medical care, a goal of oncofertility is to continually reassess ethical issues as breakthroughs in the laboratory become instituted at the bedside.

References

1. Beckman CRB, Ling FW, Laube DW, et al. Chapter 39: Infertility In: Obstetrics and Gynecology, fourth edition. Lippincott, Williams, and Wilkins, 2002:494–507.
2. Assisted reproductive technology success rates for 2004. National Summary and Fertility Clinic Reports. Available at: http://www.cdc.gov/ART/index.htm. Accessed March 17, 2007.
3. American Cancer Society. Facts and figures 2003. Available at http://www.cancer.org/docroot/STT/stt_0.asp. Accessed March 17, 2007.
4. Sonmezer Ml, Oktay K. Fertility preservation in female patents. Hum Reprod Update 2004; 10:251–266.
5. Marhhom E, Cohen I. Fertility preservation options for women with malignancies. Obstet Gynecol Surv 2007;62:58–72.
6. Ethics Committee of the American Society for Reproductive Medicine. Fertility preservation and reproduction in cancer patients. Fertil Steril 2005;83:1622–1628.
7. Practice Committee of the American Society for Reproductive Medicine and the Committee of the Society for Assisted Reproductive Technology. Ovarian tissue and oocyte cryopreservation. Fertil Steril 2006;86:S142–S147.

8. Wallace WHB, Anderson RA, Irvine DS. Fertility preservation for young patients with cancer: who is at risk and what can be offered? Lancet Oncol 2005;4:209–218.

9. Robertson JA. Cancer and fertility: ethical and legal challenges. J Natl Cancer Inst Monogr 2005;34:104–106.

10. Xu M, Kreeger PK, Shea LD, et al. Tissue engineered follicles produce live, fertile offspring. Tissue Eng 2006;12:2739–2746.

11. Oktay K, Sonmezer M. Ovarian tissue banking for cancer patients: fertility preservation not just ovarian cryopreservation. Hum Reprod 2004;19:477–480.

12. Lee SJ, Schover LR, Partridge AH, et al. American Society of Clinical Oncology recommendations of fertility preservation in cancer patients. J Clin Oncol 2006;24:2917–2931.

13. Sklar CA, Mertens AC, Mitby P, et al. Premature menopause in survivors of childhood cancer; a report from the childhood cancer survivor study. J Natl Cancer Inst 2006;98:890–896.

14. Brock DW. Funding new reproductive technologies: should they be included in health insurance benefit packages? In: Cohen CB, editor. New ways of making babies: the case of egg donation. Bloomington: Indiana University Press, 1996:213–230.

15. Robertson JA. The presumptive primacy of procreative liberty. In: Children of choice: freedom and the new reproductive technologies. Princeton: Princeton University Press, 1994:23–42.

16. Patrizio P, Butts S, Caplan A. Ovarian tissue preservation and future fertility: emerging technologies and ethical considerations. J Natl Cancer Inst Monogr 2005;34:107–110.

17. Crockin SL. Legal issues related to parenthood after cancer. J Natl Cancer Inst Monogr 2005;34:111–113.

18. Grundy R, Gosden RG, Hweitt M, et al. Fertility preservation for children treated for cancer (1): scientific advances and research dilemmas. Arch Dis Child 2001;84:355–359.

19. Robertson, JA. Procreative liberty, harm to offspring, and assisted reproduction. Am J Law Med 2004;30:7–40.

20. Department of Health and Human Services. 45 CFR §46.401–408. Revised June 18, 1991.

21. Whittle A, Shah S, Wilfond B, et al. Institutional review board practices regarding assent in pediatric research. Pediatrics. 2004:113;1747–1752.

22. Shah S, Whittle A, Wilfond B, et al. How do institutional review boards apply the federal risk and benefit standards for pediatric research? JAMA 2004;291:476–482.

23. American College of Obstetricians and Gynecologists. Ethics in Obstetrics and Gynecology. 2nd ed. Available at: http://www.acog.org/from_home/publications/ethics/. Accessed March 17, 2007.

24. Dudzinski DM. Ethical Issues in fertility preservation for adolescent cancer survivors: oocyte and ovarian tissue cryopreservation. J Pediatr Adolesc Gynecol 2004;17:97–102.

25. Weithhorn LA, Scherer DG. Children's involvement in research participation decisions: psychological considerations. In: Grodin MA, Glantz LH, editors. Children as research subjects: science, ethics and law. New York: Oxford University Press, 1994:133–179.

26. Reichenberg A, Gross R, Weiser M, et al. Advancing paternal age and autism. Arch Gen Psychiatry. 2006;63:1026–1032.

27. Chandra AJ, Martinez GM, Mosher WD, et al. Fertility, family planning, and reproductive health of U.S. women: data from the 2002 National Survey of Family Growth. Vital Heath Stat 2005:23.

28. Edwards R, Steptoe P. A matter of life: the story of a medical breakthrough. New York: William Morrow and Co., 1980.

29. American Academy of Pediatrics, Committee on Drugs. Guidelines for the ethical conduct of studies to evaluate drugs in pediatric populations. Pediatrics 1995;95:286–294.

Chapter 13
The Psychosocial Context of Cancer-Related Infertility

Matthew J. Loscalzo, MSW and Karen L. Clark, MS

The Social Context

Fertility has always been associated with awe, curiosity, and magical thinking. Since the beginning of time, fertility has been deeply imbedded in the human experience and expressed throughout the ages by all cultures in symbolic art. In trying to decipher the atavistic meanings given to fertility, it is essential to consider the hostile world in which our progenitors struggled and eventually thrived. The population of the earth is an incredible success story. No species have ever so dominated the earth as have humans. Fertility has always been the central theme of our ancestors. In many ways, cancer, as a life-threatening disease, brings people back to their most basic and primitive selves.

Archeological findings in almost all ancient cultures establish the female (primarily in the form of goddesses) and particularly the womb and breast as the primary symbols for fertility. For the male, fertility is represented in the exaggerated erect phallus. The womb and phallus are universal symbols for fertility. Males and females fit together physically to create the miracle of new life – a life that is of them but not them. But the physical pieces are only part of the puzzle; the psychological, social, and spiritual interplay between men and women provides the synergies that truly make us human. "Mother" earth itself has been described as a womb from which all life springs. This is the magic of the ages. But fertility in men and women has always meant more than having genetic continuance and the dream of immortality. Wellness, health, strength, status, power, vitality, connection, commitment, love, family, social cohesiveness, and protection from the unknown forces in an uncontrollable future are all part of the essential fabric of trying to manage a harsh and challenging life. The promise of fertility has been the connective spiritual tissue and balm of the ages. The faces of young children reflexively move us at our very core.

Fertility mythology has had other significant implications beyond the reproductive functions. Every known culture has a creation myth explaining the existence of humankind within the context of their perceptions and level of development. For example, the ancient creation myth of Viet Nam is of the marriage of a dragon and a fairy, both having their own, but distinct, power and

T.K. Woodruff and K.A. Snyder (eds.) *Oncofertility*.

magic. The theme of two alchemizing into three is universal. It is easy to see that the creation myth is an outgrowth of and deification of the cultural perceptions of fertility. For the connections between where we come from and where we go when we die is all part of the same story. This is our story. It is a story played out every day in every country in the world with little thought until something goes wrong.

Within this greater context of fertility, it is possible to understand that even for persons who have long decided not to have children, or are much too old to do so, being deprived of the option and having the decision made for them may involve a deep sense of loss, anger, confusion, and yearning that is beyond intellectual reasoning.

The recognition that having a child of your own is no longer possible always occurs within a social context. Society reinforces guilt, especially in women, when it comes to a threat to fertility. Delaying pregnancy due to personal choice, health concerns in self or partner, finances, lack of a partner, or career advancement is guilt provoking in women trying to balance the conflicting and all too often unrealistic expectations and realities of daily living. Regardless of the cause, infertility is usually assumed to be the problem of the woman. For men, the stressors are different and shame is common: financial concerns, job insecurity, and doubts about the ability to be a good father all may conspire to delay having a child, but ultimately the sense of shame that follows when the option to have children is at-risk can be very powerful and can result in disabling distress and avoidance. When a couple is unable to conceive, even if the man is fertile, his sense of self-esteem, respect, and power is undermined.

When it comes to something as instinctual and important as the ability to have children, both women and men have the unfortunate capacity for relentless self-blame, guilt, and shame, regardless of the cause or choice. When cancer is superimposed on the ability to have children, there can be great stress on the patient, partner, relationship, and family. When fertility is openly discussed and informed joint decision making is actively supported as it relates to cancer, this dreadful situation can have great potential for the deepening of commitment and love, with or without a biological child.

All cancers, to varying degrees, due to the illness itself, treatment side-effects, or related psychosocial distress, always have the potential to significantly undermine sexual health and the ability to have children [1]. Approximately 10.5 million Americans with a history of cancer are alive today, and over one million new cancer cases are estimated to be diagnosed in 2006 [2]. Given these statistics, it is not surprising that three out of four families have been affected by cancer [3]. These statistics make apparent the need for research to identify the impact of cancer on the women and men for whom fertility is a concern. Zanagnolo et al. reported that there is little information available regarding survivors' attitudes, emotions, and choices to have children; therefore, for treatment of young patients with malignant ovarian tumors who may be cured and lead normal lives, preservation of reproductive ability has become an important

issue [4]. In this cross-sectional study of 75 women under the age of 40 with
Stage I ovarian cancer or any stage LMP tumors when at least one of the ovaries
was not or was only minimally involved, malignant ovarian germ cell tumor, or
Stage I sex cord-stromal tumor, 51% of patients feared that their ovarian disease
could have damaged their reproductive potential. An additional 66% of these
women felt anxiety about infertility. Significantly, the investigators found that
infertility increased distress in this group of survivors, regardless of their current
parental status. They also reported that counseling on infertility or pregnancy
was rarely offered or available to these patients [4].

The face of cancer has significantly changed over the past 25 years. Cancer
survivors are living longer, dying less often from the disease, and are increasingly
concerned about quality of life. For many people, the ability to conceive and deliver
a healthy baby of their own is of paramount importance. Unfortunately, in many
circumstances, and for a variety of complex reasons, health care professionals fail
to discuss fertility preservation and other options with cancer patients until it is
too late. Prognosis, survival, and the timing of diseased-focused treatments seem to
provide adequate rationale for the implicit delegation of fertility options as a second
tier concern for health care professionals.

Our clinical experience consistently demonstrates that fertility is important to all
people, regardless of age and situation, and marks a developmental milestone in
their lives. Not surprisingly, women and men who were not informed about the
option of preserving eggs and sperm manifest high levels of confusion, frustration,
and anger toward their health care professionals that is not readily assuaged. At
least in retrospect, very few women and men, if any, who wanted to have children
report that hearing their physician say that "saving your life was of paramount
importance" was an adequate reason not to discuss fertility preservation options
when they were still viable. If the patient is lesbian or homosexual, there is even
greater health care professional discomfort and the false assumption that having
children is not relevant is the convenient default.

Clearly, with the recent dramatic progress in egg preservation options now
available, open and timely communication followed by systematic referral
processes are essential to ensure quality care and to avoid unnecessary psychosocial
distress and litigation. Ultimately, any discussion of oncofertility must be integrated
into the overall medical and psychosocial care of the patient and family. One way
to introduce the conversation is through screening at the first visit. To open the
conversation about fertility, we suggest that the treating physician say something
like, "*You may be aware that cancer and or the treatments we provide frequently
interfere with the ability to have children. Many people will not be able to have
children after treatment. Can you please tell me what your thoughts are about
this?*" Timing is essential here because the window of egg harvesting or sperm
banking may be quite limited due to menstrual cycles and the urgency of cancer
treatments. Therefore, it is essential that a triage system exists that prioritizes the
needs of cancer patients in busy fertility clinics that may have long waiting lists that
extend over weeks.

Psychosocial Screening for Infertility Concerns

Cancer patients are confronted with many challenges to their sense of personal control and ability to integrate new and complex information. It is estimated that 30–50% of cancer patients are reported to have high levels of psychosocial distress at some point in the course of their diagnosis and treatment, yet only 5% ever access mental health services [5].

Psychological screening of cancer patients represents one of the solutions to the under-diagnosis of anxiety, depression, distress, and other cancer-related psychiatric morbidities [6]. However, screening is also helpful to anticipate potential non-psychiatric concerns and problems that may not be evident to the health care team. Screening is also helpful to open the conversation with frank and honest communication, normalize concerns, and to role model team work. Fertility preservation, sexuality, and intimacy are all subject areas that health care professionals tend to avoid, especially when the focus is on "survival". In a longitudinal study of 17 women diagnosed with breast cancer before the age of 41, some of the psychosocial concerns related to reproduction were fertility, contraception, pregnancy (fear and anxiety concerning passing on a breast cancer gene to an unborn child), and breastfeeding (fear and anxiety that breastfeeding will not be possible or that they feel uncomfortable with breastfeeding their baby on the breast that was infected). This study found that fertility status can change over time for young women with breast cancer, as well as their perspectives on fertility. In other words, at baseline, women stated that fertility issues were not of concern; however, by the final interview, they stated that infertility became a concern for them. In addition, regrets of not utilizing fertility-preserving choices in early diagnosis were expressed [7]. Because survival fears can mask important life-long dreams and aspirations, it is incumbent on health care professionals to anticipate and to give voice to the longer term perspectives that may not be readily apparent to cancer patients in this context-sensitive situation.

Biopsychosocial Screening Instrument: How Can We Help You and Your Family?

As a part of the standard of clinical care at the Moores University of California - San Diego (UCSD) Cancer Center, an Institutional Review Board (IRB) – approved study is prospectively collecting data from patients using the only systematic universal program of biopsychosocial screening in the United States. New patients seen at the Moores UCSD Cancer Center outpatient clinic are asked to complete the self-administered biopsychosocial screening instrument, *How Can We Help You and Your Family?* (see Fig. 13.1). This screening instrument takes approximately 2–5 min to complete and consists of 36 cancer-related problems most commonly identified by cancer patients in the physical, social, spiritual, psychological, emotional, and practical domains. Patients are asked to rate the severity of the problems listed on a scale of 1

How Can We Help You and Your Family?
By completing this form you will tell us how we can best work together with you as an effective team.
Please take a few moments to:
1. Rate each and every problem by circling a number 1^{thru} 5. [1 means this is *Not A Problem At All To Me*, 5 means this is the *Worst Problem I Could Have*.]
2. Then, please circle Yes to indicate problems you would like to discuss with a member of our staff.
Ask at the Front Desk if you would like help completing this form.

Problems	Rating [1-5]	Yes	Problems	Rating [1-5]	Yes
	Not a Problem → Worst Problem			Not a Problem → Worst Problem	
1. Transportation	1 2 3 4 5	Yes	19. Ability to have children	1 2 3 4 5	Yes
2. Finances	1 2 3 4 5	Yes	20. Being an anxious or nervous person	1 2 3 4 5	Yes
3. Needing someone to help coordinate my medical care	1 2 3 4 5	Yes	21. Losing control of things that matter to me	1 2 3 4 5	Yes
4. Sleeping	1 2 3 4 5	Yes	22. Feeling down, depressed or blue	1 2 3 4 5	Yes
5. Talking with the doctor	1 2 3 4 5	Yes	23. Thinking clearly	1 2 3 4 5	Yes
6. Understanding my treatment options	1 2 3 4 5	Yes	24. Me being dependent on others	1 2 3 4 5	Yes
7. Talking with the health care team	1 2 3 4 5	Yes	25. Someone else totally dependent on me for their care	1 2 3 4 5	Yes
8. Talking with family, children, friends	1 2 3 4 5	Yes	26. Fatigue (feeling tired)	1 2 3 4 5	Yes
9. Managing my emotions	1 2 3 4 5	Yes	27. Thoughts of ending my own life	1 2 3 4 5	Yes
10. Solving problems due to my illness	1 2 3 4 5	Yes	28. Pain	1 2 3 4 5	Yes
11. Managing work, school, home life	1 2 3 4 5	Yes	29. Sexual Function	1 2 3 4 5	Yes
12. Controlling my anger	1 2 3 4 5	Yes	30. Recent weight loss	1 2 3 4 5	Yes
13. Writing down my choices about medical care for the medical team and my family if I ever become too ill to speak for myself	1 2 3 4 5	Yes	31. Having people near by to help me or needing more practical help at home	1 2 3 4 5	Yes
14. Controlling my fear and worry about the future	1 2 3 4 5	Yes	32. Nausea and vomiting	1 2 3 4 5	Yes
15. Questions and concerns about end of life	1 2 3 4 5	Yes	33. Substance abuse (drugs, alcohol, nicotine, other)	1 2 3 4 5	Yes
16. Finding community resources near where I live	1 2 3 4 5	Yes	34. My ability to cope	1 2 3 4 5	Yes
17. Getting medicines	1 2 3 4 5	Yes	35. Abandonment by my family	1 2 3 4 5	Yes
18. Spiritual Concerns	1 2 3 4 5	Yes	36. Any other Problems you would like to tell us about (please specify):	1 2 3 4 5	Yes

PLEASE CHECKONE: **PLEASE CHECK ONE:**

Present Relationship-   Race-   Native Hawaiian/Other Pacific Islander □

Married □   Single □   African American □   Native American/Native Alaskan □   [Stick-on Patient Info Label here]
Living with Partner □   Widowed □   Asian □   Unknown □   (For Office Use Only)
Divorced □   Hispanic □   White □
                                      Multi-racial □   Other_____

Language I prefer to Speak: English □   Spanish □   Other_____
— Thankyou for taking the time to provide this information.11/16/2005

Fig. 13.1 Biopsychosocial screening instrument – how can we help you and your family?
Note: Item #19 *Ability to Have Children*

(Not a Problem) to 5 (Worst Problem) and indicate which problems they *"would like to discuss with a member of our staff?"* Significant to high levels of distress are defined as a rating ≥3. Approximately 100 new patients are screened monthly. Completed copies of the screening form are distributed to the treating physician, nurse case manager, and social worker. A unique systematic triage system in real time is in place and assistance is provided to the patient in the problem areas where they have indicated they have difficulties. Every problem is pre-assigned to a specific health care professional(s) for intervention. Some problems such as *"Ability to Have Children"* will include more than one team member (see Fig. 13.2).

At the present time, year 2 of this 4-year study has already produced important information about infertility concerns. The population thus far is comprised of cancer center outpatients ($N=2,063$) who were on average 55 years of age with 63.9% females and 36.1% males. The patient sample was composed of 70.8% Caucasian, 11.1% Hispanic, 7.5% Asian, 4.5% African American, and 1.9% other. Of the sample, 57.6% of the patients were married, 18.1% were single, 12.7% were divorced, 6.7% were widowed, and 4.9% were living with a partner, with the remainder being unknown or missing. Clearly, the large number of female patients (mostly breast cancer) is of particular importance to our interests in oncofertility and Gender Synergies (a strengths-based approach to maximizing the ability of women and men to work together in managing the challenges of cancer and its treatment, see below for further discussion).

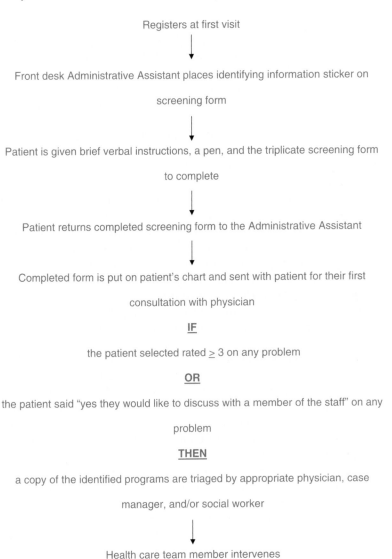

Registers at first visit

Front desk Administrative Assistant places identifying information sticker on

screening form

Patient is given brief verbal instructions, a pen, and the triplicate screening form

to complete

Patient returns completed screening form to the Administrative Assistant

Completed form is put on patient's chart and sent with patient for their first

consultation with physician

IF

the patient selected rated ≥ 3 on any problem

OR

the patient said "yes they would like to discuss with a member of the staff" on any

problem

THEN

a copy of the identified programs are triaged by appropriate physician, case

manager, and/or social worker

Health care team member intervenes

Fig. 13.2 Triage process

Preliminary Results of Screening

To access psychosocial problems related to infertility, one of the items on the screening form is *Ability to Have Children*. Almost 9% of cancer patients reported that problems with *Ability to Have Children* rated ≥3. The six most prevalent psychosocial problems reported that rated ≥3 were: *Fatigue; Finances; Pain; Feeling Down, Depressed, or Blue; Controlling My Fear and Worry About the Future*; and *Being an Anxious or Nervous Person*. See Fig. 13.1 for average distress ratings in *Ability to Have Children* for the entire population compared with those who said they would like to discuss this problem with a member of our staff and those who would not. The average distress rating for the entire population was 1.30 and for those who asked for help the average rating was 3.69, which was almost triple the distress level rating of the overall population. However, a distress score of 3 out of 5 indicates a significant level of acute stress, which warrants therapeutic intervention. It should also be noted that for an individual to indicate that they need to speak to a member of our staff about any problem is an admission of vulnerability and distress and is a high threshold to reach on any scale.

As it relates with *Ability to Have Children,* 2% of cancer patients selected the statement *would like to discuss with a member of our staff*. Since cancer is primarily a disease of the elderly, 2% can be considered a robust unmet need. The six most prevalent psychosocial problems reported *would like to discuss with a member of our staff* by this subgroup were: *Understanding My Treatment Options; Controlling My Fear and Worry About the Future; Pain; Finances; Fatigue;* and *Feeling Down, Depressed, or Blue*. The implications for undermining quality of life of these specific problems are important to all areas of psychosocial functioning, especially for emotional regulation and problem solving.

Demographic differences in problems reported in *Ability to Have Children* were explored. Surprisingly, there were no significant differences between males and females on either the frequency of *Ability to Have Children* rated ≥ 3 or indicating they *would like to discuss with a member of our staff*. However, there were significantly more single (Divorced, Living with Partner, Single, and Widowed) cancer patients (10.3%) who rated *Ability to Have Children* ≥ 3 compared with married cancer patients (7.1%, $p < 0.05$). Single cancer patients were also significantly younger than the married cancer patients ($p < 0.05$). However, there were no significant differences in marital status and if they *would like to discuss with a member of our staff*. Cancer patients under the age of 40 (21.7%) were significantly more likely to experience psychosocial distress regarding *Ability to Have Children* than cancer patients 40 and older ($p < 0.05$). In addition, younger cancer patients (younger than 40) were significantly more likely to report that they *would like to discuss with a member of our staff* problems with *Ability to have Children* than older cancer patients (40 and older, $p < 0.05$). Ethnic differences were also found: 13.6% of minorities (African American, Asian, Hispanic, Multi-racial, Native Hawaiian/Other Pacific Islander, Native American/Native Alaskan, and other) rated *Ability to Have Children* at a distress level of ≥ 3, which is significantly higher than reported by Caucasians (6.5%) ($p < 0.05$). In addition, minorities also reported that they *would like to discuss with a member of our staff* this problem (3.4%) significantly more than did Caucasians (1.7%, $p < 0.05$). See Table 13.1 for an overview of these demographic comparisons.

Table 13.1 Demographic differences in distress regarding *ability to have children*

Demographic	High distress (rated ≥3)	Requested help
Gender	–	–
Marital status		
Single	⇑	–
Married	⇓	–
Age group (years)		
<40	⇑	⇑
≥40	⇓	⇓
–		
Ethnicity		
Caucasians	⇓	⇓
Minorities	⇑	⇑
–	No significant differences	
⇑	Significantly higher distress	
⇓	Significantly lower distress	

Table 13.2 High distress in *ability to have children* also reported high distress in: ($p<0.01$)

Abandonment by my family
Being dependent on others
Controlling my anger
Controlling my fear and worry about the future
Feeling down, depressed, or blue
Finances
Losing control of things that matter to me
Managing work, school, and home life
Nausea and vomiting
Needing someone to help coordinate my medical care
Recent weight loss
Solving problems
Spiritual concerns
Talking with family, children, friends
Understanding my treatment options
*Writing down my choices about medical care for the medical team
    and my family if I ever become too Ill to speak for myself*

To explore other psychosocial problems, correlations were run between problems reported as distressing in relation to *Ability to Have Children*. The psychosocial problems that positively correlated with high distress (rated ≥3) with *Ability to Have Children* are displayed in Table 13.2.

A sum of all the problems rated ≥3 was calculated to determine an overall distress score, which ranged from 0 to 35. A score of 0 indicates that the patient did not have any problems that were rated ≥3, while on the other end of the continuum, if a patient scored a 35, the patient would have rated 35 out of a possible 36 problems ≥3. Thus, the higher the overall distress score, the more psychosocial distress a patient is experiencing. Using this sum score, significant differences were found between those patients who reported problems in *Ability to Have Children* (rated ≥ 3) (mean = 8.8) to those who did not (mean = 5.5; $p < 0.05$).

Consistent with other studies, women 40 years old and younger are more likely to report psychosocial concerns regarding fertility [8,9]; additional analyses to explore this subgroup were conducted. Two hundred and twenty-six women were included in this subanalysis. Of these 226 women, 21.6% rated *Ability to Have Children* ≥ 3 and 9.3% said they *would like to discuss with a member of our staff*. Women who reported high distress in *Ability to Have Children* were also significantly more likely to have reported high distress in the following problems: *Needing Someone to Help Coordinate My Medical Care; Understanding My Treatment Options; Managing Work, School, and Home Life; and Being Dependent on Others* ($p < 0.01$). The data indicated a statistical trend where women who reported high levels of distress regarding *Ability to Have Children* reported a higher overall distress score (mean = 7.0) than those women who did not report high levels of distress in *Ability to Have Children* ($p < 0.07$). In contrast, of the 94 men in the same age range (40 and younger), 23.2% rated *Ability to Have Children* ≥ 3, which, surprisingly, is slightly higher than the level of distress regarding *Ability to Have Children* that females within the same age range reported. It is important to note that women generally report distress and other problems at significantly higher levels than men. Therefore, it is important to recognize that the level of distress reported in this cohort requires additional exploration. On the other hand, 4.3% of the men age 40 and younger (as compared with 9.3% of women age 40 and younger) reported that they *would like to discuss with a member of our staff*. Therefore men age 40 and younger report higher levels of distress with *Ability to Have Children* but are less likely to ask for help with this problem.

Discussion and Implications

In younger women with breast cancer, anxiety and depression peak at the time of diagnosis [10], which is also the time when women and male partners may have to make complex decisions about clarifying their intentions about having children, integrating complex medical information about their options of having children, and making choices that will have an impact on the rest of their lives. Decision making is made more difficult by the need to effectively manage the emotions endemic to a cancer diagnosis: fear of death, loss of dreams and aspirations, concerns about the stability of the relationship itself, and impact on the family and close friends. A diagnosis of cancer always influences families and friends and, in turn, their responses are important to how the patient copes, solves problems, and makes important treatment decisions. Social support, larger network size, and perceived support from partners has been shown to decrease depression, especially in younger adult women with cancer [11]. However, when in crisis overall and having children specifically, it is the committed couple who bear the onus of the most far-reaching decisions of their lives.

Overall, cancer patients and their spouses report a similar level of psychological distress [12]. As it relates to women and their male partners, both clinical experience and the limited research presently available support the importance of a supportive male partner [13]. Weihs et al. provides strong support for the unique contributions of the partner relationship and of the negative impact of a "distant" partner [14]. There is an emerging literature on the importance of how males and females provide and perceive support. Kim et al. reported that men found it easier and less challenging to their self-esteem to manage the many and complex practical aspects in supporting their partners with cancer than they did in communicating with women about their emotional needs [15]. The perceptual differences may be greatly increased during the cancer diagnosis and the emotional disynchrony exaggerated by the implications of decision making around having children during the crisis of a life-threatening illness. Stress always encourages rapid action, while emotional support and wisdom come much more slowly. When fertility is at risk in a couple for whom having children is at the core of their dreams and even the implicit basis of their relationship, it is essential for the health care team to help the couple to process the information and to communicate openly their priorities in relation to having children.

Clearly, the ability to tolerate and effectively use the energy generated by the emotion-laden context of cancer and making decisions about increasing the possibilities of having a child has important implications for individual coping and for the health of the relationship. For couples, the ability to make important decisions together will also impact how and even if anti-cancer therapies will be accessed. Thus, the implications for gaining an appreciation for how women and men can best support each other are crucial. In our program, we focus on Gender Synergies, a strengths-based approach to maximizing the ability of women and men to work together in managing the challenges of cancer and its treatment. Within this model, the differences and strengths of women and men are appreciated and actively embraced to maximize mutual respect and coordinated action to a clearly defined set of values and outcomes. This strengths-based approach focuses on the resiliency, perseverance, creativity, and commitment of women and men, regardless of their relationship, to work together as they have done since the beginning of time to transcend what seem to be insurmountable obstacles.

In this on-going study, we report on 2,063 consecutive cancer patients in an out-patient setting who completed the biopsychosocial screening instrument in which one set of questions provided the opportunity to indicate if they had concerns about having children related to treatment for cancer. As reported above, problems in *Ability to Have Children* rated ≥3 were reported by almost 9% of cancer patients. Because cancer patients report that there is inadequate attention to their concerns about fertility, it is important that standardized and systematic approaches for identifying those patients who could benefit from fertility-related information and education be implemented as essential part of overall medical care.

While we were impressed that 2% of cancer patients selected the statement *would like to discuss with a member of our staff* the problem *Ability to have Children*, it is clear that many more patients could benefit from early identification of fertility-related concerns. This will only happen if health care professionals are able to comfortably address fertility concerns in an honest, open, and timely manner. The screening program described above, *Biopsychosocial Screening Instrument – How Can We Help You and Your Family?*, is a practical way to open the conversation, provide accurate and timely information, focus all energies on making informed treatment decisions, role modeling, team work, and creating a sense of direction and hope at a time when stress is high and it is difficult to manage the parallel processes of the present danger of cancer and the desire to achieve the dream of having children.

References

1. Schover LR. Sexuality and fertility after cancer. New York: John Wiley & Sons, Inc., 1997.
2. American Cancer Society. Cancer facts and figures 2006. Atlanta: American Cancer Society, 2006.
3. National Cancer Institute. Facing forward: life after cancer treatment. Washington, DC: U.S. Department of Heath and Human Services, National Institutes of Health, 2006.
4. Zanagnolo V, Sartori E, Trussardi E, et al. Preservation of ovarian function, reproductive ability and emotional attitudes in patients with malignant ovarian tumors. Eur J Obstet Gynecol Reprod Biol 2005;123:235–243.
5. Hewitt M, Rowland J. Mental health service use among cancer survivors: analysis of the National Health Survey. J Clin Oncol 2002;20:4581–4590.
6. Keller M, Sommerfieldt S, Fischer C, et al. Recognition of distress and psychiatric morbidity in cancer patients: a multi-method approach. Ann Oncol 2004;15:1243–1249.
7. Connell S, Patterson C, Newman B. A qualitative analysis of reproductive issues raised by young Australian women with breast cancer. Health Care Women Int 2006;27:94–110.
8. Partridge H, Gelber S, Peppercorn J, et al. Web-based survey of fertility issues in young women with breast cancer. J Clin Oncol 2004;20:4174–4183.
9. Thewes B, Taylor M, Phillips K, et al. Fertility-and menopause-related information needs of younger women with a diagnosis of early breast cancer. J Clin Oncol 2005;23:5155–5165.
10. Vinokur A, Threatt B, Vinokur-Kaplan D, et al. The process of recovery from breast cancer for younger and older patients: changes during the first year. Cancer 1990;65:1242–1254.
11. Hann D, Baker F, Denniston M, et al. The influence of social support on depressive symptoms in cancer patients: age and gender differences. J Psychosom Res 2002;52:279–283.
12. Baider L, Cooper C, Kaplan-DeNour A, editors. Cancer and the family. 2nd ed. New York: John Wiley & Sons, 2000.
13. Baider L, Andritsch E, Goldzweig G, et al. Changes in psychological distress of women with breast cancer in long-term remission and their husbands. Psychosomatics 2004;45:58–68.
14. Weihs K, Enright T, Howe G, et al. Marital satisfaction and emotional adjustment after breast cancer. J Psychosoc Oncol 1999;17:33–49.
15. Kim Y, Loscalzo M, Wellisch D, et al. Gender differences in caregiving stress among caregivers of cancer survivors, Psycho-oncology 2006;15:1085–1092.

Chapter 14
Childhood Cancer: Fertility and Psychosocial Implications

Karen E. Kinahan, MS, RN, APRN, Aarati Didwania, MD, and Carrie L. Nieman, BS

Having your child diagnosed with cancer is one of the most trying experiences a parent can endure. Greater than 15,000 children and adolescents under the age of 19 are diagnosed with childhood cancer each year in the United States [1]. Childhood cancer is comprised of a wide spectrum of malignancies, and outcomes are dependent upon histology type, disease origin and site, race, sex, and age at diagnosis [2]. Fortunately, advances in treatment and supportive care have led to a significant increase in survival rates for childhood cancer patients. Ries et al. reported that from 1950 to 1954 the 5-year survival rate was 20% for children diagnosed with cancer between the ages 0–14 years [3]. Almost 50 years later, by 1995–2000, the 5-year survival rate rose to 80.1%, and in the past 25 years alone this rate increased by 20% for children ages 0–19 years [4].

Approximately 270,000 Americans are childhood cancer survivors and, by 2010, an estimated 1 in every 250 adults will be living with a history of childhood cancer [5,6]. Recent studies demonstrate that while more childhood cancer patients are surviving, a high percentage of survivors are encountering serious "late effects" from their therapy. These late effects include, but are not limited to, cardiac, pulmonary and endocrine disorders, increased morbidity and mortality, as well as moderately to severely affected status in one or more of the primary domains of health (i.e., general health, mental health, functional status, limitations in activity, fear, or anxiety) [7,8]. This chapter will not go into detail on the myriad of late effects of childhood cancer treatment. Rather, we will focus on the fertility effects that adult survivors of childhood cancer may experience, including the emotional consequences of living with threatened or impaired fertility. Finally, some of the barriers to ongoing follow-up medical care will also be addressed.

Recent Research on Late Effects and Infertility

In 2006, Oeffinger et al. published data from the Childhood Cancer Survivor Study (CCSS) that investigated the health status of adult survivors of childhood cancer. The study determined the incidence and severity of chronic health conditions in adult survivors as compared with their siblings [9]. The CCSS was established

191

T.K. Woodruff and K.A. Snyder (eds.) *Oncofertility*.
© Springer 2007

in 1994 as a resource to examine the long-term outcomes of a cohort of 5-year survivors of pediatric and adolescent cancer who were diagnosed between 1970 and 1986. The CCSS consists of more than 14,000 active participants from 26 institutions in North America, including survivors of leukemia, brain tumors, Hodgkin's disease, non-Hodgkin's lymphoma, Wilm's tumor, neuroblastoma, soft-tissue sarcoma, and bone tumors. All participants provided self-reported socio-demographic and health-related information. The vast majority of the CCSS cohort is now in the second and third decades of their lives, and many years past their diagnosis of childhood cancer. The results of the research conducted from this cohort of survivors have been extremely valuable to health care professionals and survivors alike.

Based on data from the CCSS, the survivor population is at an increased risk for a broad spectrum of adverse outcomes such as early mortality, second cancers, pulmonary complications, pregnancy loss, and giving birth to offspring with low birth weights [10]. Oeffinger's compelling study consisted of 10,397 survivors who were a mean age of 26.6 years at the time of the study and an average of 17.5 years had lapsed between their cancer diagnosis and their participation in the study. The survivors' siblings ($n=3,034$) served as the study's control group, who had a mean age of 29.2 years. Oeffinger et al. found that 62.3% of adult survivors had at least one chronic condition (grade 1–4) and 27.5% had a severe, disabling, or life-threatening condition (grades 3 or 4) on the Common Terminology Criteria for Adverse Events Scale. Furthermore, survivors were 8.2 times as likely to have a grade 3 or 4 condition as their siblings. The study also noted that female survivors reported a 3.5 (2.7–5.2) relative risk (RR, 95% CI) of ovarian failure vs. their siblings. Ovarian failure was the second most common reported grade 3 or 4 condition out of ten conditions. Among female survivors, 2.79 % reported ovarian failure compared with 0.99 % of their siblings [9].

Predicting the risk of ovarian failure or azoospermia among childhood cancer survivors can be complicated. Fertility outcomes in childhood cancer depend on multiple interacting factors, namely the type of chemotherapy agents given to the patient, the site where radiation was administered, and the age of the patient at the time of treatment [11] (also see Gracia and Ginsburg, this volume). As one of the pioneer researchers in fertility effects after childhood cancer, Byrne described the incidence of infertility among childhood cancer survivors through the findings of the National Cancer Institute's Five Center Study. This study was one of the first investigations to research fertility outcomes and the health of offspring in survivors of childhood cancer by using a large cohort of patients. The study's participants were diagnosed with pediatric cancer between 1945 and 1975. Out of 1,232 married survivors of childhood cancer, there was a 15% fertility deficit among survivors. The overall treatment effects were more severe in men, who had a 15% decrease compared with a 7% decrease in female survivors. Men were more susceptible to alkylating agents such as cyclophosphamide and had less than one-half the fertility of their brothers, who served as controls. Women showed no fertility deficits following treatment with similar agents. Conversely, radiation affected both sexes similarly, with greater fertility reductions if the patient was treated below the diaphragm.

Although azoospermia and ovarian failure are the most extreme fertility threats to cancer survivors, there are also less severe but equally serious problems that survivors may encounter. For women, Byrne's study considered the risk of premature menopause, which is a risk for young women who received alkylating agents and/or abdominal radiation. With premature menopause, survivors may resume their menses after treatment and retain their fertility for several years without any overt indications of pending problems. Byrne's 1999 study provided the first data on this important complication and found that the principal risk factors for early menopause after cancer were treatment after the onset of puberty, treatment with radiation below the diaphragm, and the use of alkylating agents. Byrne found that survivors were twice as likely (RR = 2.32, $p < 0.01$) as their control siblings to reach menopause during their twenties. However, there was no excess risk during their thirties (RR = 0.78). Survivors diagnosed after puberty and treated with radiation below the diaphragm were nearly ten times more likely to reach menopause during their twenties than controls, regardless of their primary diagnosis. The RR was 9.6 for Hodgkin's disease survivors and 8.56 for all other cancers [11].

Despite the fertility issues that survivors face, most childhood cancer survivors will go on to produce healthy, live offspring [12–14]. However, studies have indicated that survivors worry about their own reproductive abilities and the health of their offspring [13,15]. Although the majority of survivors will be able to have their own children, infertility is a reality for many childhood cancer survivors. The exact number of survivors affected is unknown, but infertility is one of the most common chronic medical problems reported by childhood cancer survivors and can be a primary concern, particularly among female survivors [16,17].

Addressing the Threat of Infertility

Is the price of infertility a necessary price to pay for survival? In past decades, one would argue yes for female patients, as they lacked viable options to preserve their fertility. Sexually mature men have long had the option to cryopreserve sperm before beginning fertility-threatening cancer treatment. Without alternatives for female patients, infertility can be a considerable cost to pay; some survivors describe the loss of fertility as painful as facing cancer itself [18,19]. Recent advances in fertility preservation may soon offer potential methods for females of all ages to protect their reproductive capacity from damaging radiation and/or chemotherapy [20] (see Min, Woodruff, and Shea, this volume). Current literature focuses on the further development of preservation techniques and the numerous ethical and legal questions (see Zoloth and Backhus, this volume), but little knowledge is available on the attitudes and opinions of childhood cancer survivors and their parents regarding fertility preservation. As basic science research begins to enter the clinical arena, a large number of unanswered questions remain regarding the application of the procedures, the legal and ethical considerations involved, and the receptiveness of patients and their families to fertility preservation questions that are only recently beginning to be addressed.

Additional questions surrounding communication and decision making at the time of diagnosis are also important given that decisions about fertility preservation must be made before treatment begins. Parents, physicians, and patients are required to make a complex decision in a short amount of time during an extremely stressful situation, similar to the anxiety involved in the informed consent process of clinical cancer research trials [21]. In order for fertility preservation to become a realistic and valued addition to the treatment of childhood cancer patients, a better understanding of the decision-making process that parents and their children go through at the time of diagnosis and their interest in fertility preservation is needed (see Clayman, Galvin, and Arntson, this volume). Further, a more thorough exploration of patients' and parents' thoughts regarding the child's fertility at the time of diagnosis and later in life will be valuable in the continued advancement and eventual application of fertility preservation.

Childhood Cancer Survivors and Fertility Preservation

There are several ongoing studies that are beginning to address the perspective of survivors themselves, which will be a critical component to delivering fertility preservation in the clinic. One such study, based out of Northwestern University, was a qualitative exploratory study that consisted of four focus groups: two with adult women who were diagnosed and treated for cancer as adolescents and two with their parents (for more details, see Nieman et al., this volume). The purpose of the study was to explore and compare the attitudes towards fertility and fertility preservation among and between the survivors and parents. Eligibility criteria for survivors included diagnosis and treatment for childhood cancer between the ages of 13 and 21, English-speaking, and willingness to participate in a tape-recorded focus group. The eligibility criteria for parents of survivors included they be English-speaking and willing to participate in a tape-recorded focus group. Survivors were recruited from the Survivors Taking Action & Responsibility (STAR) Program at the Robert H. Lurie Comprehensive Cancer Center of Northwestern University in Chicago, IL, and were eligible to participate with or without a corresponding parent. Adult survivors enrolled in the study were either in ovarian failure or were at risk for infertility due to the treatment they received for their childhood malignancy. Topics addressed in the moderators' guides included (1) short- and long-term concerns at the time of cancer diagnosis, (2) attitudes about fertility at the time of diagnosis and presently, and (3) reactions to a proposed clinical research study in ovarian tissue preservation. For the third topic, participants were asked to read an educational brochure on a proposed clinical research study in ovarian tissue cryopreservation that explained the purpose of the study and the procedures involved, including laparoscopic surgery to remove an ovary.

In the first set of focus groups, four survivors and three parents participated, and in the second set, held two days later, six survivors and seven parents participated. The median age of the ten survivors was 26 years with a range of 23–36 years. Median age of survivors at the time of diagnosis was 14.5 years with a range of 13–21 years. Nine of the ten survivors were diagnosed with Hodgkin's disease and one with Ewing's sarcoma. Eight of the ten survivors received chemotherapy and all received radiation (see Nieman et al., this volume).

This study highlighted that at the time of diagnosis, most survivors reported that fertility was not an issue they considered important. However, when survivors were told that their ability to have their own children was going to be threatened, fertility gained in importance for many of them (see Nieman et al., this volume). In contrast to the time of diagnosis, survivors discussed how fertility has become a relevant issue in their lives, particularly as peers marry and have children and questions about career vs. family arise in their own lives. For many, fertility was something they took for granted until learning about the possible late effects of their treatment.

As fertility becomes an increasingly salient issue for survivors as they age, uncertainty about their fertility status remains for many. Half of the survivors in this study and other studies were unaware of their present fertility status [15,22]. At the time of diagnosis, survivors and their parents were focused on survival. Few parents remember talking with physicians about fertility at the time of diagnosis. For the majority, fertility became an issue after treatment. One parent said, "...*I wasn't thinking about fertility issues. That was a horror that was held for later.*"

With this mindset, survivors and parents were overall very receptive to learning more about the proposed fertility preservation research study. Survivors and parents agreed that infertility was not of utmost concern at the time of diagnosis and that diagnosis and treatment can be an overwhelming time period. Despite these concerns, both survivors and parents agreed that fertility preservation was something they would have considered and would at least have liked to be presented with as an option. Parents and survivors said that the research study would have given them hope that there is life beyond cancer. Participants also recognized how meaningful it is to have reproductive choices, something that male patients have with sperm banking. Many parents commented that they wished they had had something like this available to their daughters. This level of interest among survivors and parents in a research study on fertility preservation, which does not necessarily guarantee a reproductive option, underlines the importance of reproductive choices for cancer survivors and the great relevance of fertility. When asked about extending the program to younger children, survivors and parents felt that fertility preservation is an option that should be presented to everyone, regardless of age. Adolescent cancer patients and their parents echo this interest in fertility preservation. Burns et al. conducted a survey-based study of female cancer patients with a mean age of 15.5 years and their parents. The study found that patients and parents were interested in research treatments to preserve fertility, but were unwilling to delay treatment for such efforts [23].

In order for a possible late effect like infertility to be effectively addressed through fertility preservation, options must be incorporated into cancer care beginning from the diagnosis stage. Advancements should continue to be developed in the area of reproductive technologies, but health care personnel must be prepared to communicate professionally about fertility-related treatment effects with patients and their families and take a proactive and farsighted approach to comprehensive cancer care (see Nieman et al., this volume).

Male Infertility

The majority of this chapter has been focused on female adult survivors of childhood cancer. Despite this focus, many male adult survivors of childhood cancer are deemed sterile, a no less devastating late effect than female infertility, and many male survivors are at an increased risk for infertility (see also Gracia and Ginsburg, this volume and Brannigan, this volume). However, there have been much greater strides forward in addressing male infertility than with female infertility, specifically with the latest advances in in vitro fertilization (IVF) and intracytoplasmic sperm injection (ICSI) [24]. Building on these advances, research in the field of childhood cancer patients continues to address the issue of male infertility.

Kenney and colleagues studied gonadal function in 17 adult male survivors of childhood sarcomas who were treated with high dose pulse cyclophosphamide as part of a combination drug regimen. Of the 17 patients who underwent semen analysis, 58.8% (10) had azoospermia and 29.4% (5) had oligospermia, while only 11.8% (2) had a normal sperm count. The two survivors with a normal sperm count had received the lowest cumulative doses of cyclophosphamide, $<7.5 \, \text{mg/m}^2$. The chemotherapeutic exposure prior to puberty was not found to be protective for sterility and the risk of infertility increased with the higher doses of therapy [25].

Byrne et al. revealed more reassuring results from a large study of male long-term survivors of acute lymphocytic leukemia (ALL) ($n=213$) diagnosed during childhood or adolescence. Younger males, specifically those under 10 years of age, treated with cranial but not spinal radiation were less likely to become fathers than the control group. The male survivors' relative fertility was only 9% (95% CI 0.01–0.82) of the control group fertility. Byrne and her colleagues also revealed that male survivors had more concerns than study controls ($n=145$) on a number of factors related to family planning and male health conditions. One-third had been told that they might have trouble having children and many were concerned with their own health and the health of their children [26]. In the clinical setting, the assessment of male infertility is done through semen analysis. Once a young adult male survivor is ready to learn his fertility status, the health care professional can direct him to an andrology lab for testing. The results need to be discussed in a planned and private discussion, especially if results reveal azoospermia or oligospermia. The health care professional must be prepared to counsel the patient and/or their partner on reproductive technologies available to them.

Access to Care

Currently, adult survivors of childhood cancer are being studied by numerous investigators and results are being disseminated through the Internet, journals, and at medical and nursing conferences. Regardless of this growth in the field of survivorship, adult survivors are struggling to find appropriate long-term follow-up medical care. The difficulty lies in finding generalists and specialists who understand the type of therapy the survivors received and the actual or potential late effects that may arise from these treatments. Most family practice physicians or internists care for a few cancer survivors in their practice and becoming an "expert" is an unrealistic expectation. In general, we have learned that survivors themselves are not knowledgeable about the late effects of their cancer therapy [27]. This introduces an additional difficulty in dealing with this population of patients. Survivors lack knowledge about the current recommendation that they should receive systematic long-term follow-up care on a regular basis for the rest of their lives [28].

To fill this need for adult survivors, various models of care have been addressed in the literature. For example, current models include approaches like community-based programs and actual transition programs for adults to move into after "graduation" from the pediatric medical setting. Regardless of the model, the goal of each approach remains the same. By educating and empowering survivors, the hope is that they will become their own advocates, assume follow-up responsibilities, and gain access to the specialized care they need [29]. Such follow-up care is necessary to treat actual late effects like early osteopenia that can accompany ovarian failure or cardiomyopathy from treatment with anthracyclines. There is also a need to screen appropriately for other delayed effects that may take decades to present, such as secondary malignancies or coronary artery disease. Survivors and their physicians must also learn about new resources available to them, such as the Children's Oncology Group (COG). Guidelines regarding long-term follow-up care and links to health topics for survivors of childhood, adolescent and young adult cancers are available at http://www.survivorshipguidelines.org [30].

Although childhood cancer survivors face numerous late effects, results have consistently shown that the majority of adult survivors of childhood cancer are faring well in terms of adjustment, emotional state, and moving on with their lives [31,32]. However, survivors of pediatric brain tumors are not managing as well. Zebrack et al. demonstrated that pediatric brain tumor survivors have higher levels of global distress and higher depression scores, which are believed to be related to difficulties in becoming re-integrated into society, such as attaining a job and getting married after treatment [33]. Additionally, a study by Rourke et al. found that Post Traumatic Stress Disorder (PTSD) affects a subset (nearly 16%) of young adult survivors of childhood cancer. Post Traumatic Stress Symptoms (PTSS) include re-experiencing the trauma (e.g., flashbacks and nightmares), avoidance of reminders of the trauma, emotional numbing, general anxiety, and physiological arousal. Survivors with PTSS and PTSD may be less likely to follow up with medical personnel due to the distress it causes them [34]. Given the combination of physical and psychological sequelae that may afflict adult survivors of childhood cancer, the need for long-term follow-up care is great, not only for reproductive matters but also to ensure that survivors live as healthy and full lives as possible.

Conclusion

After battling pediatric cancer, many survivors endure numerous difficulties throughout their lives despite being cured of their disease. Fertility deficits are only one of the problems that they face, but the effects of being infertile or sterile can be devastating. The uncertainties of infertility and sterility do not diminish as survivors move into adulthood, rather, they shift focus. As female survivors mature into young adults, issues such as fertility status become pressing. For males, the reality of being sterile as a survivor can be difficult to accept once family planning begins. The risk and experience of infertility and sterility is closely connected to a survivor's identity, intimate relationships, plans for a family, and their concerns regarding their future and happiness. Infertility and sterility is far from a singular experience.

Connecting the pieces that make up a survivor's experience with infertility will help identify unanswered questions and, more importantly, provide guidance for clinical practice and future research. Health care professionals must now incorporate strategies to assist young adult survivors with family planning options and reproductive technologies if applicable. Since adult survivors of childhood cancer appear to lack critical information about their fertility status, efforts need to be made to equip survivors in making informed choices about family planning. A comprehensive fertility assessment of the survivor should not only include laboratory work and a health history but also consider their knowledge of their reproductive abilities as well as childbearing aspirations. Health education related to birth control practices and options and sexual behavior are an important part of a follow-up visit. Clinicians must become aware of support agencies such as Fertile Hope (http://www.fertilehope.org), Planet Cancer (http://www.planetcancer.org), and the Lance Armstrong Foundation (http://www.laf.org), which can offer important information on reproductive options and help address the psychosocial needs of survivors [15]. Although the field of oncofertility is young and growing, resources and an increasing number of options already exist. Informed, dedicated clinicians in concert with educated, empowered survivors can continue to improve the quality of life and health for childhood cancer survivors.

References

1. Ries LAG, Harkins D, Krapcho M, et al., eds. SEER cancer statistics review. 1975–2003. Bethesda, MD: National Cancer Institute, 2005. (Accessed December 27, 2006, at http://seer.cancer.gov/csr/1975_2003/.)
2. Ries LAG, Smith MA, Gurney JG, et al., eds. SEER Cancer Incidence and Survival among Children and Adolescents: United States SEER Program 1975–1995. NIH Pub. No. 99–4649. Bethesda MD, 1999.

3. Ries LAG, Eisner MP, Kosary CL, et al. SEER cancer statistics review, 1975–2001. Bethesda, MD: National Cancer Institute; 2004.

4. Hewitt M, Weiner SL, Simone JV, eds. Childhood Cancer Survivorship: Improving Care and Quality of Life. Washington, DC: National Academies Press; 2003.

5. Ries LAG, Eisner MP, Kosary CL, et al. eds. SEER Cancer Statistics Review, 1973–1999. Bethesda, MD: National Cancer Institute; 2002.

6. Bleyer WA. The Impact of Childhood Cancer on the United States and the World. Cancer 1990;40:355–367.

7. Mertens AC, Yasui Y, Neglia JP, et al. Late mortality experience in five year survivors of childhood and adolescent cancer: the Childhood Cancer Survivor Study. Journal of Clincial Oncology 2001;19:3163–3172.

8. Hudson MM, Mertens AC, Yasui Y, et al. Health status of adult long-term survivors of childhood cancer: a report from the Childhood Cancer Survivor Study. JAMA 2003;290:1583–1592.

9. Oeffinger KC, Mertens AC, Sklar CA, et al. Chronic health conditions in adult survivors of childhood cancer. The New England Journal of Medicine 2006;355:1572–1582.

10. Robison LL. The Childhood Cancer Survivor Study: a resource for research of long-term outcomes among adult survivors of childhood cancer. Minnesota Medicine 2005; Apr; 88(4):45–49.

11. Byrne J. Infertility and premature menopause in childhood cancer survivors. Medical and Pediatric Oncology 1999;33:24–28.

12. Sankila R, Olsen JH, Anderson H, et al. Risk of cancer among offspring of childhood-cancer survivors. The New England Journal of Medicine 1998;338:1339–1344.

13. Byrne J, Rasmussen SA, Steinhorn SC, et al. Genetic disease in offspring of long- term survivors of childhood and adolescent cancer. American Journal of Human Genetics 1998;62(1):45–52.

14. Nagarajan R, Robison LL. Pregnancy outcomes in survivors of childhood cancer. Journal of the National Cancer Institute Monograph 2005;34:72–76.

15. Zebrack BJ, Casillas J, Nohr L, et al. Fertility issues for young adult survivors of childhood cancer. Psycho-Oncology 2004;13:689–699.

16. Stevens MCG, Mahler H, Parkes S. The Health Status of Adult Survivors of Cancer in Childhood. European Journal of Cancer 1998;34:694–698.

17. Zeltzer LK. Cancer in Adolescents and Young Adults: Psychosocial Aspects in Long-Term Survivors. Cancer 1993; 71 (Suppl 10):3463–3468.

18. Dow KH. Having children after breast cancer. Cancer Practice 1994;2:407–413.

19. Schover L. Motivation for parenthood after cancer: a review. Journal of the National Cancer Institute Monograph 2005;34: 2–5.

20. Nieman CL, Kazer R, Brannigan RE, et al. Cancer survivors and infertility: A review of a new problem and novel answers. Journal of Supportive Oncology 2006;4:171–178.

21. Kodish ED, Pentz RD, Noll RB, et al. Informed consent in the Children's Cancer Group: Results of preliminary research. Cancer 1998;2467–2481.

22. Schover LR. Psychosocial aspects of infertility and decisions about reproduction in young cancer survivors: a review. Medical Pediatric Oncology 1999;53–59.

23. Burns KC, Boudreau C, Panepinto JA. Attitudes regarding fertility preservation in female adolescent cancer patients. Journal of Pediatric Hematology Oncology 2006;28:350–354.

24. Tournaye H, Goossens E, Verheyen G, et al. Preserving the reproductive potential of men and boys with cancer: current concepts and future prospects. Hum Reprod Update 2004;10:525–532.

25. Kenney LB, Laufer MR, Grant FD, et al. High risk of infertility and long term gonadal damage in males treated with high dose cyclophosphamide for sarcoma during childhood. Cancer 2001;91:613–621.

26. Byrne J, Fears TR, Mills JL, et al. Fertility of long-term male survivors of acute lymphoblastic leukemia diagnosed during childhood. Pediatric Blood Cancer 2004;42:364–372.

27. Kadan-Lottick NS, Robison LL, Gurney JG, et al. Childhood cancer survivors' knowledge about their past diagnosis and treatment: Childhood Cancer Survivor Study. JAMA 2002; 287:1832–1839.

28. National Cancer Policy Board, Institute of Medicine and National Research Council. Weiner SL, Simone JV, Hewitt M, eds. Childhood Cancer Survivorship: Improving Care and Quality of Life. Washington DC: National Academies Press; 2003.

29. Ryan B, Kinahan K. Models of care for childhood cancer survivors including an overview of transition of care for young adult with special health care needs. Current Problems in Pediatric Adolescent Health Care 2005;35:206–209.

30. Children's Oncology Group, Late Effects Committee, and Nursing Discipline. Long-term follow-up guidelines for survivors of childhood, adolescent and young adult cancers. Available at http://www.survivorshipguidelines.org. Accessed January 4, 2007.

31 Kazak, AE. Implications for survival: Pediatric oncology patients and their families. In A. Bearison & R Mulhurn (Eds.), Pediatric psycho-oncology. New York: Oxford University Press, 1994.

32. Kupst MJ, Natta MB, Richardson CC, et al. Family coping with pediatric leukemia. J Pediatr Psychol 1995;20:601–618.

33. Zebrack BJ, Gurney JG, Oeffinger K, et al. Psychological outcomes in long-term survivors of childhood brain cancer: A report from the Childhood Cancer Survivor Study. J Clin Oncol 2004;22:999–1006.

34. Rourke MT, Hobbie WL, Schwartz L, et al. Posttraumatic stress disorder (PTSD) in young adult survivors of childhood cancer. Pediatric Blood Cancer, 2006.

Chapter 15
Fertility Preservation and Adolescent Cancer Patients: Lessons from Adult Survivors of Childhood Cancer and Their Parents

Carrie L. Nieman, BS, Karen E. Kinahan, MS, RN, APRN,
Susan E. Yount, PhD, Sarah K. Rosenbloom, PhD, Kathleen J. Yost, PhD,
Elizabeth A. Hahn, MA, Timothy Volpe, Kimberley J. Dilley, MD, MPH,
Laurie Zoloth, PhD, and Teresa K. Woodruff, PhD

Building on 40 years of progress in cancer detection and treatment, survival rates for childhood cancers have risen from 20% to almost 80% [1,2]. Approximately 270,000 Americans are childhood cancer survivors and, by 2010, an estimated 1 in every 250 adults will be living with a history of childhood cancer [2,3]. The early and late effects of treatment are beginning to take on greater importance for survivors, their families and providers [4]. Increasing numbers of childhood cancer survivors are beginning to face a new challenge in returning to normalcy after cancer.

Infertility is one of the most common chronic medical problems reported by childhood cancer survivors [5] and can be a primary concern particularly among female survivors [6]. Female infertility has biological and psychosocial implications that cannot be easily addressed given the ethical and legal questions surrounding fertility preservation [7–9]. Recent advances in fertility preservation may soon offer potential methods for females of all ages to protect their reproductive capacity from damaging radiation and/or chemotherapy [10]. Current literature focuses on the further development of preservation techniques and the numerous ethical and legal questions, but little knowledge is available on the attitudes and opinions of childhood cancer patients and their parents regarding fertility preservation.

Progress is being made in understanding the fertility issues that women may face after treatment. Infertility as an isolated health problem can be emotionally devastating for a woman [11] and is often viewed as a loss of one's sense of femininity [12]. The risk of infertility touches on the most intimate aspects of a woman's life after cancer, particularly her relationships, future plans for a family, and concerns about pregnancy and birth [4,12–16]. For cancer survivors who may be dealing with additional physical and emotional concerns, infertility may add yet another concern to an already lengthy list of fears and worries [17]. Some survivors describe that the loss of fertility can be as painful as facing cancer itself [15,18]. The situation is further complicated by the fact that female cancer survivors, particularly pediatric cancer patients, lack clear-cut options to address their

201

T.K. Woodruff and K.A. Snyder (eds.) *Oncofertility.*
© Springer 2007

fertility that are available to their male counterparts. Advancements in semen cryopreservation and intracytoplasmic sperm injection (ICSI) have revolutionized the reproductive outlook of male patients who have reached puberty [19]. Recent advances in reproductive science are beginning to change what is possible for female survivors as well.

Traditionally, few options existed for female cancer patients who may want to have their own biological children in the future. The only two established techniques women have for fertility preservation are protecting the ovaries from radiation and emergency in vitro fertilization (IVF) [20,21]. While protecting a patient's ovaries has become common practice, emergency IVF cannot be offered to patients diagnosed with cancer before puberty because mature oocytes cannot be collected [22]. The promise for female patients with childhood cancer lies in the strides made toward ovarian transplantation and in vitro follicle maturation. Ovarian transplantation involves the removal and cryopreservation of ovarian tissue before treatment and the reintroduction of tissue after treatment, either orthotopically or heterotopically, such as in muscle or subcutaneously [23]. Researchers have demonstrated that transplantation of cryopreserved ovarian tissue has led to human embryonic development when accomplished heterotopically [24] and to a live birth after orthotopic transplantation [25]. Another promising method of fertility preservation is in vitro maturation of immature oocytes. Similar to ovarian transplantation, ovarian tissue is removed and cryopreserved before fertility-threatening treatment. Once a woman is prepared to have a child, follicles can be isolated from the thawed tissue, matured in vitro in a three-dimensional culture system, and the mature oocyte can be fertilized through IVF. Murine oocytes have been collected from in vitro grown follicles, matured, and fertilized in vitro, which has resulted in live births [26]. Human trials, where one ovary is laparoscopically removed before treatment, are being conducted on adult patients in order to begin the experimental process of perhaps one day delivering this option to female cancer patients.

As research begins to enter the clinical arena, a large number of unanswered questions remain regarding the application of the procedures, the legal and ethical considerations involved, and the receptiveness of patients and their families to fertility preservation. Thus far, very few studies have considered the viewpoints of childhood cancer patients and their parents [27]. Since decisions regarding fertility preservation must be made before treatment begins, parents, physicians, and patients are required to make a complex decision in a short amount of time during an extremely stressful situation, similar to the anxiety involved in the informed consent process of clinical cancer research trials [28]. In order for fertility preservation to become a realistic and valued addition to the treatment of childhood cancer patients, a better understanding of the decision-making process that parents and their children go through at the time of diagnosis and their interest in fertility preservation is needed. Further, a more thorough exploration of the patients' and parents' thoughts regarding the child's fertility at the time of diagnosis as well as later in the patient's life will be valuable in the continued advancement and eventual application of fertility preservation.

Methods

Study Design and Sample Recruitment

This qualitative exploratory study consisted of four focus groups: two with adult women who were diagnosed and treated for cancer as adolescents and two with their parents. The purpose of the study was to explore and compare the attitudes towards fertility and fertility preservation among and between the survivors and parents. Eligibility criteria for survivors included diagnosis and treatment for cancer between the ages of 13 and 21, English-speaking, and willing to participate in a tape-recorded focus group. Eligibility criteria for parents of survivors included English-speaking and willing to participate in a tape-recorded focus group. Survivors were recruited from the Survivors Taking Action & Responsibility (STAR Program) at the Robert H. Lurie Comprehensive Cancer Center of Northwestern University, Chicago, IL and were eligible to participate with or without a corresponding parent. All patients had received treatment that could impact their fertility. Patients were either in ovarian failure or were at risk for infertility due to treatment. This study was approved by the institutional review board of Northwestern University and all participants signed informed consent forms prior to participating.

Data Collection and Analysis

The research team (SEY, SKR, KJY, EAH) developed separate moderator's guides to facilitate the survivor and parent focus groups. The guides began with introductions, some general guidelines for conduct, and a disclaimer stating that the moderators were not involved with fertility preservation research. Topics addressed in the moderators' guides included (1) short- and long-term concerns at the time of cancer diagnosis, (2) attitudes about fertility at the time of diagnosis and presently, and (3) reactions to a proposed clinical research study in ovarian tissue preservation. For the third topic, participants were asked to read an educational brochure on a proposed clinical research study in ovarian tissue cryopreservation that explained the purpose of the study and the procedures involved, including laparoscopic surgery to remove an ovary. A mock focus group was conducted with adult female research assistants acting as survivors to provide training for the moderators and test tape-recording equipment. The focus group moderators (SEY, SKR, KJY, and TV) took turns working through the moderator's guide and interacting with the mock survivors. Two focus group moderators (SEY and SKR) are licensed clinical psychologists and another (TV) is a licensed clinical social worker.

Following the mock focus group, minor revisions were made to the moderators' guides and the actual focus groups were scheduled. A total of four focus groups were conducted; two groups of survivors (facilitated by SEY and KJY) and two groups of parents (facilitated by SKR and TV). Focus groups were conducted on June 9 and June 11, 2005. Research assistants were present during all focus groups to administer consent forms and participant intake questionnaires and to take notes and operate tape recording equipment. All focus groups were conducted at Northwestern University, Feinberg School of Medicine, Chicago, IL. Each focus group lasted approximately 1.5–2 hours. Food and beverages were provided, but no monetary incentives were offered to participants.

Audio tapes were transcribed verbatim. A 10-page section of transcripts from the June 9 survivor focus group was reviewed to standardize how important themes were to be extracted from the transcripts. Following this exercise, SEY and KJY separately reviewed the transcripts for the survivors, summarized common themes *within* each focus group and *across* the two focus groups, and then met to reconcile discrepancies and finalize the summary of extracted information. SKR and EAH followed the same procedures for analyzing the transcripts of the parents, and CLN also contributed to the summary of the parents' transcripts.

Results

Sample Characteristics

Four survivors and three parents participated in the first set of focus groups, and six survivors and seven parents participated in the second set, held two days later. The median current age of the ten survivors was 26 years with a range of 23–36 years. Median age of survivors at the time of diagnosis was 14.5 years with a range of 13–21 years. Nine of the ten survivors were diagnosed with Hodgkin's disease and one with Ewing's sarcoma (Table 15.1). Eight of the ten survivors received chemotherapy and all received radiation.

Five of the ten survivors were unaware of their present fertility status. On the other hand, three survivors attempted and successfully conceived a child (100% success rate) without reproductive medicine or procedures. Additional characteristics of the survivor group are presented in Table 15.1.

The median current age of the ten parents was 54 years with a range of 53–67 years. The median age at the time of their daughters' diagnosis was 44 years with a range of 40–51 years. Three were male and seven were female. Additional characteristics are presented in Table 15.2.

Content Analysis

The focus group data for survivors and parents followed three themes: (1) short- and long-term concerns at the time of cancer diagnosis, (2) attitudes about fertility at the time of diagnosis and presently, and (3) reactions to a proposed clinical research study in ovarian tissue preservation.

Table 15.1 Survivor characteristics

	No. of participants (Total $n=10$)
Non-Hispanic white	9
Married	3
Education	
Some college/technical degree (AA)	2
College degree (BS, BA)	7
Advanced degree (MA, PhD, MD)	1
Occupation	
Homemaker	1
Full-time employed	8
Full-time student	1
Primary diagnosis	
Hodgkin's	9
Ewing's sarcoma	1
Treated with chemotherapy	8
Treated with radiation	10
Location of radiation	
Chest	2
Chest & neck	2
Mantle	3
Head & mantle	1
Total body	1
Aware of fertility status now?	5
Ever attempted to conceive a child?	3
Successful conceiving?	3
Used reproductive medication or procedures?	0
Currently taking contraceptives	4
Why taking contraceptives?	
Birth control only	3
Both birth control & hormone replacement	1

Cancer Diagnosis: Treatment Effects and Decision Making

Following their cancer diagnosis, survivors were focused on short-term concerns, such as appearance (e.g., hair loss), feeling sick, missing out on academic and extracurricular activities in school, and the social impact of cancer (e.g., how friends would treat them). Survivors shared little consensus regarding their longer-term concerns post-diagnosis, but did mention concerns such as dying, relapse, and infertility. Despite worries of long-term health problems, many of the survivors reported being focused on "getting through" their treatment rather than

Table 15.2 Parent characteristics

	No. of participants (Total $n = 10$)
Non-Hispanic white	10
Married	10
Education	
Some college/technical degree (AA)	4
College degree (BS, BA)	2
Advanced degree (MA, PhD, MD)	4
Occupation	
Homemaker	2
Full-time employed	8
Number of living children	
2	4
3	4
4	2
Has your daughter ever attempted to conceive a child?	
Missing	1
Yes	2
No	6
Not sure	1
Daughter successfully conceived?	2
Daughter used reproductive medication or procedures?	0

contemplating the late effects of cancer and its treatment. Fertility was mentioned as a primary concern by a few survivors, while others felt it was not a prevalent concern at the time of diagnosis and treatment.

In contrast, parents concentrated mainly on their children's survival after diagnosis, which was clearly the most important concern for parents, with other issues being secondary. Short-term concerns included their children's physical symptoms such as nausea, social functioning with friends and at school, appearance (e.g., hair loss), and maintaining normal routines as much as possible. Many of these concerns, particularly appearance and maintaining normal routines, were reported by parents as their daughters' priorities. Long-term concerns included the ability of their child to maintain optimal physical functioning such as heart and lung capacity, appearance over time (e.g., scarring), the potential for increased risk of cancer later in life and infertility. Similar to survivors, some parents reported that their daughter's fertility was a concern at the time of diagnosis, while others, particularly fathers, stated that it "wasn't even on the radar screen".

Questions about the experiences of survivors and parents with their medical team and treatment decision making were also explored. All survivors felt included in discussions and informational sessions by the medical team. However, they did not feel there were any true options to be considered other than not receiving treatment, which was viewed as an unacceptable option. In addition, they felt that their parents made all of the decisions that needed to be made, which they viewed as appropriate for their age. Consistent with survivors, parents reported that little decision-making about treatment took place at the time of diagnosis. Parents viewed decisions regarding treatment as the provider's role, while their job was to select the "right provider". Like survivors, several parents said that they felt there were no choices to make. Parents said that they trusted their providers and "would have listened to whatever [they] said".

> *"I kind of felt it was either you did this or she'll die...I mean it didn't seem like there was a choice..."*

> *"And he said this...you will be fine, you will. And I never doubted that she would be fine. And maybe I was like goofy but I thought, I trust this doctor, I trust this doctor..."*

An additional aspect of the parents' experience at diagnosis was the drive to educate themselves about cancer and treatments. Parents reported that they wanted to learn as much as possible at the time of diagnosis about their child's disease and available treatment options. One parent stated, *"I just wanted to get educated immediately because I knew nothing about it."* At the same time, parents also reported that they felt overwhelmed by the amount of information coming at once, and that it was difficult to comprehend and cope with long-term issues at the time of diagnosis.

Based on discussions with the medical team, survivors reported that their physicians and nurses focused on short-term treatment side-effects, like hair loss and weight gain, at the time of diagnosis, rather than long-term consequences. Survivors felt that fertility was rarely discussed by the medical team prior to treatment. According to survivors and parents, if fertility was discussed, the issue was raised during treatment, when faced with decisions regarding location and/or additional courses of radiation, or after treatment, when describing the potential for late effects.

> *"I will just add that... I think I remember being shocked like after treatment they are like, oh well fertility is an issue, and I am like, it is? Like I was shocked."*

> *"The first time I remember them talking about it was when I was done with chemo and we started radiation...Before I went to radiation they sat me and my parents down and they talked to us about fertility issues and said that you know how it was necessary to have the radiation but that might be a consequence of it. That was the first time I remember hearing about it."*

Parents had differing experiences with medical teams, in that some recalled discussing fertility and some did not. Some parents reported that they wished they knew more about the possibility of their child's infertility and what to do before the first treatment was initiated, but acknowledged that they may not have been able to think about it at the time of diagnosis.

Importance of Fertility: Then and Now

At the time of diagnosis, most survivors reported fertility was not an issue that they considered important. As discussed above, many of the survivors first became aware of the issue when infertility was presented to them as a possible consequence of their treatment either immediately before or following treatment. Most did not remember discussing fertility with their physicians, while others remembered how disconcerting it was to learn about the risk of infertility or that they were infertile.

> *"...it was very upsetting when I was told at the onset of treatment that...my ability to conceive may or may not be affected, so even at 15 I was still very upset about that..."*

> *"I feel like I've known from a young age that I love kids...the thought of not being able to go through...that process of being pregnant was very, very scary for me."*

> *"...I didn't want to continue with treatment after they told me that I had ovarian failure. You know it was...it was very traumatic."*

When survivors were told that their ability to have one's own children was going to be threatened, fertility gained in importance for many.

> *"It made it more important. That it wasn't something I thought about really ever until they said it might be compromised. And as soon as I found out that it might be compromised, it definitely changed. It was always just something I'd take for granted and then when it may have been taken away from me that's when it became very, very important."*

Now considering fertility as adults, almost all participants endorsed the importance of fertility at the present time and three survivors already had children. Survivors discussed how fertility had become a relevant issue, particularly as their peers marry and have children and questions about career vs. family arise in their own lives.

> *"I didn't think a thing about fertility until I was 20 and people started getting married and talking about babies and stuff."*

> *"I think [fertility] is fairly important now, extremely, now that I have graduated from college and have a career and I am getting settled down."*

> *"...it is always in the back of my mind, because it is something that is important to me in the future."*

Overall, parents did not feel fertility was very important before or at the time of their child's diagnosis, although a few mothers agreed that fertility is always a concern when one has daughters, regardless of age.

> *"...I don't think that comes into play—age—really if you have a daughter...You want her to be fertile. Whether she wants to have children or not, you want them to be...capable of having a choice."*

However, most parents had not given much consideration to infertility and assumed their child would be fertile.

"I think, well, for me it was, let's get her better and we'll worry about it later."

Nearly all had daughters who were 14 or 15 years old when diagnosed with cancer, and some said that fertility might have been more important if their children were older at diagnosis. Reactions about the importance of their daughters' fertility at the present time varied between "very important" to "not that important", but the majority of parents commented that the importance of fertility is growing and has become a current issue for their daughters.

"It became more and more important as you saw them getting well..."

"...I wasn't thinking about fertility issues. That was a horror that was held for later."

As parents talked about their children and the possibility of infertility, secondary concerns related to their children's future plans and relationships also surfaced. One mother shared a concern about her daughter rushing into marriage in order to have a child, while another said that her daughter questions, *"...is anybody going to love me when they find out I can never have babies?"*

Fertility Preservation: Opinions and Reactions

The topic of fertility preservation began with a discussion of the options that survivors were aware of that are available to women who want families after cancer. Survivors demonstrated a good understanding of the available options, including adoption, IVF, surrogacy, donated eggs, and fertility drugs. Survivors appeared to have an understanding of what each option entailed, and some participants had sought out information on some of the options.

Parents also demonstrated a strong understanding of the options available to women who desire families after cancer treatment. Similar to survivors, parents were aware of currently available options as well as several experimental methods like ovarian transplantation and freezing ovarian tissue. Similar to survivors, parents appeared to both understand and be very curious about each potential option, especially the experimental techniques. Several parents also mentioned an awareness of the differences in options available for men and women.

"I do remember thinking it was just totally unfair that guys could freeze their sperm and there really were no options for women."

"If the situation were ever similar to that which it is for young males, which is to say... freeze your sperm... I think it would be outstanding. But secondarily, I think it also gives a large measure of hope and expectation to someone at the front-end of it."

After discussing their knowledge of available options to have families, survivors read the brochure describing a proposed study on preserving fertility by removing an ovary, cryopreserving it, and culturing follicles in vitro. Several of the survivors' immediate reactions were supportive of the study and indicated their own interest in the study if it had been offered to them.

"...my first reaction was had this been offered when you know I was 14, I would have been like yes, yes, just do it. And I know my mother, my parents probably, would have been absolutely with let's do it."

"Sign me up."

Parents echoed these reactions as well.

"Great idea. Something we would have considered."

"[Would have]...signed up in a heart beat."

"Very interesting. Wished this project had begun 20 years ago."

In order to determine the degree to which participants were able to understand the procedures described in the brochure, they were then asked to describe what the research entailed. In general, survivors and parents differed in their understanding of the study. Survivors acknowledged that surgery was involved in the research protocol, but lacked a clear understanding of how the ovarian tissue would be stored and later utilized. In order to address this confusion, survivors compiled a list of questions they felt were not addressed in the brochure and would be important in assessing the costs and benefits of the study. The survivors wanted additional information on an individual's fertility status and pregnancy risk before making a decision to enter the study, as well as further details on how the study would be conducted. Even with unanswered questions, several survivors believed that the benefits outweighed the costs.

"I see the benefits."

"I think the benefits you know outweigh [the costs]."

Survivors named benefits such as helping medical advancement, helping other women in the future, and the possibility that they might conceive a child. Overall, survivors found it difficult to state whether the benefits outweighed the risks; individual responses ranged from favorable to undecided and some unfavorable. Despite mixed reactions and the need for more information, however, survivors agreed that such a study on fertility preservation should be presented to others as an option, including younger patients.

"I just think you need to know your options. Even though it might seem kind of weird at first you know, I mean thinking about that when you are so young. It still has to be presented to the parents and the patient."

"It should be offered to kids younger...for sure. But I mean that's going to be...then it's going to be more the parents' decision."

Parents demonstrated a good understanding of the study's purpose and details based on the brochure. When asked about what was involved in the research protocol, parents discussed how an ovary is removed and frozen and, through continuing research, the possibility of offering an option for having a child may become available. Like survivors, parents also compiled a list of unanswered questions regarding the risk of infertility and the effect of having only one ovary. When assessing the costs and benefits of participating in the study, some parents voiced concern about exposing their young children to yet another potentially physically and emotionally harmful surgery, whereas others stated it seemed "no big deal" and very worthwhile pursuing. Despite raising these concerns, parents largely agreed that they likely would have chosen to participate in this study if it had been available at the time of their children's diagnosis, particularly if they were provided more information and answers to their questions.

"...still have one ovary and a chance...I'd go for it."

"I'd like to gamble rather than be left sterile."

"It's about options. It just gives you another option. And the more options you have in life the better off you are, you know?"

"...as a parent I would have loved to have something like this to share with her."

Parents were then asked whether or not they would have recommended offering the fertility preservation study to parents of younger children. Some stated that they believed that this study was relevant for parents of children of all ages and should be at least presented.

"If it is brought to your attention, you might say, oh wow I...I never thought of that for heaven's sakes you know...That's right they are going to grow up and you know hey thanks...for making me feel they're going to grow up here..."

"...if [doctors] are trained properly in how to present the facts to the parents of this child, they should be told in advance rather than, oops sorry I should have told you this before."

Conversely, others believed that the age of the child when diagnosed was directly related to the potential relevance of the study to parents, and that it would be far less relevant for parents of elementary school-age children and even pre-teens than for teenagers. Parents did agree that especially for parents of younger children, more information would be crucial in making a decision, as well as initial information about the need for concern about fertility in general.

Discussion

Survival rates have reached unprecedented levels and some cancers are beginning to be viewed as chronic diseases. In current literature, increasing amounts of attention are being focused on the long-term health and care of survivors. However, this farsighted view of life post-cancer diagnosis is not necessarily being translated to clinical practice at the time of diagnosis. The predominant concern of survivors in this study was "getting through" the treatment for the disease and battling short-term age-appropriate issues, such as hair loss and maintaining normalcy at school and home. At diagnosis, the majority of survivors were not aware of, much less concerned with, the late effects of cancer treatment, including infertility. For parents, late effects were also viewed as secondary when compared to the overriding fear for their daughter's survival. If fertility was a concern, most adopted a "wait and see" approach described in previous literature [4,29]. With few options available to address late effects proactively, the "wait and see" approach was appropriate. However, recent advancements in cancer care and related fields, such as reproductive technologies, make considerations about a child's future possible and critical to decision making at diagnosis and throughout the treatment process. The optimal time to intervene either to prevent possible complications and/or plan for late effects is before treatment begins. In the case of fertility preservation, ovarian tissue must be removed and cryopreserved before the ovaries are exposed to harmful radiation or chemotherapy. Survival will remain the ultimate goal of cancer treatment, but comprehensive cancer care requires planning for a patient's quality of life before and during treatment as well as years later.

Barriers exist for patients and parents to adopt a more long-term view of cancer care. As mentioned above, planning for a child's life after cancer may seem secondary to parents and physicians relative to the larger goal of keeping the child alive. In addition, parents may be overwhelmed by the diagnosis and the large amount of information they must acquire in a short period of time. Therefore, as several parents mentioned, they may be unable to think beyond fighting the disease. Furthermore, parents and patients may take their cues about late effects being less relevant or important at diagnosis and early in treatment from providers, who tend not to focus on such issues at that point. For example, many survivors reported that they did not remember their providers mentioning the issue of infertility until making decisions about additional treatment or after completion of treatment. Some parents also reported not knowing about the possibility of infertility. These responses differ from what providers report. One survey of health care providers in the pediatric hematology/oncology department at a single institution found that over 92% of providers reported that they routinely discuss the impact of cancer treatment on future fertility with all of their cancer patients and families [30]. However, only 63.3% of providers agreed with the statement that all cancer patients receiving fertility-threatening treatment at the institution are warned about the risk of infertility by a nurse or physician [30].

Such differences between the experience of patients and their families and the reported practice of providers are important, particularly given the importance of the provider in helping establish expectations and priorities regarding treatment and decision making. Based on participants' comments, both survivors and parents do not view themselves as the primary decision maker and do not feel as though there are choices to be made, which is a commonly reported feeling among parents faced with treatment decisions [31]. With this, physicians are often thrust into the role of primary decision makers and greatly influence what patients and parents know and consider important over the course of the disease. If the medical team does not emphasize late effects and infertility at diagnosis or does not do so in a memorable and manageable fashion, patients and parents may also neglect the importance of these possible complications. Additional research on the provider's perspective on decision making and the importance of late effects at diagnosis would complement this study's work with childhood cancer patients and their parents.

Another difficulty in addressing the risk of late effects at diagnosis, particularly infertility, is that the significance of late effects changes over time and the course of the disease. As discussed by participants, infertility can evolve from a seemingly secondary issue at the time of diagnosis into a complication that can negatively impact a survivor's conception of herself as a woman and her quality of life. Many participants, especially fathers, commented that they or their daughters were too young at the time of diagnosis to consider the possibility of infertility, which underlines the fact that age is a critical factor in assigning importance to fertility. Nine of ten survivors were in their early teens when diagnosed with cancer and most of them, as well as their parents, were not thinking of marriage or having families at that time in their lives. Beginning a family has become a salient question for many of the survivors, who are now in their 20s and 30s. Survivors and parents almost all agreed that fertility is an important and relevant concern. Three survivors (30%) already have children of their own. Understanding that the meaning and potential impact of late effects like infertility can change dramatically for pediatric cancer patients over time is essential to providing care for survivors that will benefit them throughout their lifetime.

As fertility becomes an increasingly salient issue for survivors, uncertainty about fertility status remains for many. Half of the survivors in this study were unaware of their present fertility status, a rate comparable to those reported elsewhere [14]. Such uncertainty complicates a survivor's ability to make decisions about having a family and assessing her need to pursue alternative reproductive options. Furthermore, survivors' uncertainty regarding their fertility status can lead to unsafe sexual behaviors, such as unprotected sex, or feelings of rejection and tension in intimate relationships [14]. As described in this study, the question of infertility can be detrimental to survivors and their relationships, as noted in one mother's hope that her daughter will find someone who will love her although she may be infertile. Such concerns about infertility highlight the psychosocial effects of the risk or reality of infertility among childhood cancer survivors. As survivors receive long-term follow-up care, sexual practices and psychosocial health must be addressed.

Fertility preservation for cancer survivors is being developed with the goal of alleviating uncertainties and restoring the reproductive choices many survivors believed they would always have. As survivors and parents discussed, fertility was something they took for granted until learning about the possible late effects of their treatment. With this mindset, survivors and parents were overall very receptive to learning more about the proposed fertility preservation research study. Although survivors and parents agreed that infertility was not a primary concern and that diagnosis and treatment can be overwhelming, both agreed that fertility preservation was something they would have considered and would at least have liked to be presented with as an option. Parents' reported eagerness to learn about fertility preservation at diagnosis follows many parents' desire to educate themselves as much as possible during their child's illness, which is a common and useful coping strategy that helps lessen the feeling of uncertainty [32–34]. Parents also mentioned the large amount of hope that the fertility preservation study would have offered their family because it focuses on their child's life beyond cancer, not simply the next round of treatment. In addition to the interest of patients and families in fertility preservation, a survey of pediatric oncology providers found that over 96% of respondents believed that all cancer patients at risk for infertility should discuss fertility preservation options [29]. Furthermore, 86.7% of providers agreed that children of any age, if developmentally appropriate, should be included in such discussions [29].

Participants viewed the fertility preservation study as an encouraging project, but several hesitations were also discussed. Such reservations must be taken into account when presenting fertility preservation to young patients and their parents. As mentioned above, parents are presented with a large amount of information at diagnosis and during treatment, in addition to the emotional burden of knowing their child's survival is uncertain. The diagnosis and the treatment process are often an overwhelmingly stressful and emotionally draining time period, during which parents often exhibit elevated levels of anxiety, depression, and posttraumatic stress symptoms [35–38]. Decisions regarding fertility preservation should occur before treatment begins, yet parents are typically naïve, unfamiliar with, and inexperienced with treatment options for their child's disease. This difficult situation underlines the importance of a well-trained and prepared medical team that can deliver the necessary facts and options that parents must consider in a comprehensive yet manageable fashion.

After reviewing the brochure participants received about the proposed fertility preservation project, several suggestions for presenting fertility options to parents of childhood cancer patients were compiled. One inference drawn from participants' comments was that how the information about the study is presented and by whom are critical elements of the decision as to whether or not to participate. Unlike merely providing families with a brochure, which was done in the focus groups, participants agreed that they would have appreciated a presentation on the project that contained personal, specific, tailored information, delivered in a sensitive and compassionate manner by a professional. Participants believed that such a presentation would have significantly enhanced their level of comfort, confidence, and ability to assess the risks and benefits of participating in such a study. Another recommendation that arose out of the focus group discussions was that parents believed that the possibility of infertility and proposal for fertility preservation should be discussed with parents by a woman due to the sensitive nature of the topic. Additionally, parents believed that for maximum acceptance, fertility preservation should be presented to parents as part of their child's treatment "package" when discussing cancer treatment options, similar to clinical trial research options. Parents also added that learning about other childhood cancer survivors' experiences with fertility would aid them in making a decision regarding fertility preservation. Parents commented that although fertility may seem of secondary importance at the time of diagnosis, hearing others' experiences would help remind them that their daughter may also grow up and one day want children.

For the majority of childhood cancer survivors, fertility will only grow in importance, which is an important consideration for parents of future patients to keep in mind who may face a decision about their young daughter's fertility.

This study focused on the opinions and attitudes of adult childhood cancer survivors who were diagnosed between the ages of 13 and 21 years, and their parents. There are some limitations. Responses may have varied if the survivors had been diagnosed earlier than 13 years, when questions about future fertility may have seemed even more distant; but, as several parents commented, a daughter's fertility will always be important to her parents if brought to their attention. Another limitation is that the study did not include any survivors who had tried to conceive and were unsuccessful; therefore, fertility concerns may have been less relevant to the study sample. Additional limitations include the small sample size, which was drawn from a single institution, and the lack of cultural diversity among participants. This study also raises questions about the unique dynamic between providers, parents, and pediatric cancer patients. Research into delivering fertility preservation that draws on the experience of patients and providers themselves must continue in order to ensure that advances in reproductive science benefit patients in substantial and meaningful ways.

Conclusion

At the time of diagnosis, survivors and their parents were focused on survival. Few parents remember talking with physicians about fertility at the time of diagnosis. For the majority, fertility became an issue after treatment. As adults, fertility took on greater importance among survivors and their parents, as peers married and began families. Survivors and especially parents said that they would have seriously considered a fertility preservation research study if it had been an option. Parents and survivors said that the research study would have given them hope that there is life beyond cancer. Participants also recognized how meaningful it is to have reproductive choices, something that male patients have with sperm banking. Many parents commented that they wished they had had something like this for their daughters. This level of interest among survivors and parents in a research study on fertility preservation, which does not necessarily guarantee a reproductive option, underlines the importance of reproductive choices for cancer survivors and the great relevance of fertility – an issue that "wasn't even on the radar screen" at diagnosis. When asked about extending the program to younger children, survivors and parents felt that fertility preservation is an option that should be presented to everyone, regardless of age. In order for a possible late effect like infertility to be effectively addressed through fertility preservation, options must be incorporated into cancer care beginning at diagnosis. Advancements must continue to be developed in the area of reproductive technologies, but providers also need to be prepared to discuss fertility with patients and their families and take a proactive and farsighted approach to comprehensive cancer care.

References

1. Bleyer WA. The U.S. pediatric cancer clinical trials programmes: international implications and the way forward. Eur J Cancer 1997;33:1439–1447.
2. Reis LAG, Eisner MP, Kosary CL, et al, editors. SEER cancer statistics review, 1973–1999. Bethesda, MD: National Cancer Institute, 2002.
3. Bleyer WA. The impact of childhood cancer on the United States and the world. Cancer 1990;40:355–367.
4. Eiser C. Practitioner review: long-term consequences of childhood cancer. J Child Psychol Psychiatry 1998;39:621–633.
5. Stevens MCG, Mahler H, Parkes S. The health status of adult survivors of cancer in childhood. Eur J Cancer 1998;34:694–698.
6. Zeltzer LK. Cancer in adolescents and young adults: psychosocial aspects in long-term survivors. Cancer 1993;71:3463–3468.
7. Robertson JA. Cancer and fertility: ethical and legal challenges. J Natl Cancer Inst Monogr 2005;34:104–106.
8. Patrizio P, Butts S, Caplan A. Ovarian tissue preservation and future fertility: emerging technologies and ethical considerations. J Natl Cancer Inst Monogr 2005;34:107–110.
9. Crockin SL. Legal issues related to parenthood after cancer. J Natl Cancer Inst Monogr 2005;34:111–113.
10. Nieman CL, Kazer R, Brannigan RE, et al. Cancer survivors and infertility: a review of a new problem and novel answers. J Support Oncol 2006;4:171–178.
11. Hammer-Burns L. An overview of the psychology of infertility: comprehensive psychosocial history of infertility. Infert Reprod Med Clinic N Am 1993;4:433–454.
12. Schover L. Psychosocial aspects of infertility and decisions about reproduction in young cancer survivors: a review. Med Pediat Oncol 1999;33:53–59.
13. Ostroff J, Steinglass P. Psychosocial adaptation following treatment: a family systems perspective on childhood cancer survivorship. In: Baider L, Cooper CL, Kaplan De-Nour A, editors. Cancer and the family. Chichester, England: John Wiley & Sons, Inc., 1996:129–148.
14. Zebrack BJ, Casillas J, Nohr L, et al. Fertility issues for young adult survivors of childhood cancer. Psycho-oncology 2004;13:689–699.
15. Schover L. Motivation for parenthood after cancer: a review. J Natl Cancer Inst Monogr 2005;34:2–5.
16. Schover LR, Rybicki LA, Martin BA, et al. Having children after cancer: a pilot survey of survivors' attitudes and experiences. Cancer 1999;86:697–709.
17. Schover LR. Sexuality and fertility after cancer. New York: John Wiley & Sons, Inc., 1997.
18. Dow KH. Having children after breast cancer. Cancer Pract 1994;2:407–413.
19. Tournaye H, Goossens E, Verheyen G, et al. Preserving the reproductive potential of men and boys with cancer: current concepts and future prospects. Hum Reprod Update 2004;10:525–532.
20. Meirow D, Nugent D. The effects of radiotherapy and chemotherapy on female reproduction. Hum Reprod Update 2001;7:535–543.
21. Sonmezer M, Oktay K. Fertility preservation in female patients. Hum Reprod Update 2004;10:251–266.
22. Wallace WHB, Anderson RA, Irvine DS. Fertility preservation for young patients with cancer: who is at risk and what can be offered? Lancet Oncol 2005;6:209–218.
23. Kim SS, Battaglia DE, Soules MR. The future of human ovarian cryopreservation and transplantation: fertility and beyond. Fertil Steril 2001;75:1049–1056.
24. Oktay K, Buyuk E, Veeck L, et al. Embryo development after heterotopic transplantation of cryopreserved ovarian tissue. Lancet 2004;363:837–840.
25. Donnez J, Dolmans MM, Demylle D, et al. Livebirth after orthotopic transplantation of cryopreserved ovarian tissue. Lancet 2004;364:1405–1410.

26. Xu M, Kreeger PK, Shea LD, et al. Tissue engineered follicles produce live, fertile offspring. Tissue Eng 2006;12:2739–2746.
27. Burns KC, Boudreau C, Panepinto JA. Attitudes regarding fertility preservation in female adolescent cancer patients. J Pediatr Hematol Oncol 2006;28:350–354.
28. Kodish ED, Pentz RD, Noll RB, et al. Informed consent in the Childrens Cancer Group: results of preliminary research. Cancer 1998;82:2467–2481.
29. Somerfield MR, Curbow B, Wingard JR, et al. Coping with the physical and psychosocial sequelae of bone marrow transplantation among long-term survivors. J Behav Med 1996;19:163–184.
30. Goodwin T, Oosterhuis BE, Kiernan M, et al. Attitudes and practices of pediatric oncology providers regarding fertility issues. Pediatr Blood Cancer 2006; [Epub ahead of print].
31. Hinds PS, Oakes L, Quargnenti A, et al. An international feasibility study of parental decision making in pediatric oncology. Oncol Nurs Forum 2000;27:1233–1243.
32. Kelly KP, Porock D. A survey of pediatric oncology nurses' perceptions of parent educational needs. J Pediatr Oncol Nurs 2005;22:58–66.
33. Pyke-Grimm KA, Degner L, Small A, et al. Preferences for participation in treatment decision making and information needs of parents of children with cancer: a pilot study. J Pediatr Oncol Nurs 1999;16:13–24.
34. Clarke-Steffen L. Waiting and not knowing: the diagnosis of cancer in a child. J Pediatr Oncol Nurs 1993;10:146–153.
35. Fife B, Norton J, Groom G. The family's adaptation to childhood leukemia. Soc Sci Med 1987;24:159–168.
36. Sawyer M, Antoniou G, Toogood I, et al. Childhood cancer: a two-year prospective study of the psychological adjustment of children and parents. J Am Acad Child Adoles Psychiatry 1997;36:1736–1743.
37. Hoekstra-Weebers JEHM, Jaspers JPC, Kamps WA, et al. Gender differences in psychological adaptation and coping in parents of pediatric cancer patients. Psycho-oncology 1998;7:26–36.
38. Kazak AE, Boeving CA, Alderfer MA, et al. Posttraumatic stress symptoms during treatment in parents of children with cancer. J Clin Oncol 2005;23:7405–7410.

Part VI
Training in a New Medical Discipline and Medical Guidelines

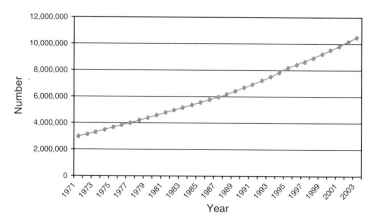

Fig. 16.1 The total number of cancer survivors in the United States has risen from 3 million in 1971 to more than 10 million in 2003. The number of young cancer survivors (<39 years of age) has also escalated to nearly 1 million individuals. Data provided above is from the NCI with original population estimates from the U.S. Bureau of the Census (most recent census data). The fertility threat of cancer treatment on women within this cohort and the impact on reproductive endocrinology has not been fully assessed by any organization. This new cohort of patients will require a new kind of physician, the "oncofertility scholar," to meet its unique set of needs (From NCI Cancer Survivorship Research [2].)

However, not all treatments result in acute gonadal failure. Instead, some treatments cause subfertility, which reduces sperm count in men and causes an accelerated loss of follicles in women. Young cancer patients are particularly susceptible to the gonadotoxic effects of certain anti-cancer agents. Beyond their role in reproduction, the gonads produce steroid hormones that impact other physiologic processes, such as bone growth and maintenance, cardiovascular health, and the development of secondary sex characteristics. For young cancer survivors, the prepubertal loss of gonadal function requires hormonal intervention to recover the beneficial effects of sex steroids as well as provide a sense of normalcy. With hormone replacement therapy, the young cancer survivor will regain these benefits and will reach the same developmental milestones as her peers; however, she may not recover the ability to conceive her own.

Infertility: An Unmet Clinical Need for Young Cancer Patients

Approximately 270,000 Americans are childhood cancer survivors, and by 2015, the NCI reports that 1 in every 250 adults will be living with a history of childhood cancer [2,7,8]. Great strides in medical therapy have improved survival rates for childhood cancers, which have risen from 20% to almost 80% [9,10]. Due to the increase in the number of survivors, the early and late effects of treatment are beginning to garner increased attention for survivors, their families, and their medical providers [11–13]. Infertility is one of the most common chronic medical problems reported by childhood cancer survivors and can be of primary concern, particularly among female survivors [14,15]. Additionally, the loss of fertility is identified as the most important concern after mortality by newly diagnosed cancer patients. Unlike other late effects, such as complications in cardiovascular or liver function, female infertility has biological and psychosocial implications that can neither be narrowly defined nor easily addressed given the number of ethical and legal questions surrounding fertility preservation [16–20]. Therefore, the hurdles associated with fertility preservation often result in the lack of meaningful discussions of the reproductive consequences of cancer therapy and the options available to women at the time of cancer diagnosis. Despite physicians' reservations, women attest that fertility is a focal point in their lives and information about fertility preservation options is a key expectation women have as part of their recovery process.

As cancer survivorship increases, the preservation of fertility in women and girls with malignancies has become an increasingly relevant unmet need. Fertility preservation for men has long been an option; post-pubertal boys and men are offered a simple process of semen cryopreservation. Although women and girls faced with a devastating cancer diagnosis have the same hope for recovery, they lack the fertility preservation options that their male counterparts are afforded. That there are fewer options for women, particularly for prepubescent girls diagnosed with cancer, holds back many medical oncologists from discussing the potential threat of cancer or its treatment to their female patients' fertility. Even more troublesome is that some physicians will not discuss options with sick women, but will talk with men [21]. For instance, seven-time Tour de France winner Lance Armstrong recalls that his oncologist recommended sperm cryopreservation at the time of his diagnosis despite facing life-threatening metastatic testicular cancer. Clearly, expanding the current menu of viable fertility-conserving options for women is necessary. However, this must be linked to a shift in a physicians' attitude about fertility and a subsequent shift in clinical practice to include future fertility as an integral part of the discussion of quality-of-life issues in the cancer remission period. Certainly, patients are vocalizing their desire to discuss fertility as a survivorship issue. In a 2000-person survey of patients at the Moore Comprehensive Cancer Center at the University of California, San Diego, fertility was of greatest concern second only to mortality, and men and women were equally concerned with how cancer treatment would impact their future ability to have children. This landmark study emphasized the importance of fertility for younger people facing cancer (see Loscalzo and Clark, this volume). Its findings underscore the urgency with which clinical centers must begin providing patients with comprehensive information regarding the potential fertility threat that cancer treatment poses and to ensure that health care professionals provide adequate fertility-conserving options for their patients. Given this unmet need, new approaches to understanding the interplay between age of diagnosis and cancer treatment and their influence on fertility outcomes are essential. It is expected that as the number of young cancer survivors increases, there will be a corresponding increase in the need for clinicians trained to meet their needs.

To further understand the barriers between patients' needs and what they are offered, a close inspection of the existing obstacles is essential. There are three main gaps that create the unmet need in fertility preservation for women and girls with cancer: the information gap, the data gap, and the option gap (see Fig. 16.2). The first gap is an information gap. In many cases, the treatment will not affect the ovaries. However, in some cases, the impact of particular treatments on fertility is not known because valid studies have not been performed on the survivors. Certainly, the ability to advise patients about the impact of a particular treatment on fertility is important. The information gap underscores the importance of the psychosocial consequences of infertility and the vital role that physicians play in allaying the concerns of cancer patients and helping them to make informed choices.

Patients are gaining appreciation that cancer treatment poses a significant fertility threat, in part due to advocacy groups such as Fertile Hope, which are dedicated to promoting fertility awareness in light of a cancer diagnosis. In response, the American Society of Reproductive Medicine offered a committee report, which outlines the pertinent issues surrounding reproduction in cancer patients for both cancer and reproductive specialists [22]. Furthermore, the Americal Society of Clinical Oncology published a review of the current literature pertaining to fertility

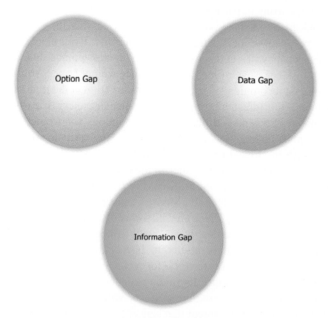

Fig. 16.2 Gaps exist that limit the number of women with fertility-threatening medical procedures from acquiring fertility preserving services. In the past, there have been few options for women, there has been poor interdisciplinary communication between internal medicine, surgery, and reproductive medicine, and there has been a paucity of data about the true impact of treatment on fertility. To fill these gaps, a new oncofertility specialist will emerge who understands the impact of treatment on fertility and can advise the medical practitioner on fertility-sparing options as well as understand and apply new technology to better serve their patients

preservation options to guide oncologists as they encounter patients of reproductive age [3]. Both organizations advocate that physicians include a discussion of the possible reproductive consequences of cancer therapy as part of the patient education and counseling prior to treatment. In order to present the full menu of options, these conversations should be initiated early in the cancer management plan. While many physicians treating young cancer patients are gaining awareness about longterm survivorship issues, oncologists traditionally have focused efforts on providing the best treatments available to improve survival. The information delivery gap still remains because many physicians are not aware of the direct correlation between the best therapies and reproductive outcomes; thus they do not discuss the possibility of treatment-induced infertility with patients [3]. Therefore, the emergence of a new scholar, one who can directly interface with practitioners and cancer patients about their fertility needs, will be necessary to meet the unique needs of cancer survivors.

Despite the best efforts of researchers, there still exists a paucity of data on the precise gonadotoxicity of cancer drugs (the data gap). Medical and surgical oncologists treat sick cancer patients. On the other hand, reproductive endocrinologists often work with healthy patients that are infertile. These two patient cohorts are dramatically different and the strategies for fertility management have not been thoroughly developed in cancer patients. The new supra-specialty of "oncofertility" exists at the intersection of these two medical arenas, and an emerging oncofertility scholar will serve to bridge this gap. This gap must be addressed by bringing the two medical disciplines together to rigorously assess the endocrinology of the cancer patient before, during, and after treatment, as well as during the remission period. Data acquisition is complicated by the fact that patients are treated at different ages and with different drug regimens. These variables make studies of gonadotoxicity more challenging and require knowledge of the treatment schedule, changes in drug regimen, and a long-term commitment to this new field. Moreover, new drugs are introduced frequently and their fertility threat must be quickly evaluated. The new oncofertility specialist will be uniquely qualified to fill this data gap.

Fundamentally, fertility preservation for men and women revolves around the common themes of gamete storage and later utilization. However, the currently available reproductive options for female survivors, as compared with their male counterparts, offer a very different prospect for future fertility (the option gap). Whereas men possess the proven success of semen cryopreservation and intracytoplasmic sperm injection (ICSI), female survivors have few established options. Options traditionally available to women, such as ovarian transposition, embryo cryopreservation, and mature oocyte cryopreservation, present unique limitations when applied to cancer patients, particularly childhood cancer patients. The promise for some female survivors lies in the strides made toward ovarian transplantation and in vitro follicle maturation (see Agarwal and Chang, this volume). The emerging scholar will fill the option gap with concrete and diverse alternatives that will result in the ability to provide authoritative answers to many of the fundamental clinical questions of oncofertility: (1) Which patients are at risk of premature loss of gonadal function? (2) Which patients should be offered fertility preserving options? and (3) Which options can provide true hope for fertility conservation?

Oncofertility and the Oncofertility Scholar

Oncofertility stems from the medical subspecialties of oncology and reproductive endocrinology and infertility (REI). With the evolution of this new complementary medical discipline comes the emergence of a new medical scholar. The purpose of the discipline of oncofertility is to address the issue of fertility preservation after cancer treatment with medical experts specifically trained to advise and treat their patients with new and emerging technologies. The long-term success of this ambitious initiative requires the well orchestrated and focused development of a physician–scientist global workforce that will implement research and clinical goals. Ultimately, the clinical investigator will spearhead the expansion and development of this new interdisciplinary field. The uncertain event horizon for the patient, the immense amount of decision-making that must occur at the time of treatment, the paucity of data about treatment-related fertility threats, and the rapidity with which an action plan must be enacted are the major clinical obstacles that must be addressed by the new oncofertility specialist.

In order to prepare this new scholar, a specialized training program will need to be created to meet the goals of the discipline. The intent of the oncofertility training program is to train and educate the first generation of new scholars and open the pipeline for the development of academic specialists in the new interdisciplinary field of oncofertility. Such education and training will provide the foundation for further development of this discipline, which exists at the intersection of oncology, pediatrics, reproductive science and medicine, biomechanics, materials science, mathematics, social science, bioethics, religion, policy research, reproductive health law, and cognitive and learning science. The goal of this training program is to prepare talented academic clinicians from the ranks of reproductive endocrinologists for investigative careers that focus on the unique reproductive and fertility needs of the female cancer patient and cancer survivor. Research will be based on molecular, cell biology, biomaterials, cryobiology and non-human primate physiology, as well as interdisciplinary training in medical oncology, bioethics, and health law or communication studies. Each of these disciplines places particular emphasis on basic and translational interdisciplinary research in order to prepare physician investigators to meet the challenges of the care of the female cancer patients and survivors.

Reproductive Endocrinology and Infertility as the Springboard to a New Oncofertility Scholar

Reproductive endocrinology and infertility is one of four subspecialty fellowships for advanced training after completion of a residency in Obstetrics and Gynecology. Formal certification for this advanced training in reproductive medicine is under the aegis of the Division of Reproductive Endocrinology and Infertility of the

American Board of Obstetrics and Gynecology, Inc. (ABOG). This board awards certificates of special competence for the practice of REI to individuals after completion of an accredited training program and subsequent passing of written and oral examinations. At present, there are over 900 REI Board certified specialists in the United States.

Training in REI has had an impressive evolution during the past three decades. This training had pursued an unstructured pathway prior to the introduction of ABOG-approved training programs initiated in 1974. The American Board of Obstetrics and Gynecology, Inc. is responsible for administration and oversight of fellowship programs. There are currently 37 approved three-year national fellowship programs, with 68 fellows in training. The majority of the programs support one fellow per year with some programs having one fellow every other year and only four programs approved for two fellows per year.

When REI fellowship programs began to proliferate in the late 1970s, two years was deemed adequate to expose fellows to state-of-the-art clinical management principles in infertility and endocrinology. The successful in vitro conception of Louise Brown in 1978 forever changed the field. An explosion in technology followed, and the clinical applicability of in vitro fertilization (IVF) and embryo transfer has expanded and remains largely within the province of the reproductive endocrinologist. Sophisticated technical advances in assisted reproductive technologies are now acquired during fellowship. This increase in required clinical competencies and the explosion in knowledge and scientific advances in molecular biology and genetics prompted ABOG to extend the required fellowship training period from two to three years, effective in 1998, by expanding the length of required research training from a minimum of 6 months to a minimum of 18 months. This additional requirement for research training by ABOG emphasizes the need and commitment for clinically trained individuals to experience an immersion in the laboratory, gain exposure to cutting edge basic research using molecular and cellular biology techniques, and complete successfully the thesis requirement. This research time also represents the opportunity to identify those fellows who are interested in reproductive research as a life-long pursuit.

Initially, the specialty was oriented towards attaining clinical competency in the field of reproductive medicine. However, research competency has always been a feature of REI training and a formal thesis requirement was instituted in 1974, concurrent with the first oral examination in the subspecialty. The thesis requirement enforces the need for exposure to scientific methods of inquiry. Fellows are required to perform and publish a study that demonstrates adequate hypothesis testing and to further defend a thesis at the time of oral examination to attain certification in the subspecialty. The Division of Reproductive Endocrinology of ABOG closely monitors the publication of this research work in peer-reviewed journals as it considers each fellowship program for continued accreditation. Formal progress reports and reviews of each program take place yearly, and formal re-accreditation reviews, which include site visits, occur at three to five year intervals.

The American Society of Reproductive Medicine (ASRM) is a multidisciplinary organization devoted to the advancement of knowledge and expertise in reproductive medicine and biology. With over 9,000 members, it is one of the premier professional associations for reproductive endocrinologists and infertility specialists. Included in its mission statement is "...a comprehensive educational program comprised of educational activities which serve to maintain, develop, or increase the knowledge, skills, and professional performance and relationships that a physician uses to provide reproductive medicine services for patients, the public and the profession" [23]. A similar mission statement can be proposed for the emerging oncofertility specialist: to provide service to the patient, to the public, and to the profession of oncofertility. The oncofertility specialist serves as the liaison between the patient and his/her options, between the medical disciplines of reproductive endocrinology and oncology, and between the scientific advances at the laboratory bench and the practical applications at the bedside.

It is expected that as the number of young cancer survivors increases, there will be a corresponding increase in the need for clinicians trained in oncofertility to meet their needs. One of the primary functions of the oncofertility specialist is to assume the role of patient advocate. In this role, the physician must acquire the most up-to-date, authoritative information and convey that information effectively to allow the patient to make a fully informed decision. The specialist must also convey authoritative information to fellow medical colleagues. Second, the emerging scholar will serve the patient as well as the public as a clinical investigator. A number of areas for investigative research, both in the basic sciences and the clinical realm, are proposed below. For instance, a greater understanding of ovarian physiology, structure, and function may help solve the complex puzzle of human in vitro follicle maturation. In addition, the direct impact of cancer treatments on reproductive capacity remains unanswered. Advancements at the bench can be translated to bedside as new technologies for fertility preservation are developed. Thus, the new scholar will contribute greatly to the field of reproductive medicine while contributing to the expansion of fertility conservation options for the public. Lastly, the oncofertility specialist will provide service to the profession of oncofertility, reproductive medicine, and oncology. As the emerging scholar, the new oncofertility specialist functions as the vanguard, thus inaugurating the discipline. It is the charge of the original scholars to create the scope of the discipline, to help shape the future directions, and to serve as mentors to the next generation. The new scholarship will expand the training of selected REI specialists into the new discipline of oncofertility through a rigorous educational, laboratory, and research curriculum (see Fig. 16.3). Reproductive endocrinology and infertility is a relatively new subspecialty, begun in the mid 1980s soon after the birth of Louise Brown and in response to the human need for fertility options. The development of the oncofertility specialist represents the next major paradigm shift for the discipline and one that will be embraced by research scientists, clinicians, and teachers of the next generation.

The first generation of oncofertility specialists will be fellowship-trained, Board certified Reproductive Endocrinologists who have:
- ➤ Completed additional educational training programs on the:
  - Effects of radiation and chemotherapeutic protocols on cells and reproductive tissues
  - Cryopreservation of oocytes, ovarian follicles and ovarian tissue
  - Cancer genetics and cancer pharmacology
  - Bio-psychosocial impact of a cancer diagnosis
  - Reproductive bioethics and reproductive health policy
- ➤ Completed additional laboratory training in the in vitro maturation of ovarian follicles
- ➤ Developed a basic research program relevant to the in vitro generation of competent oocytes, or, developed a clinical research program evaluating the outcomes and safety of fertility preservation laboratory methods

Fig. 16.3 Proposed oncofertility specialist training

Research Directions

Research is a central feature of REI fellowship programs and of subsequent academic careers. The scope of research spans both basic and clinical inquiries and covers an array of topics within reproductive medicine (see Fig. 16.4). Board-approved REI training programs are academically rigorous and require a major commitment of time to research. This is the only formalized time during the training of Obstetrician/Gynecologists that such a rigorous commitment to an academic research exercise is required. More importantly, the fellowship years represent a unique time when physicians in training have the opportunity to develop a lasting interest in, and hopefully a passion for, research. In this way, the REI fellowship programs serve as a pipeline for the development of academic reproductive medicine specialists.

Basic science research
- ➤ Structure-function relationships of the ovary
- ➤ Follicle and oocyte health
- ➤ Follicle and oocyte maturation
- ➤ In vitro follicle culture systems
- ➤ Effects of chemotherapy on the ovarian follicle in vitro
- ➤ Embryo/oocyte/ovarian tissue cryopreservation
- ➤ Methods of cryopreservation

Clinical research
- ➤ Fertility risk assessment
- ➤ Cancer therapy effects on ovarian function in vivo
- ➤ Patients' attitudes about fertility in the face of cancer diagnosis
- ➤ Patient awareness and utilization of fertility preservation options
- ➤ Barriers to access of reproductive services
- ➤ Providers' attitudes toward fertility preservation

Fig. 16.4 Research scope for the emerging clinical investigator

Future Directions

It is anticipated that in the future other physicians who develop an interest in oncofertility, such as medical and pediatric oncologists or medical endo-crinologists, will be able to participate in this or similar training programs. Moreover, a number of other diseases and surgical procedures that impact female fertility could be addressed using methodology developed through oncofertility research and clinical activities. For example, fertility is reduced after restorative proctocolectomy with ileal–anal anastomosis [24]. Restorative proctocolectomy is the gold standard operative therapy for patients with mucosal ulcerative colitis and familial adenomatous polyposis, which results in 69% infertility rates in women. In patients who receive intraoperative blood transfusions [24] a further decrease in fertility rates has been observed. The pelvic pouch procedure tends to be performed in young women. Little work has been done on linking gastroenterologists with fertility specialists, but the threefold increased risk of becoming sterile when treating inflamma-tory bowel diseases suggests that this interaction should occur. Women with autoimmune diseases such as lupus, scleroderma, and rheumatoid arthritis also have an enhanced risk of infertility, not from the disease, but from the drug cyclophosphamide, a powerful immunosuppressive drug. Women treated with cyclophosphamide after age 30 are 66% more likely to become infertile [25]. Women with chronic renal disease also have impaired fertility that can be rectified by kidney transplant [26]. Smoking, abnormal nutritional status (either morbid obesity or anorexia), and excessive exercise are known to con-tribute to infertility and these links are usually addressed by behavior modifi-cation and IVF [27]. In vitro fertilization is not successful in all cases. For instance, IVF does not efficiently produce viable offspring in women older than 42 years of age, in women resistant to exogenous hormone therapy, or in women who fail to produce viable embryos after multiple cycles. In addition, women with polycystic ovarian disease and type II diabetes represent a subset of candidates likely to fail IVF [28]. Methods to intervene in failed cases have not been well developed and new technologies could provide hope to those who face infertility after attempted IVF [29]. Indeed, if the technology works, a role may emerge for ovarian tissue banking by young women prior to entry into professional tracks, ensuring that eggs of good quality will be available at any time she is ready to have a family. As more drugs are introduced to the cancer and wider-health care markets, the impact on fertility may not be the first parameter tested. The point of this work is not to limit the access of women to vital drugs, rather, to provide health care providers and patients with infor-mation about the fertility implications of treatment and the ability to conceive and bear a pregnancy after treatment. Helping physicians understand what secondary effects treatment will have on their patients and the options available will substantially improve health care delivery.

Conclusion

Since the late 1970s, treatments for infertility have undergone a tremendous change that is as substantial as the rise in the number of cancer survivors. Not all cancer treatments cause the acute loss of ovarian function and infertility; thus, patients must be informed that their treatment may not significantly impact fertility. However, for some patients, life-saving cancer treatment may permanently influence their reproductive capacity. Therefore, the oncofertility specialist must be present to help patients and health care providers consider fertility conservation at the time of initial diagnosis. Frank discussions about fertility impairment as a consequence of treatment have not been a priority for the medical oncologist. There are a number of reasons for this. First, the main goal of the oncologist and the patient is to eliminate the cancer with the use of the best available therapies. This scenario provides a unique niche for the new oncofertility specialist to apply their unique knowledge and training. Second, the impact of the improving and constantly changing landscape of cancer drugs on fertility has not been directly assessed. Therefore, it is difficult for the oncologist to know what to advise their patients. It is the role of the new oncofertility specialist to examine this question and provide a means for informed dialogue with the patient. Finally, for women, there have been so few viable options to preserve fertility that patients may not be able to find a fertility specialist until it is too late.

The current method of coordination and implementation of fertility care in women with cancer consists of a series of communications between a cancer specialist with limited knowledge of reproductive biology and a reproductive specialist who has little understanding of how cancer treatment impacts oocyte health. Therefore, a comprehensive approach to provide patients and their families with a full overview of reproductive options is necessary. Moreover, there is no single specialty in physiology or medicine that can provide all the elements of such a service. The emerging oncofertility training program will directly address this void by providing reproductive specialists with the necessary knowledge and skills to fulfill this unmet need. To that end, the curriculum is broad and highly focused in selected areas. In particular, there is a heavy emphasis on research, not only to learn more about the impact of cancer treatment on follicle and oocyte health, but also for the purpose of conveying the latest information to patients and their health care providers. In addition, it will provide the budding oncofertility specialist the opportunity to become familiar with emerging technologies for in vitro follicular growth and for cryopreservation of ovarian tissue, follicles, and oocytes. Moreover, this research experience will provide a springboard for fellows to pursue an academic career in this specialty. The comprehensive nature of the training will introduce bio-psychosocial, ethical, and policy considerations that arise during an emotionally difficult time for patients and their families, which will improve the ability of health care providers to give counsel.

Infertility is one condition that transgresses the realm of pure science and medicine into the social sciences. It causes significant emotional and financial stress for those it affects. Thus, attempts to prevent iatrogenic infertility require an approach that involves the social sciences as well as the physical and medical sciences. Infertility resulting from cancer therapy in women is particularly complex due to the limited options for its prevention. It requires understanding how to maintain the life potential of the female gamete in its immature state and how to harness that potential when the time is appropriate. It also requires an understanding of the social and emotional impact of cancer therapy on affected individuals, as well as on society, in the face of uncertainty. Overcoming such a complex challenge necessitates the interaction of many individuals with varying expertise.

Oncofertility recognizes that fertility and cancer combine to create a unique set of issues to be addressed. Oncofertility is not a multidisciplinary field allowing for scholarship on a problem from different perspectives, rather it is an interdisciplinary field that brings together scholars from diverse fields to collaboratively ask new questions and develop new measures and research paradigms, resulting in a new way of looking at the problem of cancer and infertility. This involves more than identifying a generic menu of reproductive options that may be applied to all cancer patients. Rather, the aim is to develop novel technologies that take into account the unique circumstances of cancer patients and to bring together insights from a broad range fields including gynecology, oncology, and endocrinology into a new area of scholarship. Moreover, education, ethics, and the social sciences are constitutive parts of oncofertility because understanding the social dynamics that envelop emerging technologies are not secondary research issues but require careful empirical inquiry as well. This comprehensive and interdisciplinary approach will ensure that the medical discoveries of oncofertility are both robust in their scientific base but also that these technologies can be moved from the bench to the bedside. The newly trained oncofertility scholar will therefore have unparallel opportunities that will contribute to solving the gaps in fertility preservation for women and girls facing a cancer diagnosis. The aim of this interdisciplinary approach is to fill in the "gaps" in our current knowledge and promote understanding of the intersection between fertility and cancer. Filling in these gaps in information exchange (e.g., how do physicians learn about the latest oncofertility techniques?) and data (e.g., what is the precise gonadotoxicity of cancer drugs?) will ultimately result in the ability to provide new fertility-preserving options for women diagnosed with cancer so they can take proactive steps to help safeguard their future ability to have biological children.

Although malignancy remains a critical health concern, significant medical advances in cancer detection and treatment have improved survival rates for patients. As patients live longer, the immediate and long-term consequences of cancer management are assuming greater importance for survivors, their families, and their providers. Traditionally, cancer patients had few choices for fertility preservation. However, recent advances employing a three-dimensional alginate scaffold system for the in vitro maturation of murine follicles provides a promising new technology that may one day be applied clinically to the maturation of human ovarian follicles (see Xu, Woodruff, and Shea, this volume). Restoration of fertility and hormonal function would substantially improve the quality of life for women of reproductive age after surviving cancer and the exposure to potentially gonadotoxic cancer therapies. The oncofertility training program is vital to the goals of this pursuit by ensuring the creation of a new generation of specialists who will help to merge fertility-conserving options into conventional cancer care.

References

1. American Cancer Society. Cancer facts and figures 2007. Atlanta: American Cancer Society, 2007.
2. National Cancer Institute. Cancer Survivorship Research–2005. Bethesda, MD: National Cancer Institute, 2005.
3. Lee SJ, Schover LR, Partridge AH, et al. American Society of Clinical Oncology recommendations on fertility preservation in cancer patients. J Clin Oncol 2006;24:2917–2931.
4. Wallace WH, Thomson AB, Kelsey TW. The radiosensitivity of the human oocyte. Hum Reprod 2003;18:117–121.
5. Wallace WH, Thomson AB, Saran F, et al. Predicting age of ovarian failure after radiation to a field that includes the ovaries. Int J Radiat Oncol Biol Phys 2005;62:738–744.
6. Wallace WH, Anderson RA, Irvine DS. Fertility preservation for young patients with cancer: Who is at risk and what can be offered? Lancet 2005;6:209–218.
7. Bleyer WA. The impact of childhood cancer on the United States and the world. CA Cancer J Clin 1990;40:355–367.
8. Reiss U, Cowan M, McMillan A, et al. Hepatic venoocclusive disease in blood and bone marrow transplantation in children and young adults: incidence, risk factors, and outcome in a cohort of 241 patients. J Pediatr Hematol Oncol 2002;24:746–750.
9. Bleyer WA. The U.S. pediatric cancer clinical trials programmes: International implications and the way forward. Eur J Cancer 1997;33:1439–1447.
10. Bhatia S, Meadows AT. Long-term follow-up of childhood cancer survivors: future directions for clinical care and research. Pediatr Blood Cancer 2006;46:143–148.
11. Eiser C. Practitioner review: long-term consequences of childhood cancer. J Child Psychol Psychiatry 1998;39:621–633.
12. Eiser C. Repressive adaptation in children with cancer: It may be better not to know. Child Care Health Dev 1998;24:243–244.
13. Kopel SJ, Eiser C, Cool P, et al. Brief report: Assessment of body image in survivors of childhood cancer. J Pediatr Psychol 1998;23:141–147.
14. Zeltzer LK. Cancer in adolescents and young adults psychosocial aspects. Long-term survivors. Cancer 1993;71:3463–3468.
15. Stevens MC, Mahler H, Parkes S. The health status of adult survivors of cancer in childhood. Eur J Cancer 1998;34:694–698.
16. Crockin SL. The "embryo" wars: at the epicenter of science, law, religion, and politics. Fam Law Q 2005;39:599–632.
17. Crockin SL. Reproduction, genetics and the law. Reprod Biomed Online 2005;10:692–704.
18. Crockin SL. Legal issues related to parenthood after cancer. J Natl Cancer Inst Monogr 2005;34:111–113.
19. Patrizio P, Butts S, Caplan A. Ovarian tissue preservation and future fertility: emerging technologies and ethical considerations. J Natl Cancer Inst Monogr 2005;34:107–110.
20. Robertson JA. Cancer and fertility: ethical and legal challenges. J Natl Cancer Inst Monogr 2005;34:104–106.
21. Schover LR, Brey K, Lichtin A, et al. Oncologists' attitudes and practices regarding banking sperm before cancer treatment. J Clin Oncol 2002;20:1890–1897.
22. The Ethics Committee of the American Society for Reproductive Medicine. Fertility preservation and reproduction in cancer Patients. Fertil Steril 2005;83:1622–1628.

23. American Society of Reproductive Medicine Mission Statement. Birmingham: American Society of Reproductive Medicine, 2005.
24. Waljee A, Waljee J, Morris AM, et al. Threefold increased risk of infertility: a meta-analysis of infertility after ileal pouch anal anastomosis in ulcerative colitis. Gut 2006; 55:1575–1580.
25. Janssen NM, Genta MS. The effects of immunosuppressive and anti-inflammatory medications on fertility, pregnancy, and lactation. Arch Intern Med 2000;160:610–619.
26. Holley JL. The hypothalamic–pituitary axis in men and women with chronic kidney disease. Adv Chronic Kidney Dis 2004;11:337–341.
27. Kelly-Weeder S, O'Connor A. Modifiable risk factors for impaired fertility in women: what nurse practitioners need to know. J Am Acad Nurse Pract 2006;18:268–276.
28. Boomsma CM, Eijkemans MJ, Hughes EG, et al. A meta-analysis of pregnancy outcomes in women with polycystic ovary syndrome. Hum Reprod Update 2006;12:673–683.
29. Jordan C, Revenson TA. Gender differences in coping with infertility: A meta-analysis. J Behav Med 1999;22:341–358.

Chapter 17
Oncofertility Consortium Consensus Statement: Guidelines for Ovarian Tissue Cryopreservation

Leilah E. Backhus, MD, MS, Laxmi A. Kondapalli, MD, MS, R. Jeffrey Chang, MD, Christos Coutifaris, MD, PhD, Ralph Kazer, MD, and Teresa K. Woodruff, PhD

In vitro fertilization (IVF) and storage of the resulting embryos is currently a proven method of fertility preservation for women who face an immediate threat to their future fertility. This method, however, is suitable for a fraction of patients and depends on a number of factors that may include her diagnosis, age, partner status, willingness to accept donor sperm, desire to freeze embryos, and ability to pay for these services. As fertility preservation techniques evolve, it is critical that physicians continue to evaluate practice guidelines in order to offer a wider menu of fertility preservation options tailored to each patient's specific clinical scenario, to the risk-benefit ratio and takes into consideration the patient's values.

Practice guidelines and consensus statements for fertility preservation for oncology patients reflect the current evidence based and ethical practices in the related disciplines of oncology and reproductive endocrinology. Both the American Society of Clinical Oncology (ASCO) and the American Society of Reproductive Medicine (ASRM) recently published guidelines to describe the circumstances under which fertility preservation should be discussed and to describe patients for which experimental methods, such as ovarian cryopreservation, may be suitable [1–3]. Taken together, these documents are comprehensive in their description of:

1. The need for discussion with patients about impaired fertility resulting from cancer treatment,
2. The need for early referral to a reproductive specialist to improve fertility outcome and minimize the delay of cancer treatment,
3. Malignant and benign conditions that render a patient a potential candidate for IRB approved protocols for ovarian cryopreservation.
4. The current established and experimental options available to preserve female fertility, and
5. The difficulty in providing and accurate estimate of the degree of future impaired fertility.

International interdisciplinary committees have also produced consensus statements to describe practice guidelines for offering experimental fertility preservation options to patients. Although both domestic and foreign guidelines illustrate the importance of offering fertility preservation to cancer patients, the interpretation of these guidelines that influences clinical practice may ultimately reflect the clinician's bias of "good candidates"

T.K. Woodruff and K.A. Snyder (eds.) *Oncofertility.*
© Springer 2007

for experimental options based on his or her experience, values, or availability of resources. Researchers in the United Kingdom have offered distilled interpretations of the interdisciplinary committee guidelines for candidates for ovarian cryopreservation [4], which suggests that clinicians would appreciate a relatively short "list" of criteria to consult prior to referring or offering ovarian tissue cryopreservation (see Fig. 17.1).

We find, however, the Edinburgh guidelines are inconsistent with criteria that would be used to offer reproductive assistance to patients in the United States. We propose new criteria for candidates for ovarian tissue cryopreservation that is consistent with the ASCO and ASRM consensus statements [1–3]. These guidelines could be used to identify potential candidates for ovarian cryopreservation in cases where a woman is at risk for iatrogenic infertility as a result of surgical or medical treatment for a benign or malignant condition. Due to the experimental nature of ovarian cryopreservation, in vitro maturation of follicles, and ovarian transplantation, these recommendations are not currently applicable for patients who desire fertility preservation in the absence of an immediate or iatrogenic threat.

Proposed criteria for candidate selection

1. Age <42 years
2. Cannot or chooses not to undergo an IVF cycle, regardless of partner status
3. Demonstrated or assumed pre-menopausal ovarian function
4. Risk of significant acceleration of anticipated loss of ovarian function
5. Informed consent from adult patient
6. Informed assent from patients <18 years, and informed parental/guardian consent
7. Meets criteria to be an appropriate candidate for an elective surgical procedure
8. Would consider having a child in the future
9. In the case of hormone-sensitive malignancy in which ovarian stimulation or oocyte retrieval are contraindicated.

Edinburgh Criteria for Selection for Ovarian Cryopreservation

1. Age <30
2. No previous chemotherapy or radiotherapy (patients <15 considered with previous low risk chemotherapy)
3. Realistic chance of long-term survival
4. High risk of treatment induced immediate ovarian failure (estimated at >50%)
5. Informed consent from patient or (in the case of and incompetent child) from parents
6. Negative HIV and hepatitis serology
7. No existing children

Fig. 17.1 Edinburgh criteria for selection of candidates for ovarian cryopreservation. Criteria are based on multidisciplinary discussion and working group report of the Royal College of Obstetricians and Gynaecologists [4]

The above criteria uses the age and testing of the potential reproductive status of the woman to be consistent with the criteria that would be used to identify the patient as a candidate for IVF if her ovary were to remain in situ. If time constraints prohibit testing at the appropriate time in her cycle, it should be assumed the patient is currently fertile in the absence of evidence to the contrary. After the process of informed consent, patients have the right to refuse to delay their own cancer treatment in service of IVF or to decide this method is not acceptable to them. Patients should be extensively counseled that IVF and embryo cryopreservation is an established method of fertility preservation and that ovarian cryopreservation is experimental, however counseling patients concurrently about IVF, oocyte cryopreservation, and ovarian tissue cryopreservation would eliminate the risk that a patient would choose IVF because she did not know about other options.

Any patient who is at risk of accelerated ovarian failure significantly earlier than the norm for the population as a result of her treatment should be counseled about this risk and offered fertility preservation. Although the patient may not undergo immediate ovarian failure, a shift in her reproductive life span such that her ability to have her own genetic children may end by her early 30s instead of her early 40s is a significant factor that could significantly change her range of choices and quality of life. Current infertility practice allows healthy women to receive donor eggs up to their early 50s, thus a woman who is 40 today may still be able to use her own gametes in the future. The patient's estimated long-term survival should not be applied as a criterion since this is often difficult to predict, and cancer survivors may elect to have children in the future. Ethical analysis has not yielded arguments to use length of survival of parents or risk of recurrence as a criterion to restrict access to fertility preservation [5].

Informed consent of both adult and pediatric patients must be in compliance with the institutions IRB protocols. A minor who is able to understand the procedure presented must give her assent. The procedure cannot be done with parental consent alone. If the patient is too young to give assent, then the procedure cannot pose more than minimal risk to the patient and the benefit must be clear. In the case of both adults and children, the surgery cannot pose additional significant risk to the patient in the judgment of the health care team, and the risks are clearly explained to the patient in the consent process. Patients should meet the same criteria for fertility preserving surgery that they would need to meet for other elective surgical procedures of roughly equivalent invasiveness and duration.

The discussion of fertility preservation for the patient with hormone-sensitive malignancy is controversial – it not a clear-cut issue and there are conflicting opinions. Breast cancer is a classic model of a hormone-dependent malignancy. Some experts believe that women with breast cancer should not be offered embryo or oocyte cryopreservation prior to chemotherapy. Since the drugs used for ovulation induction as part of IVF treatment increase the levels of endogenous gonadal hormones to a supraphysiological level, concerns have arisen regarding, at least theoretically, the potential for stimulation of malignant cell growth in a patient with a hormonally sensitive tumor. Therefore, some oncologists do not recommend traditional ovarian stimulation regimens because the markedly elevated, albeit transient,

Part VII
Patient Stories and Oncofertility

Chapter 18
Personal Accounts of Cancer and Infertility

Provided by Fertile Hope

The following personal accounts, provided by the patient advocacy group Fertile Hope, demonstrate how cancer and possible associated infertility can influence cancer patients' and survivors' sense of self and their life plans and goals. As research continues in the area of oncofertility, we hope to add to this base of knowledge of the impact of cancer-related infertility on the survivorship experiences of those diagnosed with cancer.

A New Generation of Hope: Antoinette's Story

For Antoinette, a bright 25-year-old California woman, life couldn't have been better. She was starting off on a great career path and had just received an exciting job transfer to San Francisco. However, Antoinette's excitement changed to shock in May 2005 when she was unexpectedly diagnosed with Stage 3 Hodgkin's Lymphoma.

> *"Just like everyone faced with cancer, it couldn't have come at a worse time. I was young and just starting a wonderful new career. I was moving to a new city, single and now faced with the reality of being very sick and losing my hair. What guy is going to want to date a 25-year-old woman with no hair?"*

While speaking with her oncologist, Antoinette learned that infertility was another possible side effect of her upcoming chemotherapy. The news was devastating because she had always wanted to have a family. Her mother had been diagnosed with cervical cancer and had a hysterectomy, leaving Antoinette an only child. In a cruel twist of fate, a nurse from the hospital where Antoinette was born called one year later to inform her mom that files had surfaced and that she had been misdiagnosed – she didn't have cancer and never needed a hysterectomy after all.

> *"When I was first diagnosed with cancer, my friends couldn't believe how well I took the news. But the one fear that continued to haunt me was the thought that I might become infertile. My mother had always wanted to have a big family and was unable to do so because of her hysterectomy. I was now staring infertility in the face, just like my mother had, and it just didn't seem fair."*

T.K. Woodruff and K.A. Snyder (eds.) *Oncofertility*.
© Springer 2007

Antoinette discovered Fertile Hope and the Sharing Hope financial assistance program while researching her fertility options on the Internet. She learned that the program provides financial assistance for cancer patients to increase access to sperm banking and egg and embryo freezing. This was particularly important to Antoinette because her health insurance would not pay for fertility treatments and she couldn't afford the procedures on her own.

> *"I quickly called Fertile Hope, filled out the paperwork, and was approved and enrolled in Sharing Hope. Fertile Hope allowed me to take control of my own destiny and provided me with the opportunity to make decisions that were right for me."*

Antoinette has undergone three months of chemotherapy and is currently in remission. She had 19 eggs frozen and is looking forward to one day getting married and realizing her dream of starting a family.

> *"Freezing my eggs allowed me to focus on getting through treatments without the added stress I felt about infertility. The success I've had so far is because my primary concern had been taken care of and that gave me the ability to focus on the biggest battle of my life."*

Starting a Family One Day: Adriane's Story

In the summer of 2004, life couldn't have been better for Adriane, a 27-year-old third grade teacher in suburban Atlanta. Adriane had recently purchased her first home and she was excited about starting work on her master's degree. However, in August 2004 Adriane's world came to a halt when she was diagnosed with Chronic Myelogenous Leukemia.

> *"I couldn't believe the news. I didn't know anyone else my age with cancer and I was really scared because I had always equated cancer with death."*

Adriane received more bad news when her oncologist told her that she could become infertile as a result of her chemotherapy treatments. The news was frightening because Adriane loved children and had dreams about one day having a large family with as many as nine children.

> *"Initially, I was devastated when I learned that I might not be able to have children. I was single and the one thought that kept entering my mind was that no one would ever want to marry me if I couldn't have children."*

Before she began her chemotherapy treatments, Adriane's oncologist and stem cell transplant doctor told her about an organization called Fertile Hope. She called Fertile Hope and learned that financial assistance was available through the organization's Sharing Hope program. The program would help to defray some of the costs of potentially fertility-sparing reproductive procedures and, therefore, she could have her eggs frozen.

"I contacted Fertile Hope and the Sharing Hope Program and instantly felt better about my chances to start a family of my own. The financial assistance helped immensely and the paperwork was easy to complete. I was approved almost immediately."

A short time later Adriane had 12 eggs frozen and she is excited about starting a family in the future. She underwent chemotherapy and received a stem cell transplant in March 2005.

"Through my experiences I learned that there is life after cancer and thanks to Fertile Hope, my life will include lots of babies!"

An Improvised Script: Beverley's Story

It would be hard for Beverley to have scripted a better story. She had a great career as a producer for Bravo's hit series *Queer Eye for the Straight Guy* and she was a happy newlywed, having just married her husband in November 2005. However, on December 1st, just over 2 weeks after her wedding, Beverley's life took an unexpected turn – she was diagnosed with Stage 2 Hodgkin's Lymphoma.

"I had a plan for where I wanted to be in life, but spending the first year of my marriage bald and infertile was not something that I'd considered! When my physician spoke to me about treatment, I got a lump in my throat and my eyes welled with tears as I realized that the chemo was about to destroy my ability to have children. It was a very empty feeling."

Beverley's feeling of emptiness was replaced with optimism when she and her husband learned about Fertile Hope's Sharing Hope financial assistance program from her physician. After learning about the program's benefits, Beverley and her husband agreed to participate and immediately filled out the paperwork.

"Our experience was great and the approval process was simple and uncomplicated. I was able to fax the information and received a response on the same day. In short, it couldn't have been faster or more efficient."

The couple had 15 eggs harvested, but Dr. Noyes, their endocrinologist, felt their best hope for future pregnancy lay in freezing embryos rather than eggs. They ended up with nine viable embryos and are looking forward to starting a family in the future.

"We are hopeful that we will have our own biological child in the future. And hopeful that one day, I will sit across the table from one or two small children who eat their corn on the cob just the way my husband does."

Beverley had surgery in December to remove a lymph node from her neck. She is currently receiving ABVD chemotherapy and will more than likely require a course of radiation after her chemotherapy. However, after her experience with Fertile Hope's Sharing Hope program, Beverley is looking forward to having children and experiencing the next chapter in her life.

Life is Worth Living: Brian's Story

In today's fast paced world, many 18-year olds deal with problems such as peer pressure, dating issues, and deciding whether to attend college or enter the workforce. For Brian, an 18-year-old young man in Southern California, those issues seem minor after being diagnosed with Stage 3 Hodgkin's Lymphoma during his junior year of high school.

> *"During my exam, the doctor's found numerous small tumors in my waist, neck, and armpits, as well as a seven-inch tumor in my spleen and a six-inch tumor wrapped around my heart. I was shocked to hear the news about my tumors and then completely devastated when the oncologist told me that I might become sterile as a result of my cancer treatment."*

While the doctors were deciding the best treatment options, Brian's grandmother came across information on Fertile Hope and the Sharing Hope program. She took the steps to sign Brian up for the program and he was approved immediately. For the first time in many years the family began to believe that with programs like this life might actually be worth living.

> *"I had a tough life growing up in a group home. When I learned about Fertile Hope and the Sharing Hope program, I felt that something positive was about to happen to me for the first time in my life."*

Brian's life has made a dramatic turn for the better in a short period of time. After meeting with his endocrinologist, he made the decision to have his sperm banked for future use, giving him the opportunity to someday start a family of his own.

> *"Cancer affects everyone whether they are rich or poor and everyone should have the opportunity to have a family regardless of their income. One day, when I'm looking at my little girl or boy, I want them to know about my tough upbringing, my battle with cancer, and that they were able to be brought into this world because I discovered Fertile Hope's Sharing Hope Program."*

Brian underwent six months of chemotherapy and four weeks of radiation treatment and he is now cancer free. He plans on moving to Hollywood to pursue his dream of becoming an actor.

Young and Hopeful for the Future: Dorothy's Story

For Dorothy, a 26-year-old Austin woman, 2005 was off to a great start. Dorothy was beginning to do well after being employed at the same company for four and a half years and she was considering moving to New York City later in the year. Dorothy's life changed dramatically one month later when she was diagnosed with breast cancer.

> *"When my oncologist told me that I had cancer, I was in shock. As far as I knew I was a healthy 26-year-old woman. The thought that I might have cancer had never entered my mind."*

Dorothy's friend accompanied her to an appointment with her oncologist, and it wasn't until he asked about side effects that she learned about the possibility of becoming infertile as a result of chemotherapy.

> *"I was terrified when I learned that I might not be able to have children. I was adopted as an infant and I knew what it's like to still feel somewhat out of place in the home you love, even in the presence of family who love you. I knew I wanted my own children not only for those reasons but also to fill the void of not having my own family."*

Dorothy's reproductive endocrinologist informed her about an organization called Fertile Hope. After more research, Dorothy discovered that through Fertile Hope's Sharing Hope program she would qualify for financial assistance and therefore be able to preserve her fertility.

> *"I knew that I wanted to have my own children, but until I came in contact with Fertile Hope and the Sharing Hope program I didn't think it was a possibility due to the financial obligations. The Sharing Hope program gave me hope for obtaining my most precious desire in life – to have a family."*

Dorothy made the decision to have her eggs frozen and has since completed all of her chemotherapy and radiation treatments. She is looking forward to one day having her own family.

> *"I can't imagine what the end result would've been without the help I received from Fertile Hope. The stress of fertility preservation would've been tenfold and it wouldn't have been possible to even think about having my own children."*

Hope, from Texas to Panama: Elia's Story

Elia, a 34-year-old Austin-based Sales Manager, had just returned from a business trip to Panama in October 2004. The trip had gone well and Elia was excited because her boss had asked her to return to Panama the following month to lead a sales team. However, Elia's return trip was abruptly placed on hold when she was diagnosed with Stage 2 Hodgkin's Lymphoma.

> *"I was in shock when I heard the news about my cancer. At the time, I loved my life and I was at a point where my career was really taking off. I knew that I would probably lose my hair during chemotherapy but I had no idea that I could become infertile until my oncologist told me during our meeting. That's when I began to cry."*

Elia had always wanted to raise children of her own and she loved the idea that her children would be able to one day meet their grandparents. Elia's parents lived in Mexico and she was frightened about the possibility of facing cancer by herself and ending up alone for the rest of her life.

> *"I was sure I would end up single forever and die alone because no man is going to want to marry a 34-year-old woman who can't have a baby, right? After a couple of weeks of depression I went to see a reproductive endocrinologist and my outlook on life began to change when I learned about Fertile Hope and the Sharing Hope program."*

Elia was elated to learn that as a cancer patient she had access to fertility options through the Sharing Hope financial assistance program. She filled out the paperwork and was approved almost immediately. One month later, Elia had a number of eggs frozen for future use.

> *"There are different stages that people go through when cancer is involved. Initially, I went through depression and anger about my diagnosis, followed by an overwhelming sense of relief once I learned about Fertile Hope's Sharing Hope program. As a woman in her prime childbearing years, I'm not sure I would have gotten beyond my depression if it hadn't been for this program. I'm thankful for all of the support I received and I encourage anyone who has cancer and wants children to take advantage of the program's benefits."*

After undergoing chemotherapy and radiation treatment, Elia's cancer is in remission and she is excited about the possibility of one day starting a family. In the next couple of months, nearly a year and a half after first being diagnosed with cancer, Elia will be returning to Panama to lead her sales team.

Appendix A: Oncofertility Options

Provided by Fertile Hope

Options for women

Method	Timing	Definition	Medical status	Time requirement	Success rates	Cost	Pubertal status	Special considerations
(1) Embryo freezing	Before or after treatment	Harvesting eggs, fertilizing them in the lab with sperm (in vitro fertilization) and freezing the resulting embryos	Standard	10–14 days of ovarian stimulation from the first day of our period Outpatient surgical procedure	Varies based on age, your fertility status and expertise of your center Approximately 40% per three embryos transferred in women under 35; lower in older women Thousands of babies born	$8,000/cycle, plus $.3500–$5,000 for medications Long-term storage fees average $500/year Approximately $2,500/cycle to use the embryos later to become pregnant	After puberty	Requires partner or donor sperm Experimental protocols exist for patients with hormone sensitive cancers (e.g. breast and gynecological)
(2) Egg freezing	Before or after treatment	Harvesting and freezing of unfertilized eggs	Experimental	10–14 days of ovarian stimulation from the first day or your period	Approximately 21.6% per embryo transfer	$8,000/cycle, plus $3,500–$5,000 for medications	After puberty	My be particularly desirable for sing women or those opposed to embryo creation

(continued)

Options for women (continued)

Method	Timing	Definition	Medical status	Time requirement	Success rates	Cost	Pubertal status	Special considerations
				Outpatient surgical procedure	Approximately 3–4 times lower than embryo freezing 180 live births reported to date	Long-term storage fees average $500/year Approximately $5,000/cycle to use the embryos later to become pregnant (this is higher for egg freezing because the eggs have to be fertilized with sperm)		Experimental protocols exist for patients with hormone sensitive cancers (e.g. breast and gynecological)
(3) Ovarian tissue freezing (reimplantation)	Before treatment	Freezing of ovarian tissue and reimplantation after cancer treatment	Experimental	Outpatient surgical procedure	Case reports of 2 live births reported	$12,000 Long-term storage fees average $500/year $20,000 to use the tissue later to restore hormone function and/or try to achieve pregnancy	Before puberty	Not suitable when the risk of ovarian cancer involvement is high
(4) Ovarian tissue freezing (in vitro development)	Before treatment	Freezing of ovarian tissue and in vitro follicle development	Experimental	Outpatient surgical procedure	Live births in mouse	$12,000 Long-term storage fees average $500/year $20,000 to use the tissue later to restore hormone function and/or try to achieve pregnancy	Before or after puberty	Potentially only good option for pre-pubertal women

250

	Timing	Procedure	Status	Procedure type	Evidence	Cost/insurance	Puberty	Notes
(5) Ovarian transposition	Before treatment	Surgical repositioning of ovaries away from the radiation field	Standard	Outpatient procedure	Large cohort studies suggest approximately 50% chance of success due to altered ovarian blood flow and scattered radiation	Unknown Generally covered by insurance	Before or after puberty	Important to work with a physician who has expertise in transposition
(6) Radiation shielding of gonads	During treatment	Use of shielding to reduce the dose of radiation delivered to the reproductive organs	Standard	In conjunction with radiation treatments	Only possible with selected radiation fields and anatomy (e.g. pelvic region)	Generally included in cost of radiation	Before or after puberty	Important to choose a physician who has expertise in shielding. Does not protect against chemotherapy
(7) Trachelectomy	During treatment	Surgical removal of the cervix while preserving the uterus	Standard	Inpatient surgical procedure	No evidence of higher cancer recurrence rates in appropriate candidates	Generally included in the cost of cancer treatment	After puberty	Limited to early stage cervical cancer. Offered at a limited number of centers

(continued)

Options for women (continued)

Method	Timing	Definition	Medical status	Time requirement	Success rates	Cost	Pubertal status	Special considerations
(8) Ovarian suppression	During treatment	Use of Gonadotropin Releasing Hormone (GnRH) analogs or antagonists to protect ovarian tissue during chemotherapy	Experimental	In conjunction with chemotherapy	Unknown: small randomized studies and case series report conflicting results. Larger randomized trials in progress	$500/monthly injection	After puberty	Does not protect from radiation
(9) Donor embryos	After treatment	Embryos donated by a couple	Standard	Varies; is done in conjunction with IVF	Unknown; higher than that of frozen embryo IVF transfers	$5,000–$7,000 in addition to IVF ($8,000, plus $3,500–5,000 medications)	After puberty	Several reproductive centers have informal programs. Donor embryo agencies are also available. Patient can choose donors based on several characteristics
(10) Donor eggs	After treatment	Eggs donated by a woman	Standard	Varies; is done in conjunction with IVF	40–50%	$5,000–$15,000 in addition to OVF ($8,000, plus $3,500–$5,000 medications)	After puberty	Patient can choose donor based on various characteristics

(11) Gestational surrogacy	After treatment	Woman carries a pregnancy for you	Standard	Varies; time is required to match you with a surrogate as well as perform IVF	Similar to IVF – approximately 30%	$10,000–$100,000	After puberty	Legal status varies by state Known surrogates (e.g. friend or family member) are usually less expensive
(12) Adoption	After treatment	A legal proceeding that creates a parent–child relation	Standard	Depending on the type of adoption the process can take months to more than a year	Varies greatly	$2,500–$35,000	After puberty	Can be difficult for cancer survivors given negative medical history

(continued)

Options for men

Method	Timing	Definition	Medical status	Time requirement	Success rates	Cost	Pubertal status	Special considerations
(1) Sperm banking (masturbation)	Before treatment	Sperm is obtained through masturbation, then frozen	Standard	Outpatient procedure	Generally high – success depends on sperm quality and quantity as well as your female partners age and fertility status The most established technique for men	$1,500 for 3 samples stored for 3 years Future storage fees average $500/year	After puberty	Can be as performed as often as once a day
(2) Sperm banking (alternative collection methods)	Before treatment	Freezing sperm optained through testicular aspiration, extraction, or electroejaculation under sedation	Experimental	Outpatient procedure	If sperm is obtained, success rates are similar to standard sperm banking	Varies greatly based on collection method	After puberty	Can be used when you cannot ejaculate
(3) Testicular tissue freezing	Before treatment	Testicular tissue is obtained through surgical biopsy and frozen for either reimplantation or in vitro maturation of sperm cells	Experimental	Outpatient procedure	No available human success rates	$500–$2,500 for surgery $300–$1,000 to freeze tissue Storage fees average $100–500/year	Before or after puberty	Important to choose a physician with expertise in this area Still experimental, may be the only option for pre-pubescent boys

(4) Testicular sperm extraction	Before or after treatment	Use of biopsy to obtain individual sperm from testicular tissue	Standard	Outpatient procedure	30–70% in postpubescent patients; Unknown in prepubescent patients	$6,000–$16,000 in addition to costs for IVF	Before or after puberty	Important to work with a center that can freeze any sperm found at the time of the biopsy
(5) Radiation shielding of gonads	During treatment	Use of shielding to reduce the dose of radiation delivered to the testes	Standard	In conjunction with radiation treatments	Success rates high in terms of reducing damage to testes; Only possible with select radiation fields and anatomy (e.g. pelvic region)	Generally included in the cost of radiation treatments	Before or after puberty	Important to work with a physician who has expertise in shielding; Does not protect against chemotherapy
(6) Donor Sperm	After treatment	Sperm donated by a man for artificial insemination	Standard	Donor sperm is readily available for purchase; If you use a known donor a quarantine time of 6 months is required	50–80%	$200–$500 per vial in addition to costs for IUI or IVF	After puberty	Patient can choose donor based on wide range of characteristics
(7) Adoption	After treatment	Legal proceeding that creates a parent–child relation	Standard	Depending on the type of adoption the process can take months to more than a year	After puberty	$2,500–$35,000	Varies greatly	Can be difficult for cancer survivors given negative health history

255

Index

Cancer Treatment and Research (continued from p. ii)
Steven T. Rosen, M.D., Series Editor

Figlin, R.A. (ed.): *Kidney Cancer.* 2003.   ISBN 1-4020-7457-3.

Kirsch, M., Black, P. McL. (ed.): *Angiogenesis in Brain Tumors.* 2003.
ISBN 1-4020-7704-1.

Keller, E.T., Chung, L.W.K. (eds): *The Biology of Skeletal Metastases.* 2004.
ISBN 1-4020-7749-1.

Kumar, R. (ed.): *Molecular Targeting and Signal Transduction.* 2004.
ISBN 1-4020-7822-6.

Verweij, J., Pinedo, H.M. (eds): *Targeting Treatment of Soft Tissue Sarcomas.* 2004.
ISBN 1-4020-7808-0.

Finn, W.G., Peterson, L.C. (eds.): *Hematopathology in Oncology.* 2004.
ISBN 1-4020-7919-2.

Farid, N. (ed.): *Molecular Basis of Thyroid Cancer.* 2004.   ISBN 1-4020-8106-5.

Khleif, S. (ed.): *Tumor Immunology and Cancer* Vaccines. 2004.   ISBN 1-4020-8119-7.

Balducci, L., Extermann, M. (eds): *Biological Basis of Geriatric Oncology.* 2004.
ISBN

Abrey, L.E., Chamberlain, M.C., Engelhard, H.H. (eds): *Leptomeningeal Metastases.*
2005.   ISBN 0-387-24198-1.

Platanias, L.C. (ed.): *Cytokines and Cancer.* 2005.   ISBN 0-387-24360-7.

Leong, S.P.L., Kitagawa, Y., Kitajima, M. (eds): *Selective Sentinel Lymphadenectomy for*
Human Solid Cancer. 2005.   ISBN 0-387-23603-1.

Small, Jr. W., Woloschak, G. (eds): *Radiation Toxicity: A Practical Guide.* 2005.
ISBN 1-4020-8053-0.

Haefner, B., Dalgleish, A. (eds): *The Link Between Inflammation and Cancer.* 2006.
ISBN 0-387-26282-2.

Leonard, J.P., Coleman, M. (eds): *Hodgkin's and Non-Hodgkin's Lymphoma.* 2006.
ISBN 0-387-29345.

Leong, S.P.L. (ed): *Cancer Clinical Trials: Proactive Strategies.* 2006.
ISBN 0-387-33224-3.

Meyers, C. (ed): *Aids-Associated Viral Oncogenesis.* 2007.   ISBN 978-0-387-46804-4.

Ceelen, W.P. (ed): *Peritoneal Carcinomatosis: A Multidisciplinary Approach.* 2007.
ISBN 978-0-387-48991-9.

Leong, S.P.L. (ed): *Cancer Metastasis and the Lymphovascular System: Basis for rational*
therapy. 2007.   ISBN 978-0-387-69218-0.

Raizer, J., Abrey, L.E. (eds): *Brain Metastases.* 2007.   ISBN 978-0-387-69221-0.

Woodruff, T., Snyder, K.A. (eds): *Oncofertility.* 2007.   ISBN 978-0-387-72292-4.